Tinnitus

This second edition is dedicated with love to Sheila and Bridget Baguley, Ebba, Edvin and Elsa Andersson, Tanya McFerran and Anne O'Sullivan

Tinnitus

A multidisciplinary approach

Second Edition

David Baguley PhD MBA
Consultant Clinical Scientist
Head of Audiology
Cambridge University Hospitals
Visiting Professor
Anglia Ruskin University
Cambridge University Hospitals NHS Foundation Trust
Cambridge, UK

Gerhard Andersson BSc MSc PhD
Professor in Clinical Psychology
Department of Behavioural Sciences and Learning
Linköping University
Clinical Psychologist
Department of Audiology
Linköping University Hospital
Guest Researcher
Department of Clinical Neuroscience
Karolinska Institute
Stockholm, Sweden

Don McFerran MA FRCS
Consultant ENT Surgeon
Colchester Hospital University NHS Foundation Trust
Colchester, UK

Laurence McKenna M.Clin Psychol PhD
Clinical Psychologist
Royal National Throat Nose & Ear Hospital
University College London Hospitals
Clinical Psychologist
South London and Maudsley NHS Trust
Honorary Lecturer
UCL Ear Institute
London, UK

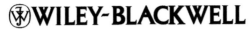

WILEY-BLACKWELL

A John Wiley & Sons, Ltd., Publication

This edition first published 2013 © 2013 by David Baguley, Gerhard Andersson, Don McFerran, Laurence McKenna

Blackwell Publishing was acquired by John Wiley & Sons in February 2007. Blackwell's publishing program has been merged with Wiley's global Scientific, Technical and Medical business to form Wiley-Blackwell.

Registered Office
John Wiley & Sons, Ltd, The Atrium, Southern Gate, Chichester, West Sussex, PO19 8SQ, UK

Editorial Offices
9600 Garsington Road, Oxford, OX4 2DQ, UK
The Atrium, Southern Gate, Chichester, West Sussex, PO19 8SQ, UK
111 River Street, Hoboken, NJ 07030-5774, USA

For details of our global editorial offices, for customer services and for information about how to apply for permission to reuse the copyright material in this book please see our website at www.wiley.com/wiley-blackwell.

Library of Congress Cataloging-in-Publication Data

Tinnitus : a multidisciplinary approach / David Baguley ... [et al.]. – 2nd ed.
    p. ; cm.
  Includes bibliographical references and index.
  ISBN 978-1-4051-9989-6 (pbk. : alk. paper)
I. Baguley, David (David M.)
  [DNLM: 1. Tinnitus. WV 272]
  617.8–dc23

                                   2012032714

A catalogue record for this book is available from the British Library.

Wiley also publishes its books in a variety of electronic formats. Some content that appears in print may not be available in electronic books.

Cover image: © Fotolia/philhol
Cover design by Meaden Creative

Set in 10/12.5pt Times by SPi Publisher Services, Pondicherry, India

1   2013

Contents

Foreword

Clinicians and researchers who accept the challenge of helping patients suffering from tinnitus must be prepared to implement management strategies that are as varied and diverse as the population they serve. The notorious abundance of tinnitus 'cures' suggests that there are (at least) as many tinnitus causes, triggers and mechanisms. It will probably always be the case that no one-size-fits-all approach to tinnitus management will succeed, but it is equally likely that a variety of interventions may, in many cases, produce some amelioration of the patient's distress. Most researchers and practising clinicians report that a combination of sound therapy and counselling facilitates the patient's ability to manage the tinnitus experience. Psychotropic agents produce mixed success from which we infer that, at a minimum, such drugs work well for some patients regardless of whether the influence is upon the tinnitus sound, the patient's psychological health or both. Herbal supplements, vitamins and alternative therapies such as acupuncture, biofeedback and hyperbaric oxygen therapy have produced mixed results that must be weighed against the potential, and substantial, risks associated with their use. What is the practitioner who answers the call, and decides to work with tinnitus patients, to make of this situation?

The second edition of *Tinnitus: A multidisciplinary approach* promotes tinnitus management strategies built upon the collaborative care for suffering patients and the preparation of clinicians for such practice. We have a set of authors uniquely qualified to tackle thorny tinnitus problems, and it is clear that their work as clinicians and researchers has crystallised in the group the certainty that our patients more often than not require care that knows no borders. The centrepiece of this text is its dispensing of practical, evidence-based information from the fields of audiology, otology, psychology, psychiatry and auditory neuroscience. Tinnitus distress may derive from several different factors simultaneously, and the authors remind us to weigh the potential risks and benefits of action and inaction. Throughout, they provide thorough and current reviews of material germane not just to clinical practice but to the educating of individuals who will conduct the practice.

The reader will find resources that facilitate the essential task of interacting with patients and determining a tinnitus management plan. To address the likelihood that all tinnitus patients present unique challenges to the clinician, the authors provide guideposts, evidence and thoughtful rationales for selecting a course of action tailored to each patient's needs. For example, some tinnitus programmes focus on modifying a patient's concept of tinnitus and its effects, thereby facilitating a change in the patient's behaviour and approach to the problem (i.e. Cognitive Behavioural Therapy). Others utilise particular protocol-driven therapy, specifying more consistent application of sound levels and specific counselling components (i.e. Tinnitus Retraining Therapy). Others (i.e. Neuromonics) couple sound or music filtered specifically to account for each patient's hearing sensitivity and loudness tolerance to counselling that varies little across patients. The reviews of these and other management protocols are of great value not only to present practitioners but also to the student or professional who considers working with tinnitus patients.

It is admittedly difficult to report clinical success when the approach to patient management is idiosyncratic and driven more by the patient's needs than by a cookbook plan of action. Particularly at this time, when clinical success is defined in the context of evidence-based practice, an eclectic approach to management of a potentially disabling condition may provide benefit to patients but may be difficult to sell to peer reviewers and other clinicians. Yet, when we observe improvements in our patients, it is undeniable, and when we measure a patient's self-assessment of handicap, we may measure statistically significant changes in the patient's tinnitus experience. While it is difficult to define precise tinnitus distress or tinnitus relief, clinicians working with tinnitus patients see their share of both.

A clinician's experience with suffering patients provides the impetus to adapt and adjust strategies in order to facilitate the patient managing the condition effectively. As the authors point out, some of these 'real time' adjustments may lead to novel methods for use with other patients. However, the clinician's experience with tinnitus patients likely influences their willingness and ability to adapt clinical approaches with which they are comfortable. It is therefore important to gain, or help others achieve, the experience and confidence required to implement starkly different strategies for different patients. The authors have provided a rich inventory of management strategies that should foster a clinician's flexibility in order to meet the diverse needs and challenges associated with the tinnitus patient population.

Unfortunately, as the professional training of individuals to join the ranks of tinnitus clinicians lags far behind the need for such providers, it is also the case that the need for multidisciplinary patient care goes unrecognised too often. In this second edition, the authors stress the need for professionals across the disciplines of neuroscience, psychology, medicine and audiology to collaborate in the clinic and the lab in order to meet patient needs. Audiologists and otologists have for years recognised that tinnitus is frequently complicated by psychological co-morbidities. It is imperative for hearing health care professionals to seek out practitioners from related clinical areas to whom patients whose tinnitus is complicated by other factors may be referred. Medical issues must also be acknowledged and managed. Recognising the signs that would trigger such referrals is the first step to providing comprehensive patient care. The authors provide the means by which tinnitus clinicians can place the patient's needs in a broader context than would be available through the inherently limited view of tinnitus as exclusively an auditory problem. Because the needs of tinnitus patients are difficult to meet in many cases, clinicians must be versed in the literature and practice of related disciplines. Tinnitus distress is multidimensional and this book does not purport to solve the myriad problems that derive from that fact. However, it is hoped that a forthright discussion of the state of the art of tinnitus management will inspire clinicians across medicine, audiology and psychology to embark upon the journey of tinnitus therapy in concert.

Professor Marc Fagelson
East Tennessee State University
Johnson City, TN, USA

Preface

The field of tinnitus is resurgent, with very significant streams of research activity into mechanisms and treatments now in place. This is not restricted to the traditional themes of cochlear hair cells, and of sound-based and counselling-based therapies, but also involves robust pharmaceutical research, and also the design, implementation and evaluation of novel approaches to treatment.

Additionally there are indications that a multidisciplinary ethos is permeating the tinnitus world, with voices from neuroscience, pharmacology, psychology and audiology interweaving as we investigate this fascinating and sometimes debilitating symptom. Once characterised by opinion and a few isolated expert voices, the tinnitus community now look for evidence and consensus when it comes to both basic research and clinical perspectives.

With this in mind, the four of us thought it time to prepare and present a second edition of *Tinnitus: A multidisciplinary approach*. New findings abound, and there are new treatments to describe and novel perspectives through which to consider tinnitus. While the magic pill continues to elude us, there are indications that progress is being made in effective intervention and that many more patients are accessing clinical services.

The distinctive perspective of this book is that each of the four authors is a practising clinician while also involved in research. The emphasis for each of us is different, but being able to inhabit both worlds gives, we hope, insight into the translational nature of tinnitus work: that is, that the clinic must influence the research agenda and that research should underpin and inform clinical practice. Seeing tinnitus patients in the clinic on a regular basis also gives an authenticity to what one believes about tinnitus and how it can best be treated. Some of the insights in this book have been hard won.

Our Editors at Wiley-Blackwell are to be thanked, not least for the patience they have shown to four authors who have been weighed down at times with administrative and clinical responsibilities. Our colleagues too have been patient and supportive, but most of all our families and friends have been mainstays of support. We hope that the current vitality of the tinnitus field continues and that this second edition may help guide the interested scientist and/or clinician into the wealth of knowledge that is available about tinnitus.

David Baguley
Gerhard Andersson
Don McFerran
Laurence McKenna

Chapter 1

Introduction

Tinnitus and hyperacusis continue to intrigue patients, scientists and clinicians alike. That so many people can have some experience of these symptoms and not be distressed, while others are troubled to the point that they are no longer able to perform their normal daily activities remains paradoxical. Furthermore, researchers have reported that when tinnitus is matched in intensity in this troubled group of people, it has been indicated to match to sound of low intensity (though the complexities of such experiments will be discussed below). Despite this apparent low intensity the intrusiveness of the symptom in patients with severe tinnitus is remarkable. Given these paradoxes, it is unsurprising that no single approach to tinnitus and hyperacusis has been shown to be overwhelmingly stronger than any other in terms of understanding and managing these symptoms.

The aim of this book is to present a multidisciplinary approach to tinnitus and hyperacusis, incorporating insights from Audiology, Otology, Psychology, Psychiatry and Auditory Neuroscience. It is hoped that this will inspire a collaborative approach to tinnitus and hyperacusis management that will benefit patients and clinicians alike. There is already good evidence that such collaborative and multidisciplinary initiatives in other fields, such as chronic pain, have increased the efficacy of treatments.

Definitions

The word tinnitus derives from the Latin verb 'tinnire' meaning 'to ring', and in common English usage is defined as 'a ringing in the ears' (*Concise Oxford English Dictionary*, Allen, 1990). The first recorded use of the word occurred in 1693 in *Blanchard's Physician's Dictionary*, second edition as follows (Stephens, 2000):

> Tinnitus Aurium, a certain buzzing or tingling in the Ears proceeding from obstruction, or something that irritates the Ear, whereby the Air that is shut up is continually moved by the beating of the Arteries, and the Drume of the Ear is lightly verberated, whences arises a Buzzing and a Noife (p. 201).

Tinnitus: A Multidisciplinary Approach, Second Edition. David Baguley, Gerhard Andersson, Don McFerran and Laurence McKenna.
© 2013 David Baguley, Gerhard Andersson, Don McFerran and Laurence McKenna.
Published 2013 by Blackwell Publishing Ltd.

At the time that this Dictionary was compiled there were many conditions that were thought to be due to trapped air, and procedures were developed to address that. It is interesting that the Blanchard definition fits well with the experience of pulsatile tinnitus, where an individual becomes aware of the sound of arterial or venous blood flow (see Chapter 5).

Some other languages have a variety of words to describe the phenomenon of tinnitus (Stephens, 2000), notably French, where five words are in regular use, each describing a particular timbre or quality of sound. In Swedish the word for tinnitus used to be Öronsus, which in direct translation stands for ear breeze. Few patients would agree that their tinnitus sounds like a breeze and this word does not catch the emotional impact experienced by some. There have been various attempts at a scientific definition. McFadden (1982) considered that:

> Tinnitus is the conscious expression of a sound that originates in an involuntary manner in the head of its owner, or may appear to him to do so.

This definition has been widely adopted (e.g. Coles, 1987; Davis and El Rafaie, 2000; Stephens, 2000) and has the benefit of brevity. Møller (2011b) distinguishes between *objective* tinnitus (which can be heard, measured or recorded by an external observer) and subjective tinnitus, which can be heard by the person alone. As will be shown below, this distinction was made in the work of Itard (1774–1838). Møller defines subjective tinnitus as follows:

> Subjective tinnitus is a broad group of sensations that are caused by abnormal neural activity in the nervous system that is not elicited by sound activation of sensory cells in the cochlea (Møller, 2011b, p. 9).

This definition has some insights, as it implies that tinnitus can be varied, both within and between individuals. One might question whether *anomalous* might be a better word than *abnormal*, and this will be unpacked when we consider the neuroscience of tinnitus.

Definitions of hyperacusis have tended to illustrate the perspective of the author. For instance, Vernon (1987a) proposed an open definition as

> … unusual tolerance to ordinary environmental sounds.

For Vernon the emphasis may have been upon the *unusual*, as he could only recall four such cases, having seen over 4000 persons with tinnitus. Modern epidemiology indicates that hyperacusis is a more common experience than that. A more pejorative view is that of Klein et al. (1990):

> … consistently exaggerated or inappropriate responses or complaints to sounds that are neither intrinsically threatening or uncomfortably loud to a typical person.

Many persons with hyperacusis may have seen clinicians who would ascribe to this view and not been helped by the implied criticism. A less negative definition was proposed by Baguley and Andersson (2007):

> … abnormal lowered tolerance to sound.

Attempts have been made more recently to differentiate between those individuals who have a general hypersensitivity to sound that most other people can tolerate (hyperacusis) and those who find specific sounds uncomfortable, perhaps because of emotional associations with that sound. In an initial differentiation between these two the second experience was entitled phonophobia, a term that is commonly used in neurology (Woodhouse and Drummond, 1993), in particular in association with migraine attacks. However, the inference that this phenomenon was essentially phobic in nature can be unhelpful to some patients. Definitions of hyperacusis are further explored in Chapter 10.

Historical aspects

The experience of the perception of sound generated internally has been mentioned in many historical medical texts. These original sources have been reviewed by Stephens (1987, 2000) and Feldmann (1997), and while these authors have many detailed issues upon which they are at variance, they are in broad agreement on the interest expressed in tinnitus by medical authors from historical times. A series of ancient Babylonian medical texts, inscribed upon clay tablets, were housed in the library of King Assurbanipal (668–626 BC) in Ninevah. These were translated by Thompson (1931) and were found to include 22 references to tinnitus, described variously as the ears 'singing', 'speaking' or 'whispering'. Treatments are described, including whispered incantations, the instillation of various substances into the external auditory meatus and the application of charms (such as the tooth of a female ibex): specific treatments were advised for each experience of tinnitus as described above (Feldmann, 1997). The involvement of ghosts and spirits in the generation of tinnitus was described, and in particular a quiet incantation method of treatment was largely concerned with driving away such affliction, this being described as the basis of much human disease (Stephens, 1987).

Tinnitus has six mentions in the *Corpus Hippocratum*, a second century AD compilation of the works of Hippocrates of Kos (460–377 BC): each mention relates to a description of ear disease rather than of tinnitus as an experience in its own right. Other authors writing in Graeco-Roman times mentioning tinnitus include Celsus (25 BC–50 AD) who described treatments with diet and abstinence from wine and Pliny the Elder (23–79 AD) who advocated the use of wild cumin and almond oil in cases of tinnitus (Stephens, 2000). The use of sedative medication to treat persons suffering with tinnitus, still in common use in the United States of America and Western Europe, was first described by Galen (129–199 AD), who considered the benefits of opium and mandrake.

Dan (2005) considers a report that the Roman Emperor Titus (39–81 AD) experienced tinnitus. This is found in the Babylonian Talmud, and the tinnitus was considered to be punishment for the destruction of the Second Temple in Jerusalem (70 AD), though the report that at post mortem Titus was found to have a large intracranial tumour offers another perspective on this. Titus is said to have enjoyed some short-lived relief from sound therapy:

A gnat entered his nostril and pecked at his brain for seven years. One day Titus was passing by a blacksmith. He heard the noise of the sledgehammer and the gnat became silent. Titus

thus said: 'Here is the remedy'. Everyday he brought a blacksmith to bang in his presence....
For thirty days this worked fine but then the gnat became accustomed and resumed pecking
(quoted in Dan, 2005).

There are mentions of tinnitus in texts within the Islamic medical tradition from the
period following the decline of medicine in Rome (Stephens, 1987, 2000, and Feldmann,
1997). These include the first mention of the coincident complaint of tinnitus and hyperacusis (described as an 'increased sensibility') by Paul of Aegina (625–690 AD) (Stephens,
2000, after Adams, 1844).

Advances in the understanding and treatment of tinnitus were not to be seen until the
seventeenth century, with the publication of the first text entirely dedicated to the ear
and hearing. The *Traite de l'Organe de l'Ouie* by DuVerney (1683) was translated from
the original French into Latin, German, Dutch and English and is recognised as a
milestone in Otology (Weir, 1990). The insights into tinnitus represented a move away
from the concept that tinnitus may arise from trapped air in the ear, this having persisted
since Roman times, towards a model of tinnitus arising from diseases of the ear and
disorders of the brain. The implication of the influence of the brain over the ear is
prophetic of later concepts of the function of the efferent auditory system in humans. The
treatments for tinnitus that are advocated by DuVerney are limited to treatment of the
underlying disorder.

A further advance in understanding occurred in 1821 with the publication of *Traite
des Malades de l'Oreille et de l'Audition* by Itard. This comprehensive text was based
upon 20 years of experience in working with the deaf, and contained numerous case
studies, including that of Jean-Jacques Rousseau (1712–1778), the eminent philsosopher
who became afflicted by tinnitus in later life (Feldmann, 1997). Itard made the
distinction between tinnitus experiences arising from sound, thus 'objective tinnitus'
such as that caused by somatosounds, and that arising without any acoustic basis, 'false
tinnitus' (now described as 'subjective' tinnitus). This distinction is still in use today.
In addition to such medical insights Itard described the effect of tinnitus upon an
individual: 'an extremely irksome discomfort which leads to a profound sadness in
affected individuals' (translation by Stephens, 2000, p. 443). The treatment of tinnitus
was, as with previous authors, based upon treatment of the underlying otological
condition, though when such treatment failed, however, Itard advocated attention to the
behavioural manifestation of tinnitus and in particular to sleep disturbance, when the
use of external environmental sounds (such as a watermill for low-pitched tinnitus or
an open fire burning damp wood for high-pitched tinnitus) to mask the tinnitus was
suggested.

In the late nineteenth century the medical specialty of Otology underwent a renewal of
interest and effort, and several individuals have been identified as leaders in this field.
Joseph Toynbee (1815–1866) and William Wilde (1815–1876) (the father of Oscar Wilde)
were pre-eminent in this regard and wrote extensively on ear disease, including consideration of tinnitus arising from such conditions. Toynbee experienced distressing tinnitus himself and died during an experiment in which he attempted to determine 'the effect of inhala-
tion of chloroform upon tinnitus, when pressed into the tympanum' (Feldmann, 1997,
p. 18). MacNaughton Jones (1981) has been credited (Stephens, 2000) with producing

the first book in English on tinnitus alone, which contained a classification of tinnitus based upon the site of origin and a review of contemporary treatments.

The ability to use electronic instruments to measure hearing thresholds accurately by audiometry, and the consequent ability to determine hearing status in patients with a complaint of tinnitus, was developed in the early twentieth century, and became widespread in Western Europe and the United States of America from the 1940s (Weir, 1990). At this time Fowler (1941) considered the characteristics of tinnitus and is credited with the first comprehensive attempts to determine the matching and masking characteristics of tinnitus (Stephens, 2000). Among the insights gleaned by Fowler were that subjectively loud tinnitus is often matched to a low-level stimulus, that tinnitus may be masked by a broadband noise and that it is not possible to generate beats between tinnitus and externally generated tones (Fowler, 1941). In subsequent writings Fowler collaborated with his son, also an Otologist, and formulated a protocol for the examination of tinnitus patients considering the qualities of the sound, the distress associated, as well as the otological health of the patient (Fowler and Fowler, 1955).

In the late twentieth century there was little scientific or clinical interest in tinnitus and the field was kept alive by a small number of dedicated individuals. The work of Jack Vernon has already been cited: Vernon was a Professor of Audiology working for most of his career in Oregon, USA, and developed the first practical wearable masking devices for tinnitus. In the United Kingdom, Ross Coles was a prolific tinnitus researcher, clinician and teacher, and his influence and mentorship is still felt to this day. Coles worked as a Consultant Physician and academic at both Southampton and Nottingham Universities, and was the founder of the long-running European Tinnitus Course. Also from a medical background, though working as a surgeon rather than a physician, Jonathan Hazell specialised in tinnitus, and in his collaborations with Pawel Jastreboff (a neuroscientist) developed an influential model of tinnitus and a concomitant treatment protocol (Tinnitus Retraining Therapy). From an Audiology perspective, Richard Tyler, working at the University of Iowa, has written, researched and taught extensively on how tinnitus can be managed and has been extremely influential. In the early 1980s Richard Hallam, a psychologist working in London, proposed that the natural history of tinnitus is characterised by the process of habituation and pointed out the influence of psychological factors on this process. His work has had a major influence on the clinical management of tinnitus, particularly by psychologists.

Thus there has been evidence of input to tinnitus research from otology, audiology, and to some extent neuroscience. What has been missing until recently, however, has been substantial input from pharmacology, from psychiatry and from auditory neuroscience. There are indications that this is now underway and that the field is becoming characterised by collaboration and teamwork rather than a small number of experts.

Given the existence of tinnitus throughout history and the wide prevalence of tinnitus experience (see Chapter 11 for details), one should expect mentions in art and literature. In fact these are sparser than would be expected. A comprehensive survey of such mentions will have to await another day, but some can be considered here as examples. The Czech composer Smetana (1824–1884) suffered progressive, and eventually profound, hearing loss and associated tinnitus. He wrote his tinnitus into his string quartet 'From my life' (1876) as a prolonged sustained high violin note towards the end.

Thomas Hardy (1840–1928) has a character named William Worm, in his novel the *A Pair of Blue Eyes* (1873), speak of tinnitus:

> I've got such a noise in my head that there's no living night nor day. 'Tis just for all the world like people frying fish…. God A'mighty will find it out sooner or later, I hope, and relieve me (Chapter 4).

More recently, Woody Allen has the male lead, played by himself, in the film *Hannah and Her Sisters* (1986) experience unilateral tinnitus and hearing loss, and is investigated for an acoustic neuroma. The asute listener may pick up upon references to tinnitus in the lyrics of modern music: artists as diverse as Radiohead, Bob Dylan and the Broken Family Band mention the experience of tinnitus.

This short review of the historical understanding of tinnitus has three underpinning elements. The first is that any consideration of tinnitus and formulation of possible treatment should consider the otological status of the patient and thus involve the treatment of ear disease where indicated. The second is that this otological focus does not obviate the clinician of the responsibility to consider the distress caused by the tinnitus experience and, where significant behavioral manifestation of this is present, to treat that distress. The third is that the understanding and treatment of tinnitus is a changing and developing science.

Summary

From the above it is evident that concern with tinnitus is not new, and in fact is demonstrated throughout written human history. Many scientists, clinicians and artists have considered tinnitus and the involvement of systems of reaction, arousal and emotion. The indications are that a holistic view of tinnitus must consider the involvement of such systems.

Chapter 2

Prevalence and natural history

Knowledge of the epidemiology of tinnitus is fundamental to tinnitus clinicians' and researchers' understanding of the subject. Studies tell us that tinnitus is one of the most common physical symptoms experienced by humans, which inevitably leads to the question of why it is so common. One of the greatest challenges facing the tinnitus community is to understand why, if it is so common, do only some people suffer as a consequence of tinnitus? This question will be dealt with in other chapters, but knowledge of the epidemiology of tinnitus provides a backdrop against which to understand this fundamental issue. It also helps us to consider what health care services might be commissioned for persons who complain of tinnitus.

The epidemiology of tinnitus has been investigated in several studies over the years; these studies will be outlined and the implications of them considered.

Is tinnitus a universal phenomenon?

If the definition of tinnitus is expanded to include internal sounds that are perceived in silence, tinnitus becomes an almost universal experience. In the famous experiment by Heller and Bergman (1953), subjects were asked to enter a soundproof booth and to report all the sounds they could hear; 94% reported some form of tinnitus-like perception, using terms like *buzz, hum* and *ring*. Unfortunately, the conditions in which the Heller and Bergman (1953) study was conducted were not well controlled. It has been even suggested (Graham and Newby, 1962) that they did not assess subjects' hearing audiometrically; the idea that the subjects had normal hearing is therefore only an assumption. Attempts to replicate the study have not revealed the same proportion of subjects reporting tinnitus-like experiences. A replication by Graham and Newby (1962) found that only 40% of their normal hearing subjects reported tinnitus. Levine (2001) found that 55% of his normal hearing subjects had ongoing tinnitus when they were placed in a low-noise room. In a study of 120 persons with normal hearing, Tucker et al. (2005) found that 64%

Tinnitus: A Multidisciplinary Approach, Second Edition. David Baguley, Gerhard Andersson, Don McFerran and Laurence McKenna.
© 2013 David Baguley, Gerhard Andersson, Don McFerran and Laurence McKenna.
Published 2013 by Blackwell Publishing Ltd.

reported tinnitus-like perceptions in silence: the proportion was slightly higher in persons of Afro-Carribbean heritage than Caucasians. This latter finding has not been replicated. In a variation upon a now familiar theme, Del Bo et al. (2008) placed 53 normally hearing Caucasian individuals in a soundproofed room and asked them to listen hard for two 4 minute sessions. When a (disconnected) loudspeaker was not present, 83% of the group reported tinnitus-like perception: this rose to 92% when the loudspeaker was present in the second session.

Regardless of the correct figures of tinnitus in normal-hearing individuals when placed in a silent room, it is still apparent that tinnitus is a very common experience in silence, but it is often not noticed as soon as some environmental sound is present to mask that tinnitus.

Prevalence studies

The prevalence of tinnitus refers to the number of individuals within the general population who experience it at a given time. On the face of it, working out how many people have tinnitus experiences at any given moment in time might seem straightforward, but it is, in fact, a difficult thing to do. There are considerable variations in the way that people experience tinnitus and in the way that they talk about it. Furthermore, there is no objective test that can be relied on. Formal definitions of tinnitus can be complex and not easily understood by the general population. Prevalence studies have tended to rely on simplified definitions that can be open to interpretation and different studies have used slightly different definitions. The result is therefore somewhat varying prevalence figures. Nonetheless, an overview of the studies does create a useful impression.

The history of epidemiology research into tinnitus starts in the UK:

- In an early study, Hinchcliffe (1961) studied 800 individuals randomly recruited from two locations in the UK (Wales and Scotland). Participants were interviewed in their homes and asked 'Have you at one time or another noticed noises in your ears or head?' The prevalence of tinnitus showed a tendency to increase with age as follows 21% (18–24 years), 27% (25–34 years), 24% (35–44 years), 27% (45–54 years), 39% (55–64 years) and 37% (65–74 years). The average was approximately 30%.
- A follow-up study to this by the Office of Population Census and Surveys (1983) revealed a general prevalence of tinnitus of 22%.
- The UK has also produced the most robust and comprehensive study into the prevalence of tinnitus. This was carried out by the Medical Research Council's Institute of Hearing Research and reported by Davis and El Rafaie (2000). In this study questions about tinnitus were incorporated into the National Study of Hearing, a longitudinal study that sampled a very large number of the population ($n = 48\,313$) in four major cities (Cardiff, Glasgow, Nottingham and Southampton). The first part of the study involved a postal survey of 48 313 randomly selected people, with a response rate of over 80%. The questions used were 'Nowadays do you get noises in your head or your ears?' and 'Do these noises last longer than five minutes?' In this way these researchers used the concept of prolonged spontaneous tinnitus (PST). Davis and El Rafaie (2000) reported

that 10.1% of adults experienced PST. This tinnitus was reported to be moderately annoying by 2.8% of people and to be severely annoying by 1.6%. In 0.5% tinnitus was said to have a severe effect upon the ability to lead a normal life. The postal survey was followed up by a clinic examination of a sample (3234) of respondents; this part of the study also revealed a prevalence rate of 10.1%.

- Palmer et al. (2002) studied the self-reported responses of 21 201 subjects recruited from 34 general practices and members of the armed services. Ages ranged between 16 and 64 years. Questionnaire items were modelled on the National Study of Hearing (Davis, 1989). Tinnitus was defined by the question, 'During the past 12 months have you had noises in your head or ears (such as ringing, buzzing or whistling) that lasted longer than five minutes?' One additional common restriction was that only tinnitus reported to occur most or all of the time was defined as persistent tinnitus (cf. Coles, 1984). Palmer et al. (2002) found a strong relation between self-report of tinnitus and hearing difficulties. For men, the age-standardised prevalence of persistent tinnitus was 16.1% in those who reported severe hearing difficulties, whereas for those men with slight or no hearing problems the prevalence was only 5%. For women, the corresponding figures were 33.1% and 2.6%, respectively.

- In Scotland, Hannaford et al. (2005) sent out a postal questionnaire to 12 100 households, asking whether people experienced various ENT symptoms. They received a response rate of 64.2%, with 20% answering 'yes' to a question about experiencing noises in their heads or ears lasting more than 5 minutes. Tinnitus was reported to be slightly annoying by 55.7% of those who experienced it, to be moderately annoying by 17.4% and to be severely annoying by 7.3%.

A number of studies have also taken place elsewhere in Europe.

- Sweden: Axelsson and Ringdahl (1989) investigated the prevalence of tinnitus among a random sample of adults in the city of Gothenburg. They asked 3600 people 'Do you suffer from tinnitus?' They also asked people how often they experienced ear noises and asked questions about localization and severity. They had a response rate of 71%. Their results revealed that 14.2% reported tinnitus 'often' or 'always'. Just over 21% of older people reported tinnitus. In this study, tinnitus was more common in men than women. Scott and Lindberg (2000) approached a random sample of 2500 Swedish citizens from a population register (in which all citizens are registered). Responses were obtained from 1538 subjects (62%) and among these 15.8% responded 'yes' to the question, 'Have you heard buzzing, roaring or tones, or other sounds which seem to come from inside the ears or the head and that have persisted for five minutes or longer (so-called tinnitus)?' In addition, tinnitus was graded by use of the Klockhoff and Lindblom (1967) severity definition of *mild, moderate* or *severe* tinnitus, where it is masked by environmental sound, not masked but not affecting sleep or not masked and affecting sleep, respectively . As results were analysed separately for help-seeking and non-help-seeking people with tinnitus (with additional participants recruited from a clinic), no exact estimate of severe tinnitus in the general population can be derived. As only a minor proportion of subjects in the population survey had sought help ($n=7$), however, the figures for the population-derived non-help-seeking group provide an estimate of the proportion of severe (grades II–III) tinnitus. Slightly below 50% had tinnitus of grades II–III, with only a few (12.2% of the tinnitus sample) having tinnitus of grade III. Hence, a conservative estimate is that about one person in ten has severe tinnitus in the general population.

- In another study, Johansson and Arlinger (2003) studied 590 randomly selected subjects from the province of Östergötland. The prevalence of tinnitus was 13.2%, using the five minutes' definition. Andersson et al. (2012) distinguished current, 12-month and lifetime tinnitus in a random sample. The figures were 25.4% for lifetime, 21.5% for 12-month and a 17.8% point prevalence. Approximately 60% of the point prevalence group had tinnitus often or always. In common with the findings in the National Study of Hearing (Davis and El Rafaie, 2000), only a minority reported that tinnitus had a severe effect upon their ability to lead a normal life.
- Germany: In a small study with data from the city of Ulm, Nagel and Drexel (1989) found that, of their 270 participants, 11.5% reported 'longer lasting' tinnitus, corresponding to the 5-minute criterion. As many as 31%, however, had noticed tinnitus at some point in time and 19.5% had temporary tinnitus lasting not longer than five minutes. It is uncertain if this was a random sample (average cross-section) and severity of tinnitus was not clearly outlined. In a large-scale study by Pilgramm et al. (1999) 3049 people were interviewed by telephone, which comprised 41% of the eligible people initially approached. This study was published as a conference proceedings report and therefore the results were not described in much detail. The authors derived that 13% of the German population has, or once had, noise in the ears lasting longer than five minutes. They also provided an estimate of those having tinnitus at the time of the investigation, which was 3.9% of the population. They also estimated that approximately 50% of those with ongoing tinnitus considered the effect of their tinnitus as moderately serious or unbearable. This would lead to a prevalence figure of 2% for severe tinnitus.
- Denmark: Parving et al. (1993) studied 3387 males with a median age of 63 years (range 53–75 years). A prevalence of 17% of tinnitus of more than five minutes' duration was found; 3% indicated that their tinnitus was so annoying that it interfered with sleep, reading or concentration.
- Italy: Quaranta et al. (1996) studied 2170 people from the cities of Bari, Florence, Milan, Padua and Palermo, with ages ranging between 18 and 80 years. Prolonged spontaneous tinnitus was found in 14.5%. The authors reported that the prevalence increased with age up to 79 years and that manual work, dyslipidosis, hypertension, liver diseases, cervical arthrosis and alcohol consumption were statistically significant risk factors. The report was brief and it is uncertain to what extent participants were bothered by their tinnitus.
- Poland: In a conference report Fabijanska et al. (1999) found that, of a sample of 10 349 people aged 17 years or older, 20.1% reported tinnitus (defined as lasting more than five minutes). Severe annoyance was reported by one-tenth of the tinnitus population. Increasing age was associated with increased annoyance. The authors also reported constant tinnitus, which was perceived by 4.8% of the population.

A number of studies have also been carried out in the United States:

- Leske (1981) carried out a study for the FDA. She reported data from a national health examination survey dating back to 1960–1962 with a total of 6672 subjects. Respondents were asked, 'At any time over the past few years, have you ever noticed ringing (tinnitus) in your ears or have you been bothered by other funny noises?' Given this very broad definition, it is not surprising that as many as 32.4% of adults aged 18–79 years said that they did. Only 5.6%, however, considered tinnitus severe. This figure is closer to the prevalence figures of severe tinnitus found in other studies. Interestingly, a linear association was found between age and presence of both mild and severe tinnitus. In common with many other studies, a strong association was found between severity of tinnitus and hearing impairment.

- Almost a decade later Brown (1990) explored the prevalence of tinnitus in older adults using data from the 1982–1987 USA Health Interview Survey together with the supplement on ageing to the 1984 Health Interview Surveys and the first Health and Nutrition Examination Survey 1971–1975. The index question was 'Does anyone in your family now have tinnitus or ringing in the ear?' From responses to this question he estimated the prevalence of tinnitus to be 4.5% of the population; this figure rose to 12.3% for people over 55 years of age.
- Cooper (1994) reported data dating from 1971 to 1975 with 6342 subjects from the US. Participants were asked: 'At any time over the past few years have you ever noticed ringing …', so providing information about prevalence over a period of time. They found that the overall prevalence of 'bothersome tinnitus' (participant bothered 'quite a bit' or 'just a little') was 14.9%.
- Shargorodsky et al. (2010) interviewed and examined participants from the National Health and Nutrition Examination Surveys (1999–2004); this was regarded as a nationally representative data base. Participants were asked: 'In the past 12 months, have you ever had ringing, roaring, or buzzing in your ears?' and 'How often did this happen?' They found that 25.3% of their respondents reported having experienced tinnitus. Frequent tinnitus (at lest daily) was reported by 7.9% of people. These figures rose to 31.4% and 14.3% among people aged 60 to 69 years old. Non-Hispanic white people had higher odds of experiencing tinnitus than other racial/ethnic groups.

Some data are available from older adults living in Australia:

- In the Blue Mountain Study of Hearing, Sindhusake et al. (2003) examined the prevalence of tinnitus among people over the age of 55 years. They asked one question about tinnitus: 'Have you experienced prolonged noises, buzzing or any other sounds in your ears or head within the past year that last more than five minutes?' Just over 30% of respondents said they had and it was judged as moderately to severely annoying by 67% of them.

It is only recently that some data on the prevalence of tinnitus in non-Western societies has emerged:

- Egypt: Khedr et al. (2010) carried out a door-to-door survey, using a semi-structured interview, of 8484 people (700 households) living in the city of Assuit and the surrounding rural area. They also administered the Tinnitus Handicap Inventory and the Hamilton Anxiety and Depression Scale. They found that 5.17% of people reported tinnitus. This figure rose to 17.66% among people over 60 years of age. There were significant correlations between the severity of tinnitus and the extent of self-reported hearing loss and the Hamilton depression score.

- Japan: Michikawa et al. (2010) interviewed 1320 older adults (≥ 65 years) in Kurabuchi township (100 km north of Tokyo). Interviews were carried out in people's homes. The questions used to identify tinnitus were: 'In the past year have you experienced any ringing, buzzing or other sounds (tinnitus) in your ears?' and 'Have these sounds interfered with your concentration or ability to sleep?' They found that tinnitus was reported by 18.6% of people (15.5% for mild tinnitus; 3% for severe tinnitus).
- Nigeria: Lasisi et al. (2010) assessed the prevalence of tinnitus among 1302 older adults (≥ 65 years) living in the community. Tinnitus was reported by 14.1% of people.

It can be concluded from theses studies that tinnitus is a highly prevalent symptom. In fact tinnitus is one of the most prevalent symptoms experienced by humanity. While it is clear that not everyone with tinnitus is troubled by it, tinnitus-related suffering represents a major health challenge. The studies reviewed do point to slightly different prevalence figures. It can be argued that the variation stems mainly from the different questions used and the differing definitions of tinnitus employed, although most studies have excluded temporary tinnitus. When considering which prevalence figure to accept two factors need to be taken into account. The first factor is that data derived from a local population are likely to be the most relevant to a service. The second consideration is the robustness of the study. Careful methodology is an obvious consideration here. So too will be the size of the data set and the response rate. There are many reasons why a person might or might not respond to a survey. For example, it could be that people with tinnitus are more likely to respond to a tinnitus survey than those who do not have it. There is therefore a risk of overestimating the prevalence of tinnitus. The larger the response rate in a study the less likely it is that there will be errors in the data. The response rate in the national study of hearing and the size of the data set make that the study of choice in the UK. It is apparent that the proportion of sufferers versus nonsufferers is not a static figure and, for example, publicity can influence the report of tinnitus as a significant problem (Baskill et al., 1999). This was clearly seen in Sweden in 1999 after a national campaign to raise money for tinnitus research. It should be noted, however, that many people benefit from publicity and knowing that they are not alone with their tinnitus.

Incidence

Few studies have investigated the incidence of tinnitus, that is the number of new tinnitus cases for a predefined time period. A study by Nondahl et al. (2002, 2010) followed the residents of Beaver Dam in Wisconsin over a number of years. People aged 43–84 years at the start of the project were invited to take part in a study looking at hearing and vision. Tinnitus was identified by a questionnaire asking if the person had *buzzing*, *ringing* or *noises in the ears* in the past year. The prevalence of tinnitus at baseline was 8.2%, when mild cases were excluded. Those who reported no tinnitus at the time were followed for 5 and 10 years to determine the cumulative incidence of developing tinnitus. The 5-year incidence of tinnitus was 5.7%; the 10-year incidence was 12.7%. Interestingly, participants with tinnitus at baseline were more likely to report changing from mild tinnitus to no tinnitus ($n = 135/341$; 39.6%) than from mild to moderate or severe tinnitus ($n = 67/341$; 19.6%).

The approximate incidence of 5% in older adults was also found in a Swedish longitudinal study aged between 70 and 79 years (Rubinstein et al., 1992). Pilgramm et al. (1999) estimated that, for each year, 0.33% of the German population aged over 10 become chronic tinnitus patients (with subtraction of mean mortality rate and therapy success rate). Data from the National Study of Hearing (Davis and El Rafaie, 2000) indicate that 7.1% of the sample had sought the opinion of their doctor about tinnitus and that 2.5% had attended a hospital for this purpose. Clearly, there is a need for further studies of tinnitus incidence and help-seeking behaviours.

Prevalence of tinnitus in childhood

The prevalence of tinnitus in children is discussed in detail in Chapter 18. To make some generalizations, the prevalence of tinnitus awareness in children seems similar to that in adults. The prevalence of tinnitus distress, however, seems much lower in children. By and large tinnitus seems more prevalent in children who have hearing impairment, whether conductive or sensorineural. The degree of tinnitus distress broadly follows the degree of hearing impairment, though interestingly significant tinnitus is seen less frequently among children who have profound hearing loss compared to those with moderate or severe loss.

Tinnitus in older adults

Tinnitus in older adults has received some interest from researchers. A number of studies (Sindhusake et al, 2003; Michikawa et al., 2010; Lasisi et al., 2010) have focused on an assessment of the prevalence of tinnitus in older adults and found prevalence rates that are slightly higher than some of the general population rates reported elsewhere. Alone, however, they cannot be taken as evidence of a higher prevalence of tinnitus in older adults. The varying methodologies and definitions of tinnitus used in differing studies make it difficult to draw firm conclusions about the variation in prevalence rates across the ages. A few studies, however, have used the same definitions and asked the same questions of younger and older adults and these offer a comparison of the different age groups, although here too the different studies have used different age bands to stratify people. The data from the National Study of Hearing suggested an increase in the prevalence of tinnitus with age. Similar findings were reported by Brown (1990). Pilgramm et al. (1999) reported 'a pronounced increase' in the prevalence of tinnitus among people of 50–80 years compared with younger groups; unfortunately they do not report the exact figures. Shargorodsky et al. (2010) reported that the prevalence of tinnitus increased with increasing age until the age of 60–69 years. After that it declined with increasing age. The authors speculate that tinnitus may be associated with other conditions that confer a selective mortality disadvantage. Michikawa et al. (2010) reported that no age group trends were observed in a group of older adults; again these findings appear to support the idea that the prevalence of tinnitus plateaus in older adults.

Overall, it is clear that tinnitus is more prevalent in older adults than it is in younger age groups. A few studies have given precise figures; these studies are listed in Table 2.1. The

Table 2.1   The prevalence of tinnitus (%) in the general population and in younger and older adults.

Study	General prevalence	Younger adults	Older adults
Hinchcliffe (1961)	29		37
Leske (1981)	32.4		44
National Study of Hearing (1984) (see Davis, 1989)	10.1		22
Axelsson and Ringdahl (1989)	14.2		21
Brown (1990)	4.5	1.6	8.9
Quaranta et al. (1996)	14.5		
Fabijanska et al. (1999)	20.1	9.7	52.8
Hannaford et al. (2005)	17.1	7.1–13.3	23.6–34.1
Shargorodsk et al. (2010)	7.9		14.3
Khedr et al. (2010)	5.71	2.35	17.66

increased prevalence of tinnitus in older adults is perhaps not surprising given that the prevalence of hearing loss also increases with age; it is interesting to note that within the Blue Mountain Study the correlation between hearing loss and tinnitus was greater among people over the age of 65 years.

While it does seem reasonable to conclude that tinnitus is more prevalent in older age groups a separate question is whether it causes more problems in older age groups. This issue is highlighted in the tinnitus clinic when patients ask: 'Will it get worse as I get older?' Hazell (1991) found that disability resulting from tinnitus did not increase with age, but this conclusion was based on clinical data and not findings from random samples. In their population-based study, Axelsson and Ringdahl (1989) found no age effect for the men, while older women experienced tinnitus worse than younger women. Rubinstein et al. (1992) studied patients at the ages of 70, 75 and 79 years and noted that for most people tinnitus severity decreased or remained the same. These authors reported that severity increased in only a minority of people; the increase was evident more in women than men. These observations highlight the importance of considering gender differences, even among the elderly. More recently, Davis and El Rafaie (2000) reported a tendency for moderate and severe annoyance to increase by age, using data from the National Study of Hearing. A similar trend can be observed in Andersson et al.'s (2012) study of Swedish people.

In the context of an ageing society, the fact that tinnitus is very prevalent among older adults and the possibility that it is experienced as more distressing by some older adults than by younger age groups presents a major health service challenge.

Other risk factors

A number of risk factors have been identified for tinnitus. The issues of age and gender have been discussed above, the headline news being that tinnitus prevalence increases with age, and that tinnitus has often been reported to be more common, and more complex, in women than men. Other risk factors that have been identified include hearing loss, noise exposure and general health issues, and we shall consider each of these in turn.

It might seem that there is a clear and unambiguous link between hearing loss and tinnitus, and this underpins the concern of many people with troublesome tinnitus that they will imminently lose their hearing. In fact the relationship is more complex that and in several respects the information we have at present is sparse. Firstly, considering conductive hearing loss, the indications are that the presence of an air–bone gap is a risk factor for tinnitus and the greater the air–bone gap, the higher the possibility of tinnitus (Davis, 1995). Secondly, it has been demonstrated that sensorineural hearing loss is the dominant factor in predicting the occurrence of tinnitus (Coles et al., 1984; Davis and El-Refaie, 2000; Sindusake et al., 2003; Gopinath et al., 2010) and this association is especially strong for high-frequency hearing loss. It should be borne in mind that there are patients with normal audiograms who report troublesome tinnitus: the strength of the association between hearing loss and tinnitus is such that some are led to propose that such patients have either a hearing loss in higher frequencies than those routinely tested audiometrically (Kim et al., 2011) or some subtle cochlear dysfunction undetectable by audiometry (Lindblad et al., 2011) or that some form of hidden hearing loss is present in the auditory brainstem (Schaette and McAlpine, 2011). While these ideas are plausible, it is also possible that the ignition site for such tinnitus is within the central auditory pathways (see Chapter 4).

Another risk factor is that of noise exposure. Self-report studies of tinnitus consistently indicate a higher prevalence in those who identify themselves as having been exposed to noise (Nondahl et al., 2011). Such exposure can be leisure or occupational, and within these broad categories there lies a significant range of experience: for instance, the leisure noise category includes classical musicians, the person on the train playing their iPod inordinately loud and the Do It Yourself enthusiast. Similarly, occupational noise can include the factory worker, bar staff in nightclubs and combat troops (see Chapter 19 for detailed consideration of this latter group). There are also complex associations between noise and other suggested risk factors (Davis and El-Refaie, 2000) such as smoking and socioeconomic class.

A further area of risk factors for tinnitus that has been proposed is that of general health. Building upon observations that in population data there are indications that reduced cochlear function can be associated with hypertension and cardiovascular disease, similar thoughts have concerned tinnitus. Once again, however, there are possible links between such issues and gender, age, noise and smoking, and the reality is that this is multifactorial and complex. This is an area requiring large-scale and well-designed longtitudinal studies, and while there are some such studies underway (the Blue Mountains Study in Australia being an example; see Gopinath et al., 2010) until such data are available the situation is not entirely clear.

One issue raised by many patients is whether tinnitus is heritable. While there are monogenic disorders associated with tinnitus (such as Neurofibromatosis II and familial paragangliomas; for example see Sand et al., 2007), the question is more along the lines of 'I have troublesome tinnitus: are my children likely to follow suit?' Data from Kvestad et al. (2010) indicates that while there is an additive genetic component to the likelihood of experiencing troublesome tinnitus, this is very low. Further work is keenly anticipated on this theme.

Longitudinal studies

Unfortunately, there are relatively few studies on the natural history of tinnitus, and in particular the natural history of untreated tinnitus. Most of the research that has been conducted on the long-term outcome of tinnitus has been retrospective. For example, Stouffer et al. (1991) concluded that tinnitus loudness and severity increased as a function of years since onset. The study was cross-sectional, however, and therefore no definite conclusions could be drawn; the authors recommended that longitudinal studies be conducted. Smith and Coles (1987), in contrast, concluded that the severity of tinnitus was likely to decrease over time. This was an epidemiological study and did not focus just on clinical tinnitus. The data collected, however, were retrospective. Since 25 of their subjects actually stated that tinnitus had disappeared, it is clear that tinnitus may be of a temporary nature. Davis (1995) reported from the National Study of Hearing that, from onset to middle time, 25% of sufferers reported an increase in loudness, which was the same from middle to recent time. He noted, however, that for most people loudness did not change. The ratings of annoyance decreased for 31% of the respondents from onset to middle, but the decrease was smaller (10%) from middle to recent time.

Retrospective studies of patients with vestibular schwannoma (acoustic neuroma) have been published, showing that tinnitus may arise, worsen, remain or disappear following surgery for the condition (see Chapter 5). However, this aetiology is rare and the results cannot be extrapolated to individuals with the more common causes of tinnitus, such as noise-induced hearing loss. More is known about the natural history of tinnitus in older adults. Rubinstein et al. (1992) found substantial longitudinal fluctuations in tinnitus and a high occurrence of spontaneous remission. Patients were studied at the ages of 70, 75 and 79 years, and results showed that tinnitus had increased in severity in 25% of the women and decreased in 58%, leaving 17% unchanged. For the men, tinnitus increased in 8% and decreased in 39%, with a larger proportion unchanged (53%). Although the long-term outcome of tinnitus in Ménière's disease has been studied (Green et al., 1991), gradings of tinnitus severity have seldom been reported, vertigo being the symptom drawing most attention.

In a longitudinal study, data were collected for an average period of five years post treatment in a sample of tinnitus patients who had received cognitive behavioural therapy (Andersson et al., 2001). Results showed decreases in annoyance and an increase in tolerance of tinnitus. Maskability of tinnitus at the commencement of treatment was a predictor of tinnitus-related distress at follow-up. Folmer (2002) studied 190 patients who returned follow-up questionnaires, on average, 22 months after their initial tinnitus clinic appointment. The group exhibited significant decreases of tinnitus distress, depression and anxiety.

Localization of tinnitus

Numerous studies have reported the site of tinnitus and a common observation is that tinnitus is most commonly bilateral (at least 50%), followed by unilateral on the left side and then unilateral on the right side. There are other cases in which tinnitus is localised in the head and a few cases in which tinnitus is perceived as an external sound. The observation that tinnitus is more common on the left side is interesting. One possible cause for this asymmetry could be that hearing loss is more common in the left ear. However, Meikle and Greist (1992) found that noise exposure in the left ear (for example by gun shooting) could not explain the difference.

Another potential cause could be neural imbalance at a cortical level and indeed Min and Lee (1997) noted that somatic symptoms overall tend to be lateralised to the left rather than to the right. There is no clear evidence that left-sided tinnitus is more annoying than right-sided tinnitus, nor that it is associated with greater degrees of hearing loss (Cahani et al., 1984; Budd and Pugh, 1995). Tyler (1997) questioned if there are true cases of unilateral tinnitus. Firstly, the auditory pathway has many cross pathways and, secondly, patients with supposedly unilateral tinnitus may report tinnitus on the previously unaffected side when the contralateral tinnitus is masked. However, Tyler (1997) concluded that it is common for tinnitus to be dominant in one ear, but that does not prove that tinnitus originates from that ear. Davis and El Rafaie (2000) suggested that the concept of left versus right ear differences needs more detailed research studies. Interestingly, Erlandsson et al. (1992) found that multiple localizations of tinnitus were associated with more distress, again a finding that merits further investigation.

Seeking help

It is far from the case that all people with tinnitus seek any help. Davis (1995) reported that despite the frequency of the symptom in the population, only 7.1% of the population had consulted any doctor for their tinnitus and only 2.5% had sought specialist advice from an otologist. In a Swedish study, 13% of the respondents with tinnitus had been to a physician for tinnitus during the past 12 months (Andersson et al., 2012).

Summary

Prevalence studies indicate that tinnitus is a common problem in the general population. Recent studies indicate that this is true for non-Western as well as for Western societies. Different studies suggest slightly different prevalence rates; differing definitions and methodologies almost certainly play a major role in producing this variation. An approximate prevalence of 10–15% is a reasonable conclusion from the literature. The majority of people who experience prolonged spontaneous tinnitus are not severely distressed by the symptom, but tinnitus does constitute a significant problem for 0.5–3% of the population. The natural history of tinnitus is only partly known, but there are indications that the perception of tinnitus becomes less annoying over time, at least for a significant proportion of people. Tinnitus experience is common among children, but the mechanisms and natural history of tinnitus in children remain unknown to a large extent. Older people often have tinnitus and studies suggest that their tinnitus is perceived as particularly annoying. The incidence of tinnitus is not known, apart from a 5.7% estimate for a five-year period and a 12.7% estimate for a ten-year period. Tinnitus localization is well known, but there are no strong explanations for why tinnitus is more prevalent in the left ear. Characterization of annoyance in relation to tinnitus is not clearly defined in behavioural terms. Most studies to date have used questionnaire assessment. In contrast, major studies on psychiatric disturbances commonly use structured interviews, which could be an alternative in future epidemiological work on tinnitus.

Chapter 3

Anatomy and physiology

Initial views regarding the pathogenesis of tinnitus unsurprisingly focused on the ear. While the ear undoubtedly is involved in the process, tinnitus cannot be satisfactorily explained without considering the central auditory pathways of the brain and other nonauditory neural systems, particularly the limbic, autonomic and reticular systems.

Anatomy of the ear

By convention the ear (Figure 3.1) is divided into outer, middle and inner sections.

Outer ear

The outer ear consists of the pinna, the external auditory meatus and the tympanic membrane. The pinna, or auricle, has a fibrocartilaginous skeleton, which is attached to the head by ligaments and muscles. In humans the muscles attached to the pinna that are innervated by the facial nerve are largely vestigial in function. The pinna helps to collect sound and contributes to sound localisation abilities. The external auditory meatus, or ear canal, is between 2 cm and 3 cm long, is 5–9 mm in diameter in adult humans and is roughly oval-shaped in cross-section. The lateral portion, comprising one-third of the length, is a cartilaginous tube lined with squamous epithelium, which is rich in cerumen and sebum-producing glands and hair. The secretions produced by the glands together produce ear-wax. The medial portion of the canal, comprising two-thirds of the length, is bony and lined by stratified squamous epithelium. This medial portion of the ear canal does not generate wax. The epithelium of the ear canal is continuous with the external layer of the tympanic membrane and together they demonstrate the unusual property of skin migration: maturation of new skin cells on the surface of the tympanic membrane pushes existing cells towards the margin of the tympanic membrane and then outwards down the ear canal. This process removes dead skin and excess earwax. The external auditory meatus in adults is

Tinnitus: A Multidisciplinary Approach, Second Edition. David Baguley, Gerhard Andersson, Don McFerran and Laurence McKenna.
© 2013 David Baguley, Gerhard Andersson, Don McFerran and Laurence McKenna.
Published 2013 by Blackwell Publishing Ltd.

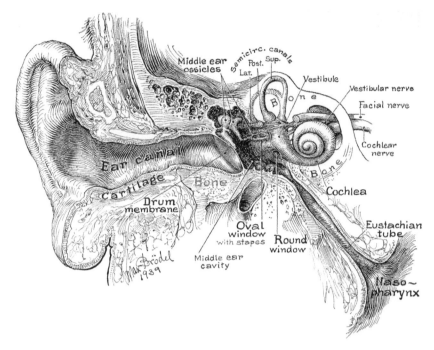

Figure 3.1 The human ear. (Reprinted with permission from Brodel (1946). Three unpublished drawings of the anatomy of the human ear, WB Saunders.)

curved in a slight antero-inferior direction, meeting the tympanic membrane obliquely so that the posterior wall is shorter and shallower than the anterior wall. The external auditory meatus has a resonant frequency approximating 3000 Hz in the adult human, enhancing the amplitude of sounds around this frequency by 10–20 dB (Rosowski, 2010).

Tympanic membrane

The tympanic membrane has three layers comprising: an outer layer continuous with the epithelium of the external auditory meatus; a fibrous middle layer of crossed collagen fibres, which are arranged both radially and circumferentially; and an inner layer of mucous membrane. The rim, or annulus, of the tympanic membrane is a fibrocartilaginous structure, approximately circular in shape (diameter 8–10 mm). The tympanic membrane itself is shaped like a shallow cone (Figure 3.2), drawn in medially to a connection with the malleus. The small central upper portion of the tympanic membrane, above the lateral process of the malleus, is called the 'pars flaccida' and, unlike the remaining larger 'pars tensa', does not possess a middle fibrous layer.

Middle ear

The middle ear or tympanum is an impedance-matching transformer; its function is to change the characteristics of sound vibrations that have passed through air into vibrations

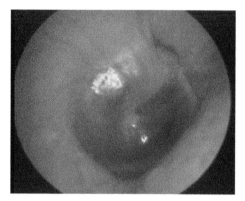

Figure 3.2   Right tympanic membrane.

that are suitable for passing through the aqueous medium of the inner ear. In structure it is an air-filled space, bounded by the tympanic membrane laterally and medially by the bone covering the inner ear. The upper part of the middle ear, which is known as the attic or epitympanum, is connected via a short tunnel, the aditus ad antrum to the mastoid antrum, a honeycomb of air cells within the mastoid bone. The tympanum is bridged by the ossicular chain, comprising the malleus, incus and stapes, connected to the tympanic membrane by the malleus and to the labyrinth at the footplate of the stapes. The ossicular chain is suspended within the tympanum by folds of mucous membrane, and two of the three bones are attached to muscles: the malleus is attached to the tensor-tympani muscle, which is innervated by the trigeminal nerve and contracts in conjunction with palatal movement; the stapes is attached to the stapedius muscle, which is innervated by the facial nerve and contracts in response to loud sound, producing the stapedial reflex. The impedance matching process is achieved in three ways: the tympanic membrane has a much larger surface area than the footplate of the stapes, thereby increasing the pressure into the cochlea at the oval window; the tympanic membrane deforms or buckles slightly; and the ossicular chain acts as a mechanical lever. The middle ear is ventilated by the Eustachian tube, which runs upwards, backwards and outwards from the space at the back of the nose, the nasopharynx. The Eustachian tube opens with swallowing and yawning, and allows nasally inhaled air to replenish air in the tympanum, which is continuously absorbed by the mucous membrane lining.

Cochlea

The human cochlea consists of a coiled tube within the temporal bone, deriving its name from the Latin *coclea* (snail). In humans there are 2.75 turns (33 mm in total length), dimensions that vary in other mammal species. The bony shell of the human cochlea coils around the modiolous, a central bony pillar containing the cochlear ganglion. The cochlear labyrinth contains three channels: the scala vestibuli (filled with perilymph and to which the stapes is connected at the oval window via the stapes footplate), the scala media (filled with endolymph and thus sometimes entitled the endolymphatic space) and the scala tympani (again filled with perilymph). The scalae vestibuli and tympani communicate at the apex of the cochlea via an opening called the heliocotrema. The scala

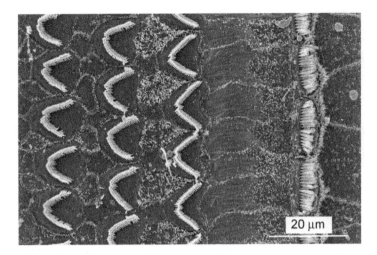

Figure 3.3   Scanning electron micrograph of the reticular lamina showing the three rows of
outer hair cells with W-shaped hair bundles and the single row of inner hair cells with more
linear bundles. The hair cells are separated by supporting cells. (Micrograph supplied by
D. N. Furness, Keele University and C. M. Hackney, University of Wisconsin-Madison.)

media is separated from the scala tympani by the basilar membrane, which is a thin mobile
membrane that becomes progressively wider towards the apex of the cochlea. Sound conducted via the middle ear causes pressure changes at the oval window, which in turn
causes the basilar membrane to move. The peak amplitude of movement of the basilar
membrane is determined by the frequency of sound: high-frequency sounds cause the
basilar membrane at the base of the cochlea to vibrate most whereas low-frequency sounds
act on the basilar membrane at the apex. The scala media is separated from the scala vestibuli by Reissner's membrane, giving the scala media a triangular shape in cross-section.
Reissner's membrane has no mechanical function but it is an important ionic barrier keeping the electrically negatively charged perilymph separate from the positively charged
endolymph. Set upon the basilar membrane within the scala media is the Organ of Corti,
a complex structure whose micromechanical properties allow the transduction of sound.
This is accomplished by approximately 15 500 hair cells within a human cochlea, these
being arranged tonotopically and being innervated by a total of 30 000 afferent nerve
fibres (Figure 3.3). Of the two varieties of hair cell in the human cochlea the inner hair
cells (Figure 3.4) form a single row close to the modiolus and number approximately 3500
in a healthy cochlea. Inner hair cells are flask-shaped with a central nucleus. The innervation of the inner hair cell is predominantly afferent. Further from the modiolus the 12 000
outer hair cells are arranged in three rows (Figure 3.5), the space between the inner hair
cells and outer hair cells being bounded by pillar cells. Outer hair cells are longer than
inner hair cells in humans (30–70 µm in length) and are cylindrical in shape, with a basally
located nucleus. A distinctive feature is the large number of mitochondria sited around the
sides of outer hair cells and associated with subsurface cisternae. Isolated outer hair cells
have been demonstrated to have motile properties when subjected to electrical or mechanical stimulation. The innervation of the outer hair cells is predominantly efferent. The tips

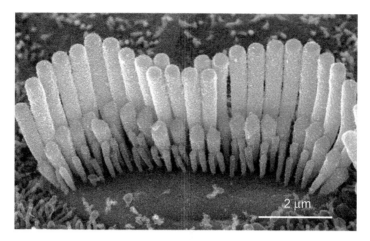

Figure 3.4 Scanning electron micrograph of a single hair bundle from an inner hair cell. (Micrograph supplied by D. N. Furness, Keele University and C. M. Hackney, University of Wisconsin-Madison.)

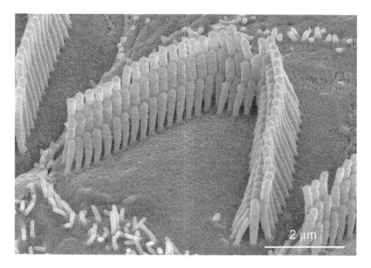

Figure 3.5 Scanning electron micrograph of a single hair bundle from an outer hair cell. Note that the stereocilia are present in three rows, the rows ranked in increasing height across the bundle. (Micrograph supplied by D. N. Furness, Keele University.)

of the outer hair cell stereocilia are embedded in the gelatinous tectorial membrane, whereas evidence suggests that those of the inner hair cells are not. The vibration of sound on the basilar membrane causes a travelling wave; the deflection at the point of that travelling wave causes sufficient motion in the inner hair cells to cause depolarization of the hair cell and hence firing of the ganglion. The outer hair cells at the point of maximum excursion of the basilar membrane change shape, producing a local amplification of the movement and therefore increased inner hair cell response.

Spiral ganglion

The spiral ganglion is contained within the modiolus and contains both Type I ganglion cells, with dendrites entitled referred to as 'radial fibres' that synapse with inner hair cells, and Type II ganglion cells with outer spiral fibre dendrites that synapse with outer hair cells. The tonotopicity of the basilar membrane is evident within the spiral ganglion, in that the fibres associated with hair cells at the apex of the cochlea are found in the centre of the spiral ganglion, while those that are associated with hair cells in the basal turn of the cochlea are found at the outside.

Internal auditory canal and cerebellopontine angle

The internal auditory canal is a bony channel for the cochlear and vestibular (VIII) nerves and facial (VII) nerves to progress to the intracranial cavity. In addition, the internal auditory canal contains the nervus intermedius and the labyrinthine artery and vein. Three regions of the internal auditory canal are identified: the fundus (abutting upon the medial aspect of the labyrinth, the lateral boundary of the fundus meeting the dura), the canal proper (the dimensions of which vary with the dimensions of the temporal bone and hence show considerable variation – mean length 8 mm, mean diameter 3.68 mm; see Gulya and Schuknecht, 1995) and the porus (located on the posterior surface of the temporal bone). At the fundus of the internal auditory canal the superior vestibular and facial nerves occupy the superior portion of the canal, with the cochlear and inferior vestibular nerves located inferiorly. The VIIth/VIIIth nerve complex undergoes a 90° rotation as it continues through the internal auditory canal and at the porus the divisions of the vestibular nerve have merged (this fusion occurring just proximal to the transverse crest) and the cochlear nerve has merged with the vestibular nerve, though the cochlear nerve fibres remain placed inferiorly. The trunks of the cochlear and vestibular nerves remain separated by a septum at the porus, although surgical specimens have shown variability in the completeness of this septum (Gulya and Schuknecht, 1995). The anastomosis of Oort (Oort, 1918) consists of a bundle of fibres running from the saccular branch of the inferior vestibular nerve to the cochlear nerve and contains efferent fibres from the medial olivo-cochlear system (Rasmussen, 1946). This vestibulo-cochlear anastomosis has been measured at 2–3 mm long and 0.1–0.3 mm wide at the base in adult humans (Arnesen, 1984) and consists of both myelinated and unmyelinated axons, with unmyelinated axons in the majority (ratio 3.0:1.0). The VIIth/VIIIth nerve complex leaves the porus of the internal auditory canal and crosses a region bounded laterally by the medial portion of the posterior surface of the temporal bone, posteriorly by the cerebellar hemisphere and the flocculus, and medially by the pons, entitled the cerebellopontine angle, containing cerebospinal fluid. In an adult human the distance from the porus to the medullary–pontine junction where the vestibulo-cochlear nerve enters the brainstem is 23–24 mm.

Central auditory anatomy

The human central auditory pathways form a complex system, with processing and feature extraction evident from a low level, but also with the maintenance of the tonotopicity set up in the cochlea to a cortical level (see Figure 3.6).

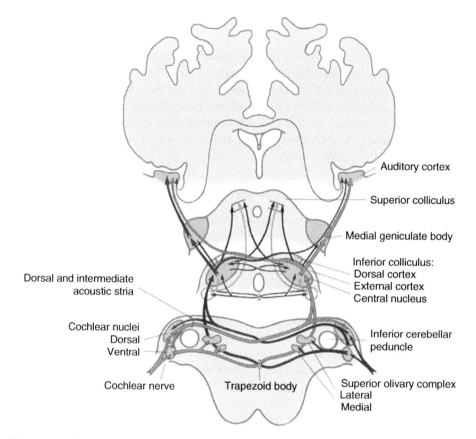

Figure 3.6 Schematic diagram of the ascending auditory pathway represented in slices of the cerebrum (upper), mid-brain and brainstem. The main nuclei between the cochlea and cerebral cortex are shown. More minor pathways are represented with finer arrows. (Reproduced from Scott-Brown's *Otorhinolarnygology* (2008), D. N. Furness and C. M. Hackney, with permission from Hodder Education.)

Cochlear nucleus

The cochlear nucleus complex spans the ponto–medullary junction and is divisible into two portions: the dorsal cochlear nucleus and the ventral cochlear nucleus. The ventral cochlear nucleus is further subdivided into the anterior ventral cochlear nucleus and the posterior ventral cochlear nucleus. Each cochlear nerve fibre divides into two main branches at entry to the brainstem, with an ascending branch to the anterior ventral cochlear nucleus and a descending branch to the posterior ventral cochlear nucleus and thence to the dorsal cochlear nucleus. In each division of the cochlear nucleus complex the tonotopicity set up within the cochlea is maintained, and such apparent redundancy is indicative of processing and feature extraction at this stage. In the anterior ventral cochlear nucleus the ascending branches of Type I spiral ganglion neurones synapse with the endbulbs of Held, large excitatory terminals with a purely relay function, ensuring the maintenance of precise tonotopicity within the arrangement of spherical bushy cells in the anterior ventral cochlear nucleus.

The axons of the spherical bushy cells are large and myelinated, and leave the anterior ventral cochlear nucleus as the ventral acoustic stria, alternatively entitled the 'trapezoid body' as it approaches the superior olivary complex. Within the posterior ventral cochlear nucleus and the dorsal cochlear nucleus lie multipolar cells that receive inputs from several cochlear nerve fibres, thus allowing frequency and intensity coding and comparison. While most of the axons from these cells project to the contralateral inferior colliculus, a number send branches to the peri-olivary region associated with the olivo-cochlear efferent system. Also within the posterior ventral cochlear nucleus are located octopus cells, which respond rapidly and have been associated with startle responses to auditory stimuli.

Inferior colliculus

The inferior colliculi are located on the dorsal surface of the mid-brain and receive branches from the contralateral cochlear nuclei running ventrally through the brainstem via the lateral lemnisci. The role of the inferior colliculi is as vital to audition as is the role of the superior colliculi in vision, and coordination of vision and audition is undertaken by connections between these two areas.

The central nucleus of the inferior colliculi is the largest brainstem auditory nucleus, and the tonotopicity seen in lower auditory brainstem structures is maintained. Within the central nuclei of the inferior colliculi, frequency and intensity maps interrelate, as does information about the temporal characteristics of sound. As described above, these maps of auditory information are integrated with visual space map information in the superior colliculi.

Medial geniculate body

Fibres from the inferior colliculi project to each of the three subdivisions (ventral, dorsal and medial) of the auditory nuclei on the surface of the thalamus, the medial geniculate body. It is the ventral division of the medial geniculate body that receives the majority of fibres. The ventral medial geniculate body is organised tonotopically and projects to the primary auditory cortices, these projections being reciprocated. In contrast, the dorsal and medial divisions of the medial geniculate bodies project to the associative auditory cortices and the medial division in particular is multimodal, containing visual, somatosensory and vestibular information – a role as a multisensory arousal system has been proposed. It has been suggested that the dorsal medial geniculate body has a more auditory-specific arousal function.

Auditory and associative cortices

In humans the primary auditory cortices are situated within the lateral fissure of the temporal lobe (Brodmann's areas 41 and 42), are binaurally innervated and a significant role in the perception of sound localization is implied. While Brodmann's area 41 has the characteristic structure of primary cortex, Brodmann's area 42, while also innervated by the ventral medial geniculate body, has a structure indicative of associative cortex. Information processed by Brodmann's areas 41 and 42 is passed to Brodmann's area 22, the most important of the association auditory cortical areas for speech processing.

Descending auditory pathways

There are many descending neural connections from the brain to the inner ear and functions including setting cochlear sensitivity, signal detection in noise and protection against loud sounds have been suggested for these circuits. There is little firm data regarding these systems apart from the olivo-cochlear system.

Superior olivary complex and medial olivo-cochlear bundle

Axons from spherical bushy cells in both ventral cochlear nuclei synapse with neurones in the superior olivary complex. Processing of these binaural inputs with regard to time differences has been associated with the medial superior olive and with regard to intensity differences with the lateral superior olive (the smaller of the two divisions), both these functions being involved in sound localization for low- and high-frequency sound, respectively. The peri-olivary nuclei are small and diffuse, surrounding the medial and lateral superior olive. The medial peri-olivary nuclei are collectively described as the medial olivo-cochlear bundle and consist of large multipolar neurones. The large majority of axons cross the mid-line and exit the brainstem as an element of the vestibular nerve, specifically within the inferior vestibular division. These efferent fibres leave the inferior vestibular nerve and join the cochlear nerve at the anastomosis of Oort (Oort, 1918) just beyond the saccular ganglion. At this point the efferent pathway consists of about 1300 fibres, 75% of which are unmyelinated (Arnesen, 1984; Schuknecht, 1993) and thence enter the cochlea via the modiolus through Rosenthal's canal to synapse with the outer hair cells. Axons from the ipsilateral olivo-cochlear bundle follow an ipsilateral inferior vestibular nerve route to the inner hair cells within the ipsilateral cochlea.

Interactions with other systems

Throughout the auditory system there are interactions with other systems; these connections integrate auditory information with that of the other senses and facilitate the response to such stimuli. Those interactions that are relevant to an understanding of tinnitus, however, are the connections between the auditory system and mechanisms of arousal and behavioural reaction to sound, as well as between audition and emotional reaction to sound. The reticular formation is located within the central core of the brainstem and is so called because of the net-like appearance of the fibre structure when seen in cross-section. This brainstem core is continuous with the intermediate grey matter of the spinal cord caudally and with the lateral hypothalamic and subthalamic regions rostrally. Many functions of the reticular formation have been identified and this, in conjunction with the diffuse structure of the formation, has led some to question the validity of the term 'reticular formation', preferring to name separate subsystems (see Heimer, 1995, and Saper, 2000, for reviews). Of interest when considering tinnitus are the functions of the medial reticular formation in mediating the sympathetic autonomic response to auditory stimulation, thus facilitating the behavioural response to alarming or unexpected stimuli (a function also involving the octopus cells of the posterior ventral cochlear nucleus) and of sleep regulation. In the latter case the rostral portion of the reticular formation (above the pons) has been implicated in wakefulness, this activity being normally inhibited by areas of the reticular formation below the pons (Rechtshaffen and Siegel, 2000).

Human emotional responses have been considered to involve a system of brain structures entitled the 'limbic system', first described by Papez (1937) and elaborated by MacLean (1955), and including the amygdala, hippocampus, fornix and septal nuclei. This initial model has been very significantly elaborated and modified (see LeDoux, 1998, for a review), and greater emphasis is placed upon the role of the amygdalae, in particular in experiences of fear and anxiety, while the hippocampus is now considered as involved in encoding short-term memory (Iversen et al., 2000). The use of auditory stimuli in experiments concerning animal models of fear conditioning has led to models of interaction between the auditory system and the limbic system, and two main pathways for interaction have been identified. The first of these pathways is that between the associative auditory cortex and the amygdala, and the second between the thalamic auditory nuclei (those being the subdivisions of the medial geniculate body) and the extralemniscal auditory pathways (LeDoux, 1998; Armony and LeDoux, 2010). These second interactions have been implicated in the experiences of tinnitus patients of anxiety, apprehension and fear about their tinnitus (Møller et al., 1992; Eggermont, 2000). Other nonauditory parts of the brain that may be associated with tinnitus include the cingulate gyrus (Mirz et al., 2000; Plewnia et al., 2007) and subcallosal areas including the nucleus accumbens (Mühlau et al. 2006; Rauschecker et al., 2010).

Plasticity

The concept that the human central nervous system can adapt structurally and functionally, which became apparent in the latter part of the twentieth century, is now fundamental to neuroscience. This ability to change is called *plasticity* and has been defined as:

> … dynamic changes in the structural and functional characteristics of neurons that occur in response to the nature or significance of their input (Irvine, 2010).

These changes can be instigated by experience during development, by injury (such as a cochlear hearing loss) or by learning. In the next chapter we will explore how this relates to the development of tinnitus.

Habituation

If human beings were not able to selectively attend to stimuli, we would be swamped by incoming information. One of the fathers of modern psychology, William James, described the world of the newborn child, who is unable to selectively attend and discriminate between sources of sensation as:

> The baby, assailed by eyes, ears, nose, skin, and entrails at once, feels it all as one great blooming, buzzing confusion (James, 1890).

The largest part of the filtering out of background sensory information is pre-conscious and occurs without intention. One mechanism of that filtering is *habituation*, which has been described as follows:

> In habituation, the simplest form of implicit learning, an animal learns about the properties of a novel stimulus that is harmless. An animal first responds to a new stimulus by attending to it with a series of orientating responses. If the stimulus is neither beneficial nor harmful, the animal learns after repeated exposure, to ignore it (Kandel, 2000).

An example would be the sea anemone that contracts when the water in the rock pool is first perturbed, but then does not after repeated waves. Humans retain the ability to habituate, a simple example being the observation that we sense the shoe on our foot when we first put it on but, for the remainder of the day, are unaware of its presence: we have habituated. In terms of hearing, friends who live close by a railway line tell us they no longer hear the trains – we might be incredulous, but this is a common experience. In later chapters the reasons why some people do not habituate to tinnitus are explored and how therapy can help to reverse that process.

Summary

A review of the complex anatomy of the human auditory system and its intimate relationship with systems of reaction, arousal and emotion indicate that a holistic view of tinnitus must consider the involvement of such systems. Also, the human auditory system cannot be regarded as a static pre-wired entity but is a highly dynamic and active structure. This malleable nature of the auditory system is critical to an understanding of why tinnitus arises and how it can be therapeutically manipulated.

Chapter 4

Mechanisms of tinnitus

There are many proposed mechanisms of tinnitus and at times the debate about these has raged fiercely. There are some challenges to our knowledge here. Firstly, it is hard to be certain about what is happening in a human auditory system in a person with tinnitus. Tests of hearing (objective and subjective) may shed some light, as may functional neuroimaging, but the situation may remain obscure. Secondly, an animal model of tinnitus may be instigated, but it is often difficult to be sure that one has initiated tinnitus in an animal. Even when this is clear, animals do not express the disappointment and perplexed demeanour seen in some tinnitus patients (and as described by Itard in Chapter 1). Thirdly, the complexity of the auditory system and the dynamic nature of auditory processing render any model wherein a discrete lesion at some point in the system causes a tinnitus, without initiating change elsewhere in the system, too simplistic. For instance, a change in cochlear function can instigate reorganisation in the primary auditory cortex and the downward (efferent) flow of information from the cortex to the cochlea can change cochlear hair cell function.

One means by which these challenges can be addressed is to make the distinction between the *ignition* point of a tinnitus, that being the most peripheral point at which the activity is generated, and then those *promoting mechanisms* that ensure that the tinnitus is prioritised by auditory and attentional systems within the brain (Baguley, 2006; Eggermont, 2006). In formulating this distinction it was hoped that when one came to design an intervention for troublesome tinnitus, some thought could be given to whether an ignition site or promoting mechanism was the intended target.

In this chapter we provide an overview of those mechanisms, both of ignition and promotion, that are presently thought to be credible. This cannot be exhaustive, but for the reader whose appetite is whetted, a wealth of literature is available in which to immerse oneself!

Tinnitus and the ear

Many cases of tinnitus seen clinically are associated with otological pathologies, encompassing the whole gamut of ear disease – from the sudden sensorineural hearing loss after

Tinnitus: A Multidisciplinary Approach, Second Edition. David Baguley, Gerhard Andersson, Don McFerran and Laurence McKenna.

a temporal bone fracture to the gradual onset of deafness in presbyacusis. Consequently, much effort has been put into trying to understand the pathophysiological events by which these otological conditions give rise to tinnitus. However, there are other forms of tinnitus in which there is no obvious otological trigger: sudden emotional stimulation in the form of a major life event such as bereavement, illness or psychological shock can precipitate the onset of tinnitus. Similarly, many cases of tinnitus arise without otological or emotional change. There is also an interesting subgroup of tinnitus patients whose trigger factors appear to arise in other sensory systems. Even if there is an otological trigger, there is good evidence that the tinnitus activity can occur at an anatomical site distant to the initial pathology. For example, tinnitus associated with a vestibular schwannoma often continues after surgical excision of the triggering lesion. Therefore it has become apparent to the scientific community that concentrating on the pathological event that triggered the tinnitus may not be very helpful in managing the condition. Nevertheless, it is still useful to examine the various suggested triggering mechanisms as, by understanding specific cases, more general understanding may follow.

Tinnitus mechanisms associated with the outer and middle ear

Most outer and middle ear pathology that gives rise to tinnitus does so by reducing the amount of auditory input, and so increasing the stark awareness of tinnitus ignited elsewhere. This is discussed in some depth in Chapter 5.

Tinnitus mechanisms associated with the cochlea

Initial theories of the pathophysiology of tinnitus understandably focused on the ear, particularly the cochlea. There was then a move away from ear-based theories of tinnitus generation because it was observed that a substantial number of people with tinnitus have normal audiograms, the presence of a hearing loss does not guarantee tinnitus and the degree of loss is not well related to the severity of any accompanying tinnitus. The argument to some extent has moved full circle because more sophisticated techniques for measuring hearing including Threshold Equalising Noise (TEN) testing (Weisz et al., 2006) and auditory evoked responses (Schaette and McAlpine, 2011) have suggested that if people with tinnitus are tested in enough depth some degree of cochlear deficit will be detected (Lindblad et al., 2011). It remains a moot point as to whether or not tinnitus can exist with a completely normal cochlea. Also, many persons with such deficits do not experience tinnitus.

Discordant damage of inner and outer hair cells

Noise and ototoxic agents, such as aminoglycoside antibiotics, typically cause maximal hearing loss in the 4–6 kHz range. This corresponds with an area of hair cell damage in the basal turn of the cochlea and outer hair cells have been demonstrated to be more susceptible to damage than inner hair cells (Stypulkowski, 1990). In the area of maximum damage both inner and outer hair cell cilia are destroyed. However, at the junction between damaged cochlea and normal cochlea there is an area where the outer hair cell cilia are destroyed but the inner hair cell cilia remain. Jastreboff (1990, 1995) suggested that this would result in imbalanced activity between the Type I nerve fibres that synapse with the inner hair cells and the Type II fibres that synapse with the outer hair cells. This results in imbalanced activity further up the auditory pathways, possibly in the dorsal cochlear nucleus, which in turn causes change at higher centres that may be perceived as tinnitus. In the normal cochlea the tectorial membrane touches the tips of the outer hair cell cilia but does not touch the inner hair cell cilia. It has been suggested that in a damaged cochlea, at the region where inner hair cell cilia are still present but outer hair cell cilia are missing, the tectorial membrane sags down on to the inner hair cell cilia causing them to depolarise. There is clinical evidence to support this theory; some authors report data indicating that patients with high-frequency sensorineural hearing loss have tinnitus that corresponds to, or is closely associated with, the pitch with the frequency at which the hearing loss begins (Hazell, 1987; Hazell and Jastreboff, 1990; Konig et al., 2006; Moore et al., 2010), though a caveat is that in other studies there was no relationship between the audiometric edge frequency and the most dominant tinnitus pitch (Sereda et al., 2011). In any case this could only be an expectation with patients with predominantly tonal tinnitus, and this is far from a universal experience. Additionally, other authors have noted that there are some central effects at the edge frequency of a sloping SNHL and specifically enhanced frequency discrimination around the edge frequency (Thai-Van et al., 2003, 2007), and that this may be associated with changes in cortical frequency maps (Eggermont, 2010, see below), though Irvine (2010) notes that this is inferential.

Jastreboff (1995) refined this hypothesis by suggesting that the brain might try to overcome what it saw as dysfunctional outer hair cells by increasing efferent neural activity to those outer hair cells. Clearly, without functioning outer hair cells this efferent activity would be futile within the cochlea but it is possible that it might alter the central perception of inner hair cell input, causing an apparent increase in activity. A recent study, however, has cast doubt on this theory: Tan et al. (in press) used a forward masking technique to measure cochlear compression and frequency selectivity in addition to hearing threshold. People with sensorineural hearing loss and tinnitus demonstrated better compression and frequency selectivity than controls who had similar sensorineural hearing loss without tinnitus. This suggests that people with tinnitus have better outer hair cell function than those who have similar hearing loss but no tinnitus rather than vice versa. Bauer et al. (2007) demonstrated in an animal model of tinnitus that both inner and outer hair cells were largely preserved after noise trauma in those rats that showed behavioural evidence of tinnitus, but there was significant loss of nerve fibres in the spiral lamina.

Discordant damage in normal hearing

As discussed above, a proportion of people with tinnitus have normal hearing as measured by pure tone audiometry. It is possible to damage quite a large proportion of outer hair cells – perhaps as many as 30% – without causing a measurable hearing loss by use of standard audiometric techniques (Clark et al., 1984). Thus, in areas of the cochlea where there are missing outer hair cell cilia there may be increased activity in inner hair cells and therefore an increase in neural activity in Type I nerve fibres carrying auditory information to the brain.

Discordant damage in profound hearing loss

If damage to both inner hair cells and outer hair cells is uniform there will be no imbalance in neural activity. Thus, a cochlea that has lost all or most of both populations of hair cells may not generate the central neural activity that is perceived as tinnitus. The clinical observation that 30% of people with profound sensorineural hearing loss do not have tinnitus (Hazell, 1996) supports this theory.

Otoacoustic emissions

Otoacoustic emissions are small sounds generated by the ear. They originate from mechanical activity in the outer hair cells of the cochlea and are then transmitted through the endolymph, oval window, ossicular chain and tympanic membrane. Otoacoustic emissions can be spontaneous or can arise in response to sound input to the ear, in which case they are known as 'evoked otoacoustic emissions'. Although it had been suggested as early as 1948 by Gold that ears could produce sound, this initial suggestion was that such sound was generated as a result of biomechanical imperfections in the auditory system. This remained a hypothesis until 1978, when Kemp described a means of measuring sound generated by the ear and went on to suggest that these sounds were generated as a normal otological function rather than a defect (see Kemp, 2010, for an overview). There was much initial excitement in the tinnitus field, with the hope that people who had tinnitus would have spontaneous otoacoustic emissions corresponding to their tinnitus. This hope was rapidly dashed: various studies showed that 38–60% of adults with normal hearing have spontaneous otoacoustic emissions (Hall, 2000). The majority of these people are unaware of this activity (Wilson and Sutton, 1981). Further work by Penner and Burns (1987) showed that even if a patient has tinnitus and spontaneous otoacoustic emissions, the perceived frequency of the tinnitus rarely matches that of the spontaneous otoacoustic emissions and these are therefore independent processes. Various studies have shown that only between 2% and 4.5% of tinnitus patients (Penner, 1990) and 6–12% of those tinnitus patients with normal hearing (Eggermont, 2010) have tinnitus that can be ascribed to spontaneous otoacoustic emissions. Additionally, Long and Tubis (1988) proposed that if tinnitus is a manifestation of spontaneous otoacoustic emissions activity, abolition of the spontaneous otoacoustic emissions would be expected to reduce or abolish the tinnitus. Treatment of troublesome SOAE is discussed in Chapter 5.

Calcium

Calcium transport is an important factor in the normal functioning of the cochlea (Marcus and Wangemann, 2010; Patuzzi, 2011). The stereocilia of inner hair cells and outer hair cells are surrounded by endolymph, which is a high-potassium, low-sodium fluid. The base of each hair cell is surrounded by perilymph, which is a low-potassium, high-sodium,

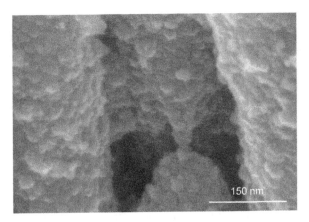

150 nm

Figure 4.1 Scanning electron micrograpgh of a close-up of the stereocilia, showing a tip link connecting the shorter stereocilium in front with the taller stereocilium behind. (Micrograph supplied by D. N. Furness, Keele Universtity.)

high-calcium solution. Incoming sound sets up waveforms in the basilar membrane which displaces the hair cell stereocilia from their resting position. This mechanical change results in the opening of ion channels on the stereocilia. Ashmore and Gale (2000) suggested that these channels are like tiny lids at the base of the tip link structures that run between adjacent stereocilia (Figure 4.1). The opening of these channels allows potassium to enter the hair cells, changing the electrical potential and thereby causing voltage-gated calcium channels to open. In inner hair cells this results in neurotransmitter release, which in turn attaches to receptors on nerve fibres and, when enough receptors have been activated, produces an action potential in the auditory nerve (Wangemann and Schact, 1996). In outer hair cells the opening of the calcium channels results in a slow motility response (Holley, 1996). The calcium that has entered the hair cells is then buffered by intracellular polypeptides, sequestered in the endoplasmic reticulum and finally returned to the perilymph via an active membrane pump which is under the control of calmodulin (Blaustein, 1988), a second messenger protein. Calcium flux is also implicated in the electrical repolarisation of the hair cell. Because calcium is so fundamental to the normal physiology of the hair cells, there have been various suggestions that defects in calcium handling could be implicated in cochlear malfunction (Zenner and Ernst, 1993). In 1990 Jastreboff suggested several mechanisms by which this might result in tinnitus. Prominent among these suggestions was the hypothesis that calcium concentrations might directly affect neurotransmitter release. Raised levels initially increase auditory nerve activity in response to mechanical stimulation of the cochlea while reducing spontaneous activity. Further increase causes reduction of both evoked and spontaneous activity. Reduction of calcium concentration conversely causes reduced evoked activity and increased spontaneous activity. Jastreboff (1990) suggested that reduced extracellular calcium concentration could alter the signal-to-noise ratio by increasing spontaneous activity and reducing evoked activity, increasing the likelihood of developing tinnitus. Both salicylates and quinine cause a rise in intracellular calcium that would be expected to have the same effect as reducing extracellular calcium. An animal model of tinnitus was developed by

Jastreboff et al. (1988) conditioning male pigmented rats to suppress licking when a background sound was turned off and the rat was in silence. Administration of quinine in ototoxic concentrations (Jastreboff et al., 1991) resulted in the rats continuing to lick in silence – behaving as if a sound was still present. Further experiments showed that the rats' response to quinine- and salicylate-induced 'tinnitus' could be abolished by administration of calcium or nimodipine, which blocks the voltage-gated calcium channels (Penner and Jastreboff, 1996).

Neurotransmitters and their receptors

Considerable research interest has been directed at the chemicals that transmit impulses between adjacent nerve cells and between nerve cells and hair cells in the auditory system. There are a wide range of these neurotransmitter chemicals including glutamate, gamma amino butyric acid (GABA), glycine, acetylcholine (Ach), serotonin (5 HT), dopamine, neurokinin (Substance P) and probably others. The effect that these chemicals have depends on the receptor that they interact with once they have been released at the synapse: this may be excitatory or inhibitory, fast or slow. Thus one neurotransmitter can interact with various different subtypes of receptors, thereby having different effects at different sites (see Sataloff et al., 2007, for a review). The main excitatory neurotransmitter in the auditory system is glutamate whereas the main inhibitory neurotransmitter is GABA. Within the cochlea the receptors that have received consideration regarding tinnitus are described below.

Alpha-amino-3-hydroxy-5-methyl-4-isoxazolepropionic acid receptors

Alpha-amino-3-hydroxy-5-methyl-4-isoxazolepropionic acid (AMPA) receptors are the main auditory nerve fibre receptors beneath the inner hair cells (Puel, 1995; Eggermont, 2010) and are important for conveying auditory information to the brain (Glowatski and Fuchs, 2002). Noise trauma causes excess glutamate to build up in the synaptic cleft, resulting in nerve fibre loss. This process is mediated by the AMPA receptors (Puel et al., 1998).

N-methyl-D-aspartate receptors

Glutamate also interacts with other receptors on Type 1 auditory fibres, including *N*-methyl-D-aspartate receptors (NMDA). These do not seem to be involved in direct transmission of auditory information but may be involved with synaptic repair after noise-induced excitotoxicity (Puel and Guitton, 2007) and have a protective function from aminoglycoside ototoxicity (Eggermont, 2011).

   Stress is well recognised as being important in both the emergence and maintenance of tinnitus in many individuals and may have a role regarding glutamate mediated tinnitus. Although it has been generally thought that the effect of stress is purely central there are suggestions that stress may have a peripheral (e.g. cochlear) role too. Dynorphins are endogenous peptides that function as selective agonists for kappa opioid receptors.

Dynorphins are released into the synaptic regions between inner hair cells and Type 1 auditory fibres by lateral efferent neurons in response to stressful situations. Sahley and Nodar (2001) suggested that dynorphins could potentiate the effect of glutamate on the NMDA receptors and postulated that chronic exposure could result in abnormal excitement in the auditory nerve. An animal model has been produced that suggests that salicylates give rise to tinnitus by activating NMDA receptors (Guitton et al., 2003). Rats were conditioned to perform a motor task in response to sound. Both salicylate and mefenamate, a nonsteroidal anti-inflammatory compound, interfered with the rats' ability to perform their task: the number of correct responses fell but the number of false positive responses in which the rats performed their task in the absence of noise rose. This was interpreted as showing that the drugs had induced tinnitus in the rats. Salicylate inhibits the enzyme cyclo-oxygenase, which prevents production of prostaglandins but causes a rise in precursor chemicals such as arachidonic acid. Arachidonic acid is known to potentiate NMDA channels so the experiment was repeated with an antagonist of NMDA receptors instilled into the perilymph. This blocked the rise in false positive responses, supporting the hypothesis that salicylates induce tinnitus by indirectly stimulating NMDA receptors.

Tinnitus and the brain

For tinnitus to be a conscious, if involuntary, perception of sound(s) there must be some representation of that percept within the auditory brain. In this section perspectives upon how that activity may arise, be organised and can be modulated by some other inputs are considered.

In considering theories of altered neural activity and tinnitus, one should bear in mind that there is always some unstructured background and stochastic electrical activity in the auditory nerve even if there is no sound input to the ear. This activity can be measured in animals and is described as the spontaneous firing rate (SFR). Initial theories of tinnitus generation were based on the hypothesis that tinnitus was caused by increase of the SFR (Evans et al., 1981). However, there was conflicting experimental evidence as to whether cochlear dysfunction caused an increase or decrease in this spontaneous neural activity. Kiang et al. (1970) studied cats that had received the ototoxic antibiotic kanamycin and discovered reduced spontaneous activity in the cochlear nerve. Evans et al. (1981) studied cats that had received salicylate at a dosage equivalent to that known to cause tinnitus in humans (400 mg/kg). They demonstrated that the cats had developed a hearing loss and found an increase in spontaneous activity in the auditory nerve. At a lower dosage of 200 mg/kg this effect was not seen. Tyler (1984) pointed out methodological differences between these two studies and pointed out that recordings from single units of the cochlear nerve might be misrepresentative of the whole nerve. Eggermont (2000) also considered these findings and suggested that, even if such animal experiments could be extrapolated to humans, it was unlikely that changes in spontaneous activity in the eighth nerve were implicated in human tinnitus experiences. There is still discussion about the extent to which cochlear SFR increases are involved in the ignition of tinnitus (Roberts et al., 2010).

Spontaneous neural activity may also be present within the central auditory pathways. In reviewing the available data regarding cochlear damage and SFR recordings in the higher auditory system Roberts and colleagues (2010) indicate that increases in SFR have been reported in association with noise trauma or cochlear ototoxicity in the following structures:

- Dorsal cochlear nucleus
- Ventral cochlear nucleus
- Inferior colliculus
- Primary and secondary auditory cortices

There have been various reports showing that intense sound exposure increases the spontaneous activity in the dorsal cochlear nucleus (DCN) of the golden hamster (e.g. Kaltenbach et al., 1996, 1999; Kaltenbach and McAslin, 1996). Similar experiments on chinchillas showed increased spontaneous activity in both the inferior colliculus (IC) and DCN (Salvi et al., 1996). There was also tonotopic reorganisation in these structures. Chen et al. (1999) exposed rats to intense sound and recorded spontaneous activity in the DCN. Although there was an increase in bursting activity there was a reduction of regular, simple spiking activity, suggesting a possible increase in auditory efferent activity.

Ototoxic agents such as salicylate were shown to produce increased spontaneous activity in the IC of both rats (Chen and Jastreboff, 1995) and guinea pigs (Jastreboff and Sasaki, 1986). Increased spontaneous activity in the cortex of gerbils after noise exposure or salicylate administration has been demonstrated using 2-deoxyglucose techniques (Wallhäusser-Franke et al., 1996) and c-fos immunochemistry (Wallhäusser-Franke, 1997). Wallhäusser-Franke and Langner (1999) demonstrated increased spontaneous activity in the amygdalae of such animals and postulated that this might represent a limbic response to tinnitus, though they could not exclude other forms of stress as the cause. Langner and Wallhäusser-Franke (1999) went on to present a computer model of tinnitus based on these results. Salicylate administration does not cause increased activity in the ventral cochlear nucleus (VCN), suggesting that the drug's effects are not due to increased afferent activity in the cochlear nerve (Zhang and Kaltenbach, 1998).

While increases in SFR may be a neural correlate of tinnitus, one should also recall that the central auditory system is indeed a system, and one with a network that can homeostatically modulate activity levels (Roberts et al., 2010). This means that any attempt to indicate that an increase in SFR at a particular level within the system is associated with tinnitus is likely to be oversimplistic. It also means that this homeostatic mechanism may be disordered by a reduction in input – so that the reported decrease in cochlear nerve SFR following cochlear injury may increase SFR in higher nuclei as the homeostatic system attempts to compensate (Schaette and Kempter, 2006; Norena, 2011). Add in the perspective that nonauditory systems can significantly influence activity within the auditory system and the complexity of the situation becomes apparent.

Abnormal synchrony

Another perspective is that it may not (only) be the amount of spontaneous activity in the auditory system that is associated with tinnitus perception, but the manner in which such activity is organised. When spontaneous activity in the auditory system is truly stochastic, no percept is elicited: it is when that activity is structured in some form that a sound perception occurs. This may involve the development of synchrony, which can occur in the time (e.g. serial synchrony as would be seen in burst firing) or frequency domains (e.g. spatial synchrony as tonotopically tuned fibres fire as correlated activity) (Roberts et al., 2010). Eggermont (2010) identifies the possibility that tinnitus may be considered as a 'hypersynchrony disorder' as an important theme in tinnitus research, though he notes that the synchronisation of spontaneous activity may be instigated by an increase in that activity and by the reorganisation of cortical frequency maps, of which more below.

One specific proposal regarding synchronous activity in the auditory system as a substrate of tinnitus regards the relationship between the auditory thalamus and the cortex (De Ridder and Vanneste, 2011). In normal hearing persons (without tinnitus) these two areas of the auditory system act in a coherent manner, meaning that the firing rhythm of each is in step with the other and that rhythm varies with the sleep/waking state and with auditory stimulation. The suggestion is that, in hearing loss, and hence reduced afferent input to the thalamus, this normal pattern of events is disrupted such that a spontaneous hyperactivity in the gamma range (>30 kHz) is instigated, such as would normally be seen in auditory stimulation, and hence is perceived as sound (tinnitus). This situation has been entitled thalamo-cortical dysrhythmia and further investigation of this proposal is underway.

Modified cortical tonotopic frequency maps

When the cochlea becomes damaged or dysfunctional, change occurs in the central auditory system. As mentioned above, changes in temporal and frequency resolution regarding frequencies at the edge of a sloping hearing loss may occur. The physiological substrate of these changes is considered to be plastic change in the tonotopic organisation by which frequency is represented in the primary auditory cortex (Robertson and Irvine, 1989). Put simply, the auditory brain musters its resources to listen to those frequencies where better auditory thresholds remain. Thus in an animal with a significant hearing loss above 2 kHz, little neural resource would attend to frequencies above 2 kHz, whereas the lower frequencies may have more cortical resources than was the case in normal hearing (Figure 4.2, Adjamian et al., 2009). This modification of the primary auditory cortex occurs due to plasticity in the mammal central nervous system – a concept that was controversial at first, but now is fundamental to modern neuroscience (see Irvine, 2010, for a review). Plastic change in the nervous system occurs during learning, but also as the nervous system attempts to recover from injury.

Salvi and colleagues (2000) proposed plastic reorganisation changes following cochlear injury as a mechanism of tinnitus. Noting that in many other sensory injuries a phantom percept may result, they considered tinnitus as a phantom auditory perception. The reorganisation of the auditory cortex may be imperfect, leading to areas of spontaneous activity. Eggermont (2010) indicated that this activity may then become synchronised, thus evoking an auditory sensation.

In an important study, Norena and Eggermont (2005, 2006) considered the effects of post-injury sound stimulation upon the reorganisation of cortical tonotopicity in kittens subjected to noise trauma. In animals raised in silence post-noise trauma the expected noise trauma-induced reorganisation of cortical tonotopicity was observed, in that the high frequencies were no longer represented. In kittens raised in an enriched auditory

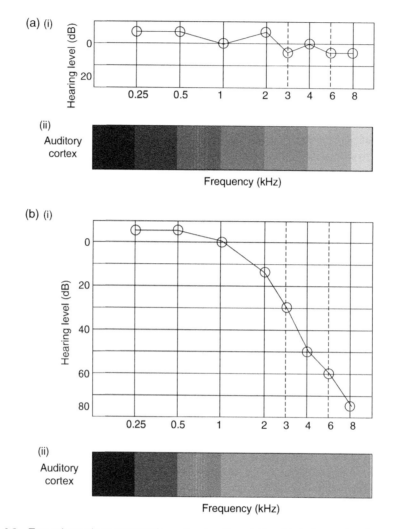

Figure 4.2 Two schematic representations showing the relationship between hearing profile and tonotopic representation of frequency in the central auditory system for normal hearing thresholds (a) and steeply sloping high-frequency hearing loss (b). In (a), a normal audiometric profile is represented cortically in bands of neurons with isofrequency tuning curves. This is schematically portrayed here with tuning shifting progressively in octave bandwidths. In (b), high-frequency hearing loss distorts this linear progression with an overrepresentation of the lesion-edge frequency. (Reproduced with permission from Adjamian, P., Sereda, M. and Hall, D. A. (2009). *Hearing Research*, **253**, 15–31.)

environment post-noise trauma, no such changes were observed: the stimulation consisted of high-frequency tonal stimulation, sounding similar to Chinese wind chimes to a human listener. The application of this study to tinnitus is inferential, as no tests of tinnitus were performed in this study, but map changes have been reported in other animal models of tinnitus. A further caveat is that the study has not been replicated, but the possible clinical implications for the importance of early auditory stimulation following noise trauma are considerable.

While the majority of studies in the field of reorganisation of the central auditory system have considered changes in tonotopicity at a cortical level, evidence is emerging that plastic change can occur elsewhere. Mulhau and colleagues (2006) used magnetic resonance imaging (MRI) and demonstrated structural changes in auditory areas of the thalamus (including the medial geniculate body) in patients with tinnitus.

Medial efferent system

Eggermont (2000) used the observation that tinnitus is often worsened by stress and can be alleviated by biofeedback techniques to propose that the medial efferent system might play a role in tinnitus perception. The efferent system is closely linked to the reticular formation in the brainstem and Hazell and Jastreboff (1990) suggested that such links would help to explain how tinnitus produces its alerting effect. Jastreboff and Hazell (1993) also suggested that the efferent system might be able to modify pre-existing cochlear tinnitus. However, experimental evidence for efferent system implication in tinnitus is not strong. Veuillet et al. (1992) performed an experiment that measured transient evoked otoacoustic emissions (TEOAE) in patients with unilateral tinnitus while noise was applied to the contralateral ear. They hypothesised that efferent dysfunction would cause less TEOAE suppression in the tinnitus ear compared to the nontinnitus ear. The hypothesis was weakly supported by the results, but there was marked intersubject variability. A similar experiment by Lind (1996) showed no statistical difference between the ears. Geven et al. (2011) compared contralateral suppression of OAE in tinnitus and nontinnitus groups and found no statistically significant differences. Baguley et al. (2002) reviewed vestibular nerve section in humans. Medial efferent auditory information runs in the inferior vestibular nerve and therefore section of the nerve would be expected to modify tinnitus. This was not the case.

Somatic modulation

It has been recognised for a considerable time that a small number of patients are able to modify their tinnitus by performing somatic tasks such as clenching their jaws (Lockwood et al., 1998) or stimulating their skin (Cacace et al., 1999a, 1999b). In 1999 Levine investigated this phenomenon by asking all patients attending the tinnitus clinic to perform a series of head and neck contractions. Over two-thirds (68%) reported a change in their tinnitus: loudness, pitch and laterality could all be affected. Decrease in tinnitus was more likely to occur if the tinnitus was unilateral. Some of the patients were also asked to perform extremity contractions. These were less likely to affect the tinnitus. The findings were used to suggest that somatic inputs could disinhibit the ipsilateral dorsal cochlear nucleus, acting via the medullary somatosensory nucleus. This disinhibition could affect spontaneous activity in the DCN altering tinnitus perception. Connections between the DCN and medullary somatosensory nucleus have been identified in cats and are thought to be important in relating pinna location and sound localisation (Nelken and Young, 1996). The anatomical evidence in humans is, however, less clear though significant research is underway (Shore et al., 2007; Møller and Shore, 2011) and the focus is upon the trigeminal nerve (Shore, 2011). Levine (1999) speculated that somatic modulation is a fundamental property of tinnitus: for others this is a specific subtype of tinnitus and should be considered separately (e.g. Sanchez and Rocha, 2011). While the fact that somatic input can modulate tinnitus may signpost a possibility for future treatments (Møller, 2011a), no such therapeutic opportunity exists at present.

Analogies with pain

Tinnitus has long been compared with pain; the initial observation of this has been ascribed to Tonndorf (Møller, 2011c). Both conditions can follow a variety of different peripheral pathologies, both can be governed by different mechanisms, both are highly subjective and both are difficult to treat (Møller, 2011c). Also, like tinnitus, chronic pain can be a sequel to a peripheral injury even after the peripheral injury has resolved. Møller (1997) concluded that both chronic pain and tinnitus are caused by central nervous system changes and that the site of this change is not the same as the perceived site of the problem. Different types of pain respond to different types of treatment, and it is reasonable to expect this to be true also of tinnitus (Møller, 1997).

Gaze evoked tinnitus

Gaze evoked tinnitus is a condition in which tinnitus can be modified by altering the direction of gaze from a neutral position. It was originally recognised as a rare sequel to surgery for cerebellopontine angle tumours (Whittaker, 1982). The phenomenon has now been recognised as being more common than previously thought (Giraud et al., 1999; Biggs and Ramsden, 2002) and may occur in as many as 20% of patients who undergo translabyrinthine surgery for removal of a vestibular schwannoma (Baguley et al., 2006b). Various suggestions have been promoted to explain the phenomenon. As it is rare for tinnitus to be gaze-evoked from silence and more common that it is a low-intensity tinnitus that is exacerbated, gaze modulated tinnitus may be a more accurate term (Baguley et al., 2006b). As it seems most commonly to follow deafferentation (for example by surgery for a vestibular schwannoma, which sacrifices any residual hearing), most theories have focused on central neural plasticity. It has variously been suggested that cross-modal neurons sprout to occupy synapses that have been denervated, previously silent synapses become unmasked or ephaptic interactions occur (Wall et al., 1987; Cacace et al., 1994; Baguley et al., 2006b).

Ephaptic coupling

Ephaptic coupling is a process in which a cell membrane can become excited due to its coming into contact with an adjacent cell membrane that is already excited. Impulses are normally passed along the auditory nerve fibres without exciting adjacent fibres, electrical transmission generally only occurring at synapses. However, in certain circumstances this insulation effect can fail, allowing signals to spread throughout the nerve, causing crosstalk. This phenomenon has been implicated in hemifacial spasm and trigeminal neuralgia (Møller, 1984). Blood vessels pressing against the facial and trigeminal nerves, respectively, are thought to be responsible for these conditions in some instances and surgical separation of the vessels has been reported to successfully control the symptoms. Møller (1984) suggested that this could apply to the eighth cranial nerve too and pressure from blood vessels or tumours such as a vestibular schwannoma could increase neural activity within the nerve, which might be perceived as tinnitus. Eggermont (1990) suggested that a space occupying lesion such as a vestibular schwannoma would cause breakdown of the myelin sheath of the auditory nerve, resulting in tinnitus. Møller (2011b) proposed that while ephaptic coupling may be an ignition site for certain specific tinnitus patients, robust evidence for this as a common mechanism for tinnitus has not been forthcoming.

Stochastic resonance

Stochastic resonance is a phenomenon in which a signal within is too weak for a sensory system to detect. However, in certain circumstances it is possible for this weak signal to resonate with noise in the system, producing enhancement and thereby enabling detection of the signal. Several animal senses use this technique as a means of detecting sensory inputs that would otherwise be too small to notice. It has been suggested that this process could also enhance the spontaneous pseudorandom firing within the auditory nerve resulting in tinnitus (Baguley, 1997; Jastreboff et al., 1996).

5HT

5HT (5-hydroxytryptamine) or serotonin is an amine produced by the hydroxylation and decarboxylation of the essential amino acid tryptophan. Receptors are found mainly in the gut and brain and exist in many forms. 5HT receptors are found in the auditory nuclei of the brainstem (Thompson et al., 1994). Increased levels of 5HT in the central nervous system generally have an inhibitory effect and have been shown to reduce the auditory startle reflex (Davis et al., 1980). Thus reduced levels of 5HT might be expected to have an excitatory effect in the central auditory pathways and this has been suggested as a cause of both tinnitus (Simpson and Davies, 2000) and hyperacusis (Marriage and Barnes, 1995). However, to date, drugs that increase 5HT concentrations, such as monoamine oxidase inhibitors and selective serotonin reuptake inhibitors, have not proved effective in tinnitus inhibition.

Auditory–limbic interactions

While there is a consensus that a person with emotional distress associated with tinnitus must have some involvement of the limbic system, a novel perspective has been suggested, proposing that the limbic system may usually have an inhibitory role for tinnitus-like signals in the brain and that troublesome tinnitus emerges as a result of failure of that function (Rauschecker et al., 2010). The ignition point of the tinnitus would be in the classical auditory system, but interaction between the auditory thalamus and the limbic system – specifically the medial geniculate body and the amygdalae – performs an inhibitory role, which the authors describe as a 'noise-cancellation system'. They postulate that this function may fail due to individual susceptibility or system overload. Clinical evidence supporting these ideas is awaited, but is said to be forthcoming (Leaver et al., 2011).

Summary

The experimental evidence supports the theory that there are multiple possible mechanisms for tinnitus generation, occurring at all levels of the auditory pathways. This diversity of causation of this single symptom may help to explain why no 'cure-all' for tinnitus has yet been discovered. In many cases it may be more accurate to talk about association with tinnitus onset rather than direct causality. In current clinical practice, treatment strategies address the distress that tinnitus generates rather than treat the underlying cause of the symptom. Hopefully, as knowledge of the pathophysiology of the condition improves more precise therapeutic tools will become available.

Chapter 5

Medical models of tinnitus

Research into tinnitus is hindered by the fact that tinnitus patients display marked heterogeneity. Although most patients with tinnitus have no more serious otological pathology than cochlear degeneration appropriate to their age and previous noise exposure, there are a few specific diseases that incorporate tinnitus as a key symptom. Such cases of tinnitus, sometimes referred to as 'syndromic tinnitus', have received much interest in a hope that understanding a few highly defined examples of tinnitus would clarify the wider picture. Similarly, there are a few drugs that induce tinnitus and much effort has been directed towards understanding the route by which this occurs.

Drug-induced tinnitus

Even a casual perusal of the internet or drug data sheets reveals that many prescription drugs have tinnitus listed as a potential side effect. Closer scrutiny reveals that, for the majority of drugs, the number of reported instances of tinnitus have occurred in a tiny percentage of the total patients taking that drug. Some of these occurrences will undoubtedly be simple coincidence, while others will be idiosyncratic unpredictable events. Furthermore, drugs are given in response to health-related problems, and both the problem that requires the treatment and the treatment itself are potent stimulants of the limbic system. This limbic system activation could account for the onset of tinnitus rather than a direct effect of the drug. There are, however, a small number of drugs that have a proven tinnitus association. Some have direct effects on the cochlea, some may act on receptors in the central auditory pathways, but in many cases the mode of action is unknown. Commonly reported drugs causing tinnitus include salicylates and some of the other nonsteroidal anti-inflammatory drugs (NSAIDs); certain antibiotics such as the aminoglycosides and ciprofloxacin; quinine and other similar antimalarial agents; loop diuretics such as furosemide; and cytotoxic agents such as cisplatin. The mechanisms of tinnitus generation are best understood for salicylates and aminoglycosides.

Tinnitus: A Multidisciplinary Approach, Second Edition. David Baguley, Gerhard Andersson, Don McFerran and Laurence McKenna.
© 2013 David Baguley, Gerhard Andersson, Don McFerran and Laurence McKenna.
Published 2013 by Blackwell Publishing Ltd.

Salicylates generally have a reversible, dose-related ototoxic effect, although permanent effects have been reported (Miller, 1985). There are several theories as to how salicylate administration results in tinnitus and there is good evidence that such compounds are active at several points in the auditory system. Mammano and Ashmore (1993) reported that salicylates affect the outer hair cells, decoupling stereocilia from the tectorial membrane. Acetyl salicylic acid (aspirin) has been shown to abolish spontaneous otoacoustic emissions (Penner and Coles, 1992; McFadden and Pasanen, 1994), adding clinical evidence that salicylates cause outer hair cell dysfunction. Salicylates reversibly interfere with prestin, the motor protein of the outer hair cells but, paradoxically, prolonged administration appears to result in an up-regulation of prestin expression (Yu et al., 2008). Jung et al. (1993) demonstrated that salicylates reduce cochlear blood flow, but as the endolymph potential remains unchanged with aspirin administration it is unlikely that reduced perfusion in the stria vascularis is very important in salicylate-induced tinnitus (Puel et al., 1990). Salicylates inhibit the enzyme cyclo-oxygenase (also known as 'prostaglandin synthetase' and 'COX'), thereby reducing prostaglandin production, reducing inflammation and exerting their beneficial therapeutic effect. However, some of the arachidonic acid that was due to be turned into prostaglandins under the control of cyclo-oxygenase can then accumulate. Some is diverted into leukotriene production but the excess arachadonic acid may act directly on N-methyl-D-aspartate (NMDA) receptors, thereby increasing activity in auditory neurons (Guitton et al., 2003). Support for this hypothesis comes from the observation that pharmacological blockade of NMDA receptors prevents the development of salicylate-induced tinnitus in an animal model (Puel, 2007). It has also been suggested that the excess leukotriene production is implicated in tinnitus generation (Jung et al., 1997). More recent work suggests that salicylates may also have an effect on central auditory pathways (Wang, 2006; Su et al., 2009). Increased serotonergic neuron activation has been demonstrated in the dorsal raphe of gerbils treated with salicylate (Caperton and Thompson, 2011).

Aminoglycoside antibiotics such as gentamicin have their antimicrobial action by acting on ribosomes and preventing polypeptide synthesis. The parentrally administered aminoglycosides have maximal effect on bacterial ribosomes and relatively little effect on mammalian ribosomes. However, if the concentration of aminoglycosides exceeds normal therapeutic limits ototoxicity can occur, and in 1981 Bernard demonstrated histopathological evidence of outer hair cell damage in cats that had been treated with gentamicin. It is thought that aminoglycosides chelate with metal ions, with the resulting compound stimulating free radical production within outer hair cells and ultimately a process of programmed cell death or apoptosis (Reiter et al., 2011). There are certain human families that display unusually high cochlear sensitivity to aminoglycosides, while the vestibular system is spared. The incidence of this susceptibility is 1:500 in the European population (Huth et al., 2011). Investigation of these families has shown a mutation of a mitochondrial gene, the small ribosomal RNA gene (12 S rRNA) (Prezant et al., 1996; Cortopassi and Hutchin, 1994). Like all mitochondrial genes, this is passed down the maternal line. The altered gene appears to make the outer hair cells less able to deal with the increased level of free radicals and hence more susceptible to aminoglycoside damage.

Many of the drugs that have a specific ototoxic effect, such as the aminoglycoside antibiotics and cytotoxic agents, are given only for life-threatening conditions and their usage is often unavoidable. To minimise the risk of ototoxicity, plasma levels of the drug should be monitored to keep the drug level within its therapeutic range. Identifying particularly susceptible individuals should also help to limit iatrogenic tinnitus. Pre-treatment genetic screening for the aminoglycoside susceptibility mutation is possible (Xie et al., 2011) but these drugs are often used in acute situations where time is of the essence, such that screening may not be feasible.

Although there have been anecdotal reports of recreational drugs such as cannabis and ecstasy either causing or relieving tinnitus, there is no good evidence to support either argument. Studies on the effect of cannabis on hearing suggest that the drug has little effect on the auditory system (Liedgren et al., 1976). The case with alcohol is confused; there have been suggestions that alcohol in large quantities can damage the cochlea (Quick, 1973) or adversely affect central auditory pathways (Spitzer and Ventry, 1980). Despite these findings, reports on the effect of alcohol on tinnitus have shown both exacerbation and relief of the symptom (Ronis, 1984; Pugh et al., 1995). The two groups of recreational drugs that do seem to be associated with increased risk of developing tinnitus are the hallucinogenic drugs and inhaled solvents (Han, 2010).

Otosclerosis

Otosclerosis is a disease of the bone of the otic capsule, which is the bone that forms the cochlea, vestibular apparatus and the footplate of the stapes. Clinically, patients present with conductive hearing loss that may start as a unilateral loss but usually eventually affects both ears. The patients may display paracusis Willisi (better hearing in noisy environment). Later in the disease sensorineural loss may occur. Tinnitus is present in the majority, most commonly with high-pitched or white noise tinnitus (Sobrinho et al., 2004). Occasionally tinnitus is the presenting symptom. In the early stages of otosclerosis the tinnitus may have a pulsatile nature. Vertigo was said to be common among people with otosclerosis but a large study found that otosclerosis patients were not over-represented in balance clinics (Grayeli et al., 2009). The tympanic membranes usually look normal, though a red flush may be apparent. This finding is referred to as 'Schwartze's sign' and is indicative of active disease. Audiology typically shows a hearing loss with an air–bone gap and a dip in bone conduction at 2 kHz called the 'Carhart notch'. There is reduced compliance on tympanometry and reduced or absent stapedial reflex. High-resolution CT scanning shows thickening of otic capsule bone with surrounding rarefaction. Estimates of the prevalence of otosclerosis vary from 0.3% (Morrison and Bundey, 1970) to 2.1% (Browning and Gatehouse, 1992) of the adult population, with most studies supplying figures at the lower end of this range. The annual incidence of otosclerosis in Sweden was reported as 12 per 100000 in 1973 (Stahle et al., 1978) and 6.1 per 100000 in 1981 (Levin et al., 1988). Clinical otosclerosis is more common in women by a ratio of 2:1 and is more common in Caucasians than other races . Onset is generally between the ages of 15 and 45 years, and the condition tends to progress in puberty and pregnancy. There have also been suggestions that administered female sex hormones, such as hormone replacement therapy (HRT), can cause progression of otosclerosis – though this is still disputed. A study by Declau et al. (2001) examined temporal bones from 118 people and found histological evidence of otosclerosis in 2.5% of 236 temporal bones. As several of the people had histological evidence of otosclerosis bilaterally the prevalence within the test population was 3.4%, demonstrating that the underlying condition is more common than the clinical disease. Hueb et al. (1991) showed that, unlike clinical otosclerosis, histological otosclerosis occurs with similar frequency in men and women. The aetiology of otosclerosis remains incompletely understood. There is often a positive family history and the condition does seem to have a genetic basis in 50–70% of cases (Levin et al., 1988). The mode of inheritance in these cases seems to be autosomal dominant with variable penetration. Various genes have been suggested as being responsible but there appears to be considerable variation between different study populations (Priyadarshi et al., 2010) and the overall picture regarding inheritance remains unclear. Arnold and Friedmann (1988) suggested that previous measles infection played a role and the number of patients requiring stapedectomy does seem to be falling following the widespread introduction of vaccination against measles (Niedermeyer and Arnold, 2008). Other hypotheses include metabolic, immune, vascular and traumatic aetiologies.

There are several theories as to how otosclerosis causes tinnitus:

- Conductive hearing loss causing deafferentation.
- Conductive hearing loss reducing the masking effect of environmental sound.
- The new bone formed has a rich blood supply, causing pulsatile tinnitus (Gibson, 1973).
- The otosclerotic process produces small arteriovenous malformations (abnormal connections between arteries and veins) resulting in pulsatile tinnitus (Sismanis and Smoker, 1994).
- Cochlear tinnitus caused by: toxic enzymes produced by the otosclerotic bone damage the cochlea; bony invasion of the cochlea; damage to the cochlear blood supply; deafferentation.

In the early twentieth century it was recognised that the hearing loss of otosclerosis had a mechanical cause and was potentially amenable to surgery. Modern microsurgical apparatus and techniques were not available and therefore surgery on the ossicles was not feasible. In the 1920s the operation of fenestration was developed and later popularised by Lempert (1938). This involved performing a mastoidectomy and then removing some of the bone over the membranous labyrinth. This allowed sound to bypass the conductive block and pass straight into the inner ear. This improved the hearing but did not return it to normal. Also, the operation produced a large mastoid cavity with all its attendant disadvantages and patients often suffered from dizziness post-operatively. Once microsurgical techniques had been developed further therapeutic options became possible, and in 1952 the operation of stapes mobilization was developed by Rosen (1953). He noticed that if one gently pressed the stapes of someone with otosclerosis, the hearing often improved – albeit temporarily. The operation worked by breaking the bony union between the stapes footplate and the round window. Unfortunately, the otosclerotic process usually began again and the stapes became fused with the round window once more. In 1958 Shea developed the operation of stapedectomy, in which the stapes is removed and replaced by a prosthesis. Initially, the whole stapes bone was removed (stapedectomy); now most surgeons remove only the superstructure and then make a small hole, or fenestra, through the footplate with microinstruments, a microdrill or laser (stapedotomy, though the term stapedectomy is still frequently used to describe this procedure).

Current treatment options include:

- Observation.
- Hearing aid amplification.
- Sodium fluoride, 50 mg daily for two years. This should be avoided in children, pregnant women, patients with rheumatoid arthritis and patients with renal disease.
- Stapedectomy or stapedotomy.

Several studies have looked at tinnitus following stapedectomy operations. Gersdorff et al. (2000) found disappearance of tinnitus in 64%, improvement in 16%, no change in 14% and worsening in 6%. Surprisingly, the outcome with respect to the tinnitus was unrelated to the hearing outcome. Ayache et al. (2003) studied 62 patients undergoing stapes surgery for otosclerosis. Pre-operative tinnitus was present in 74%. Among these patients the tinnitus ceased in 55.9%, reduced in 32.4%, remained unchanged in 8.8% and worsened in 2.9%. Among the patients who did not have pre-operative tinnitus, none developed tinnitus in the immediate post-operative period. Lima et al. (2005) looked at a small group of patients ($n=23$) who had tinnitus in association with otosclerosis. Tinnitus was abolished or reduced in 96% and a visual analogue measurement of tinnitus annoyance dropped from 8.34 pre-operatively to 1.56 post-operatively. Surgical technique has been investigated with reference to tinnitus outcome: modern small fenestra surgical techniques gave a better outcome than operations in which the footplate was removed (Gersdorff et al., 2000).

Other forms of conductive hearing loss

Conditions such as impacted wax, glue ear (secretory otitis media, otitis media with effusion), perforations of the tympanic membrane or cholesteatoma (chronic otitis media, chronic suppurative otitis media) can all be associated with tinnitus. These are all common conditions: the prevalence of chronic otitis media in the UK is estimated at 4.1% (Browning and Gatehouse, 1992). In 1984, Mills and Cherry reported a series of 66 children (aged 5–15 years) who presented to an ENT outpatient clinic with otitis media with effusion. Of these children, 29 (43.9%) reported tinnitus when asked. Forty-four children with sensorineural hearing loss were chosen as a control group: there was no use of a normally hearing control group. Among the sensorineural hearing loss control subjects 13 (29.5%) reported tinnitus. Much of the tinnitus perception in conductive hearing loss is probably due to reduction of environmental sound input, allowing better perception of sensorineural tinnitus or somatosounds. Additionally, central gain in the auditory system may increase in the presence of a conductive lesion. Some tinnitus in chronic suppurative otitis media may be iatrogenic, a consequence of using ototoxic ear drops. Theoretically, the group of patients with conductive lesions should be relatively easily treated. Wax can be removed, glue can be aspirated, grommets can be inserted, perforations can be repaired and ossicles can be reconstructed or replaced. However, if the operation is being performed specifically for tinnitus these patients need very careful counselling before undertaking surgery. Surgery is a profound stimulant of the limbic system and hence tends to increase tinnitus perioperatively. Also, tympanomastoid surgery usually increases any conductive loss in the immediate post-operative period because of swelling and haematoma in the middle ear and dressing packs in the ear canal. Patients need to be warned to expect this. Lastly, there is always a risk with middle ear surgery that the inner ear will be damaged inadvertently. Although conductive hearing loss is common, and tinnitus is common in conductive hearing loss, there is a dearth of good trials on the effect of surgery upon any tinnitus in these patients. Helm (1981) looked at the effects of tympanoplasty on patients with perforations of the tympanic membrane associated with tinnitus. Approximately one-third had less tinnitus post-operatively, one-third were unchanged and one-third were worse. Lima et al. (2007) looked at a small group of patients ($n=23$) who had tinnitus in association with perforations of the tympanic membrane. After these patients had undergone tympanoplasty, tinnitus was abolished or reduced in 83%, which was slightly better than the perforation closure rate of 78%. Patients graded their tinnitus discomfort on a 10-point scale and mean scores dropped from 5.26 pre-operatively to 1.91 post-operatively.

Ménière's disease

In 1861 Prosper Ménière described an otological disease that subsequently became eponymous. In the classical form of Ménière's disease the clinical picture is easy to recognise: episodic attacks with prodromal aural fullness and tinnitus followed by acute vertigo and hearing loss. The episodes tend to last for a period of hours and the patient then recovers. The hearing loss is characteristically maximal at low frequencies and with recurrent attacks tends to become permanent rather than temporary. Estimating the prevalence of the condition is fraught because the diagnostic criteria for Ménière's disease were originally rather loose: a study in the UK suggested a disease occurence of 157 per 100 000 (Cawthorne and Hewlett, 1954). In an attempt to facilitate accurate research on the condition, the American Academy of Otolaryngology – Head and Neck Surgery (Committee on Hearing and Equilibrium, 1995) created a set of criteria for making a diagnosis of Ménière's disease. Observing these criteria, a survey in Finland showed a disease prevalence of 43 per 100 000 with an annual incidence of up to 4.3 per 100 000 (Kotimaki et al., 1999). In 1938, Hallpike and Cairns described the histopathological findings in Ménière's disease with dilatation of the scala media and saccule, suggesting that excessive endolymph, or endolymphatic hydrops, was the cause of the condition. It subsequently became apparent that endolymphatic hydrops was a pathological condition seen in several other conditions as well as Ménière's disease (Table 5.1). By definition, Ménière's disease is primary endolymphatic hydrops and various theories have been suggested for the pathogenesis of the disease (Gibson and Arenberg, 1997):

- Congenital predisposition
- Defects of endolymph production or absorption
- Local hormones (saccin) and hydrophyllic proteins
- Systemic hormones (vasopressin)
- Autoimmunity
- Allergy

Table 5.1 Causes of endolymphatic hydrops.

- Congenital: some forms of congenital deafness such as Pendred's syndrome cochlear dysplasias (e.g. Mondini and Scheibe)
- Trauma: head injuries, surgery
- Infection: systemic syphilis, mumps, measles, otic labyrinthitis
- Neoplasia: leukaemia, Letterer–Siwe disease
- Immunological: autoimmune sudden sensorineural hearing loss, Cogan's syndrome
- Bone disease: otosclerosis, Paget's disease

Just as there is dispute about the aetiology of the condition, there is also dispute as to whether the classical microscopic appearance of the cochlea is caused by increased endolymph pressure or if this appearance represents an end stage of the process. The mechanism for tinnitus production is even more obscure. If the pressure within the organ of Corti is raised this may cause mechanical disruption and hence cause depolarization of hair cells. However, it is also possible that the process causes rupture of Reissener's membrane with consequent mixing of endolymph and perilymph. This would result in electrolyte changes that could cause depolarization of hair cells. End-stage Ménière's disease is characterised by loss of hair cells, though this is often the stage of the disease when tinnitus becomes most troublesome. A deafferentation model may explain tinnitus at this stage. The optimum management of Ménière's disease is equally unclear, with various different treatments recommended by different clinicians.

Medical treatments include:

- A low salt diet
- Betahistine
- Diuretics
- Vestibular sedatives

Surgery (conservative procedures) include:

- Endolymphatic sac surgery. Some surgeons decompress the sac whereas others insert a shunt tube or even excise it in an attempt to stabilise endolymph pressure in the inner ear.
- Sacculotomy.
- Grommet (ventilation tube) insertion. There is no logical basis for inserting a grommet in the management of Ménière's disease but the procedure is still undertaken; any benefit that does arise may well be attributed to the placebo effect.
- Grommet insertion and use of a Meniett pressure device (Mattox and Reichert, 2008).
- Intratympanic steroid injection.
- Division of intratympanic muscles.

Surgery (destructive procedures) include:

- Intratympanic gentamicin. This uses the fact that gentamicin is more toxic to the neuroepithelium of the vestibular apparatus than the cochlea to ablate residual vestibular function without damaging the hearing.

- Vestibular nerve section.
- Vestibulo-cochlear nerve section.
- Labyrinthectomy.

There are some indications that patients with Ménière's disease have specific tinnitus experiences. Stouffer and Tyler (1990) noted that patients with Ménière's disease had significantly higher ratings of tinnitus severity and annoyance than patients with other aetiologies. Douek and Reid (1968) found that patients with tinnitus as a symptom of Ménière's disease consistently matched their tinnitus to a low-frequency tone (usually in the range 125–250 Hz), unlike the majority of tinnitus patients who match tinnitus to a pitch above 3000 Hz (Tyler, 2000). Erlandsson et al. (1996) noted that those patients with anxiety and depression associated with Ménière's disease found their tinnitus intolerable.

Most research into the management of Ménière's disease has tended to concentrate primarily on the vertiginous symptoms and secondarily on the hearing loss. There is less information about the effects of the various treatments on any tinnitus. Cochrane systematic reviews have been conducted on randomised controlled trials of several Ménière's disease treatment modalities. Burgess and Kundu (2006) assessed the published research on the use of diuretics and judged that none of the available research papers had reached adequate quality to enable any conclusion to be drawn. James and Burton (2001) examined the use of betahistine and identified five studies that had looked at tinnitus, though the outcome measures chosen were weak. Mixed results were obtained in these studies though the most scientifically robust (Schmidt and Huizing, 1992) showed no difference in tinnitus outcome between betahistine and control. Overall, James and Burton (2001) felt that there was insufficient good evidence to prove whether betahistine was effective or ineffective in the management of any of the symptoms of Ménière's disease. A Cochrane review of surgical treatments for Ménière's disease (Pullens et al., 2010) reported two studies that had examined the effect of endolymphatic sac surgery on tinnitus. In one study a placebo of a cortical mastoidectomy was employed and both active and placebo groups reported improvement in tinnitus, though a nonvalidated measure was used; there was no statistically significant difference between the groups. A second study compared endolymphatic sac surgery versus grommet insertion and found no tinnitus benefit in either group. Pullens et al. (2010) assessed the literature for other surgical procedures such as vestibular nerve section, vestibulocochlear nerve section, labyrinthectomy or grommet insertion. Using the strict criteria of Cochrane reviews the authors felt that no other studies of surgical treatment of Ménière's disease were of adequate quality for consideration. Using less stringent criteria, a review article looked at the effects of vestibular nerve section on tinnitus in Ménière's disease. Overall, a mean of 16.4% had worse tinnitus post-operatively, 38.5% were unchanged and 37.2% felt their tinnitus improved (Baguley et al., 2002).

The use of intratympanic medication for Ménière's disease has been the focus of two Cochrane reviews: one examined the use of gentamicin whereas the other examined the use of steroids. The study that assessed the use of gentamicin (Pullens and van Benthem, 2011) identified two trials suitable for inclusion: the first of these did not use tinnitus as one of its outcome measures (Stokroos and Kingma, 2004); the second found no effect on tinnitus (Postema et al., 2008). Phillips and Westerberg (2011) reviewed studies on the use of intratympanic steroids in Ménière's disease. They identified one appropriate trial (Garduno-Anaya, 2005). This paper concluded that intratympanic steroids were helpful for the tinnitus of Ménière's disease but it was not apparent what result this statement was based upon. Certainly the well-validated Tinnitus Handicap Inventory questionnaire showed no statistical improvement. Phillips and Westerberg (2011) were unable to clarify this ambiguity with the original authors.

A note of caution regarding Ménières disease treatments was sounded by Vernon and Johnson (1980), who found that following vertigo control some patients with Ménière's disease focus more upon their tinnitus and hence are more distressed by it.

Vestibular schwannomas and other cerebellopontine angle lesions

As the name suggests, the cerebellopontine angle is the anatomical space between the cerebellum and pons bounded laterally by the temporal bone. It is crossed by the trigeminal, facial and vestibulocochlear nerves and the anterior inferior cerebellar artery. Caudally the lower cranial nerves also traverse the cerebellopontine angle. A wide variety of lesions can occur in this space, including meningiomas, lipomas, medulloblastomas, endolymphatic sac tumours, haemangioblastomas, secondary tumour deposits and epidermoid cysts (Bonneville et al., 2007). By far the most common lesion in this space, however, is the benign tumour popularly known as an 'acoustic neuroma'. Such tumours are more correctly called vestibular schwannomas as they are not true neuromas and normally arise on one of the vestibular nerves, usually the inferior vestibular nerve, rather than the auditory nerve. They generally start growing within the bony confines of the internal auditory meatus, pouting out into the cerebellopontine angle when they have outgrown the meatus. Patients by and large complain of unilateral hearing loss and tinnitus. Tinnitus is present in 75% of persons diagnosed with a vestibular schwannoma and is the principle presenting symptom in 11% (Baguley et al., 2001). A study by Humphriss et al. (2006) showed that in a group of 145 patients with unilateral sporadic vestibular schwannomas, 30% had tinnitus that was causing a significant handicap with Tinnitus Handicap Inventory scores of 18 or greater. Although these benign tumours arise on the vestibular nerve their growth is so gradual that the patient usually has time to accommodate to the changing vestibular input and balance symptoms are less common than hearing symptoms. However, these lesions can on occasion mimic other conditions: vestibular schwannomas have been reported with symptoms suggestive of acute vestibular failure, benign paroxysmal positional vertigo or Ménière's disease (Morrison and Sterkers, 1996). Investigation is by magnetic resonance imaging. If magnetic resonance imaging is not possible, computed tomography is a useful alternative though is not quite as sensitive. The incidence of vestibular schwannomas has shown an apparent increase but this is probably a reflection of higher indices of suspicion and the availability of better diagnostic tools such as magnetic resonance imaging scanners (Figure 5.1). A study by Moffat et al. (1995) suggested an annual incidence of 2 per 100 000 population. This figure is congruent with a Danish study that showed an annual incidence of 19.4 per 1 000 000 population in 2008 (Stangerup et al., 2010). The pathogenesis is unknown in the majority of cases. It has been suggested

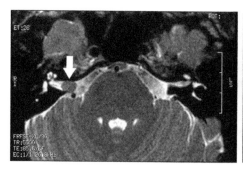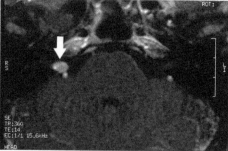

Figure 5.1   A small right-sided vestibular schwannoma: the image on the left is a T2 weighted MRI scan; the image on the right is a gadolinium-enhanced MRI scan. The white arrows point to the schwannoma.

that there is an area of cellular instability on the outer covering of the vestibular nerves that predisposes these particular nerves to develop schwannomas. There is a clear genetic cause in a small subgroup of vestibular schwannoma patients who have neurofibromatosis 2 (NF2). It has been suggested that the use of mobile telephones and other wireless devices may increase the risk of developing a vestibular schwannoma. A systematic review of this topic (Repacholi et al., 2012) showed no increased risk though as mobile phone usage is a relatively new phenomenon and vestibular schwannomas are extremely slow growing tumours this hypothesis cannot yet be completely discounted.

Although from first principles vestibular schwannomas would be expected to cause a retrocochlear or neural deafness, this is not always the case. Purely retrocochlear, purely cochlear or mixed losses can occur. There are various theories as to how vestibular schwannomas cause tinnitus (Baguley et al., 2001):

- Pressure on the auditory nerve causing a physiological breakdown of the insulating properties of the individual nerve fibres with resultant crosstalk between the fibres (ephaptic coupling) (Møller, 1984; Eggermont, 1990; Levine and Kiang, 1995). This theory is discussed in more detail in Chapter 4.
- Pressure on the auditory nerve causing an increase in the desynchronised pseudorandom firing of the auditory nerve (stochastic resonance) (Baguley, 1997; Jastreboff, 1997). This theory is also discussed in more detail in Chapter 4.
- Pressure on the auditory nerve fibres causing destruction of those nerve fibres and hence a block to auditory input. Central tinnitus then supervenes via a deafferentation mechanism (see Chapter 4).
- Pressure on the inferior vestibular nerve causing interference with the efferent nerve supply to the cochlea with resultant reduced cochlear 'damping' (Sahley et al., 1997).
- Cochlear tinnitus caused by pressure on the arterial blood supply causing atrophy of the cochlea or biochemical degradation of the cochlea and the vestibular labyrinth by polypeptides produced by the tumour.

These theories remain unproven. It is probable that the causation of the tinnitus is not the same in every patient with vestibular schwannoma and it is possible that more than one pathophysiological process may be at work in any given patient. There are several potential management strategies for patients with vestibular schwannomas:

- Do nothing because of other health considerations.
- Watch and wait and rescan, offering active treatment only if the lesion grows.
- Surgery to excise the tumour using a middle cranial fossa, suboccipital or translabyrin-thine route.
- Fractionated radiotherapy.
- Radiosurgery (gamma knife). This is very precise stereotactic radiotherapy that is usually given as a single relatively large dose.

These strategies for the management of vestibular schwannomas continue to evolve and, for smaller lesions, watch, wait and re-scan is becoming the norm. Partly because of this evolving treatment protocol the literature on management can seem confusing and at times contradictory. The first treatment option that presented good information about tinnitus outcome was the surgical option. It was observed that, intriguingly, in many cases the tinnitus persists after surgical removal of the tumour (see Baguley et al., 2001, for a review), being persistently present in 60% of patients undergoing translabyrinthine removal. Reports indicate that this post-operative tinnitus is severe in a proportion of cases, ranging from 2.5% (Baguley et al., 1992) to 6% (Andersson et al., 1997). Kameda et al. (2010) investigated 242 patients who underwent retrosigmoid excision of vestibular schwannomas; 70.7% had tinnitus pre-operatively and, of these, 25.2% had no tinnitus after surgery, 33.3% had tinnitus that was better than before, 31.6% were unchanged and 9.9% had worse tinnitus post-operatively. Interestingly, the post-operative tinnitus was unrelated to whether or not the cochlear nerve had been preserved and was also unrelated to the degree of hearing preservation that had been achieved. These findings are in contradiction to an earlier smaller study (Catalano and Post, 1996) in which hearing preservation appeared to be helpful with regard to tinnitus outcome. Grauvogel et al. (2010) used a visual analogue scale to determine tinnitus impact before and after surgery for cerebellopontine angle tumours (vestibular schwannomas and meningiomas). They reported that there was a statistically significant rise in the mean tinnitus scores. As with pre-operative tinnitus, the mechanism of post-operative tinnitus remains unclear; of the hypotheses mentioned above, that of ephaptic coupling could be applied to the post-operative situation as crosstalk has been demonstrated in damaged peripheral nerves (Seltzer and Devor, 1979). Tumour removal necessitates section of the inferior and superior vestibular nerves and so efferent dysfunction will be total because of the ablation of efferent fibres within the inferior vestibular nerve. Surgery that has resulted in increased or complete hearing loss will increase the central auditory deafferentation. There is some evidence that tinnitus after vestibular schwannoma surgery is different from idiopathic tinnitus. Cope et al. (2011) assessed a cohort of patients who had undergone translabyrinthine vestibular schwannoma removal and found that background noise tended to worsen their tinnitus compared to a control group of patients with idiopathic tinnitus for whom background noise tended to alleviate their tinnitus.

Little is yet known regarding what happens to tinnitus during a 'watch and wait policy', though anecdotally it does seem possible to help this group with standard tinnitus treatments. Lloyd et al. (2010) indicated that untreated tinnitus had an adverse influence upon patients with a conservatively managed vestibular schwannoma. Within the group being watched and serially scanned there is some evidence to suggest that the presence of tinnitus is more common among patients with growing neuromas compared to those whose lesions remain static after diagnosis. Agrawal et al. (2010) found that people with tinnitus at the time of diagnosis were more likely to show tumour growth subsequently and Breivik et al. (2012) found that people who complained of tinnitus during the period of watchful waiting were more likely to have growing tumours. Conversely, Quaranta et al. (2007) found no association between tinnitus severity and tumour growth rate.

With regard to gamma knife radiotherapy for vestibular schwannomas, several studies have compared gamma knife with surgical treatment. Coelho et al. (2008) looked at patients with small vestibular schwannomas and no useful hearing on the affected side, treated by gamma knife or translabyrinthine surgery; there was no difference with respect to tinnitus outcome. Myseth et al. (2009) compared gamma knife treatment with suboccipital approach surgery and found no difference in tinnitus outcomes. C. E. Park et al. (2011) also considered gamma knife treatment with suboccipital (retrosigmoid) approach surgery. Both groups in this study showed improvement in tinnitus after treatment but there was no difference between the groups. A longitudinal study of 59 patients undergoing gamma knife radiosurgery assessed tinnitus at various time intervals with a median follow-up of 15 months (S. S. Park et al., 2011). Tinnitus Handicap Inventory scores showed no statistical change during the study.

Pulsatile tinnitus

Pulsatile tinnitus is experienced as a rhythmical noise that may have the same rate as the heartbeat. Other forms of rhythmical tinnitus exist that have different rates, not linked to the heartbeat; these are usually due to myoclonic muscular activity and are discussed below. This section concentrates on heartbeat synchronous pulsatile tinnitus. With most forms of tinnitus it is rare to find a single identifiable cause for the problem. With pulsatile tinnitus it is also unusual to find a specific cause but the chances are greater in this form of tinnitus than in the nonpulsatile form. It therefore represents an important subgroup that merits detailed investigation. Pulsatile tinnitus is subdivided into subjective (heard only by the patient) and objective (audible to others, either directly, with a stethoscope or with a microphone in the ear canal). Pulsatile tinnitus accounts for about 4% of cases of tinnitus (Stouffer and Tyler, 1990) and can coexist with nonpulsatile tinnitus. Pulsatile tinnitus is usually caused by a change in blood flow in the vessels near the ear or by a change in awareness of that blood flow. The involved vessels include the large arteries and veins of the neck and base of the skull and smaller vessels within the ear itself. The blood flow can be altered by a variety of factors:

- Generalised increased blood flow throughout the body, such as occurs in strenuous exercise, thyrotoxicosis, pregnancy or severe anaemia. Certain drugs such as angiotensin converting enzyme inhibitors or calcium channel blockers, used in the treatment of hypertension, heart failure and angina, can cause a hyperdynamic circulation with consequent pulsatile tinnitus.
- Localised increased flow. This can occur when a blood vessel becomes blocked and other neighbouring blood vessels have to carry extra blood or when there are abnormal

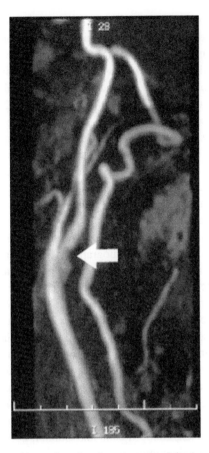

Figure 5.2 MRA of the carotid arteries showing stenosis of the internal carotid artery just above the bifurcation of the common carotid artery. The white arrow points to the stenotic portion of the internal carotid artery.

vessels, such as occurs with arterio-venous malformations. If a blood vessel is stenosed but not completely blocked, blood has to speed up to pass through the stenosed segment. This is seen in atherosclerotic disease of the carotid arteries and in fibromuscular dysplasia. An atherosclerotic stenosis of the internal carotid artery is shown in Figure 5.2. Vascular tumours such as glomus tumours can increase local blood flow. Metabolically active bone as in Paget's disease or otosclerosis has a much larger blood supply than normal bone, generating increased local blood flow.
- Turbulent blood flow. If the inside of a blood vessel becomes irregular due to atherosclerosis the blood flow will become turbulent rather than smooth.
- Awareness can be increased by several factors: conductive hearing losses associated with perforated eardrums or glue ear tend to make patients more aware of sounds inside their body (somatosounds) because they no longer have the masking effect of external sound; heightened sensitivity in the auditory pathways can alert the brain to normal noise in blood vessels in much the same way that the awareness of nonpulsatile tinnitus is generated.

In addition to the above mechanisms, pulsatile tinnitus is sometimes associated with an enigmatic condition called idiopathic intracranial hypertension or benign intracranial hypertension or 'pseudo-tumour cerebri'. This unusual syndrome is characterised by headaches, dizziness, pulsatile tinnitus, hearing loss and aural fullness; these symptoms may be exacerbated on lying down. It is more common in women of child-bearing age than men or older women and is frequently associated with obesity (Wall, 2010). Focal neurological signs are rare apart from occasional VIth or VIIth cranial nerve palsies. Papilloedema is common but not invariable. Magnetic resonance imaging scans may show the typical features of raised intracranial pressure with small cerebral ventricles and effacement of the cortical sulci, but this also is not invariable. Magnetic resonance imaging may also show an empty sella in which the pituitary gland appears to be absent from its normal location. In actuality it is present but flattened because of the increased pressure. It is easy to overlook this condition but if the condition is clinically suspected advice should be sought from neurological and ophthalmological colleagues. Various ophthalmological tests including visual field testing and optical coherence tomography (Heidary and Rizzo, 2010) may help to point to the diagnosis, but the gold standard test is to perform a lumbar puncture. In idiopathic intracranial hypertension the cerebrospinal fluid pressure is raised with an opening pressure of 200 mm H_2O or more (Sismanis, 1987). Although the condition is usually idiopathic it is sometimes seen with other disease processes, including hyperthyroidism, anaemia, Cushing's disease and several vitamin deficiencies (Fishman, 1980). It is also seen in patients taking a variety of drugs including some antibiotics, female sex hormones, some nonsteroidal anti-inflammatory drugs and steroids (Fishman, 1980; Sismanis, 1987). Treatment is by addressing any associated disease process or causative medication, encouraging weight loss and judicious use of diuretics (Sismanis and Smoker, 1994).

The investigation of patients with pulsatile tinnitus depends on the clinical history and findings (Weissman and Hirsch, 2000; Madani and Connor, 2009) but generally relies on one or more of the following modalities:

- Ultrasound, with Doppler to show the blood flow within vessels.
- Computed tomography scanning.
- Computed tomography angiography.
- Magnetic resonance imaging.
- Magnetic resonance angiography.
- Angiography. Although this is still the most accurate method of investigating the cranial vasculature it is an invasive process with an associated morbidity and mortality, and it is probably no longer justifiable to perform this as a first-line investigation.
- Haematological tests including Full Blood Count and Thyroid Function Tests. Alkaline phosphatase levels may be required if Paget's disease is suspected.

Various algorithms for the investigation of pulsatile tinnitus have been devised (Madani and Connor, 2009) but to a certain extent the investigative path will depend on the local availabilities and expertises within the radiology department. The treatment of pulsatile tinnitus clearly depends on the aetiology. High blood pressure can be treated with medication, drug-induced pulsatile tinnitus can be reduced by altering the offending medication and stenotic segments of carotid artery can be repaired surgically. Vascular tumours, such as glomus tumours (Figure 5.3) or meningiomas, can be excised or if inoperable can be

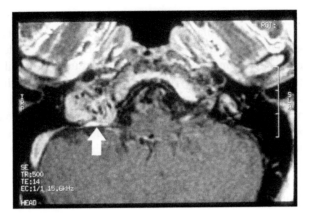

Figure 5.3 Magnetic resonance imaging scan of a right-sided Fisch Type D glomus tumour. The scan shows black flow voids that give the lesion its characteristic 'salt and pepper' appearance. The white arrow points to the glomus tumour.

partially controlled with radiotherapy. Otitis media with effusion can be treated with grommets; perforations can be closed with tympanoplasty grafts. For patients with pulsatile tinnitus who have no demonstrable abnormality, methods such as tinnitus retraining therapy or psychological treatments can be used.

Vascular loops

Compression of cranial nerves by adjacent blood vessels has been suggested as a cause of several conditions including trigeminal neuralgia, glossopharyngeal neuralgia, hemi-facial spasm and certain forms of tinnitus (Møller, 1998; De Ridder and Møller, 2011). The pressure of the vessel is thought to damage the nerve (Schwaber and Whetswell, 1992), leading to hyperactivity within the affected nerve, resulting, in the case of the vestibulo-cochlear nerve, in tinnitus (De Ridder and Møller, 2011). While this neurovascular conflict or vascular compression syndrome can occur bilaterally, it is most commonly unilateral. De Ridder and Møller (2011) suggested that the natural history of tinnitus arising from cochlear nerve compression should be of initially intermittent bursts of tinnitus becoming constant over time. In the cerebellopontine angle and internal auditory meatus the eighth nerve complex is closely related to a loop of the anterior inferior cerebellar artery (McDermott et al., 2003) and this is the usual vessel implicated in neurovascular conflicts of the vestibulocochlear nerve. It has also been suggested that the position at which the vessel touches the nerve determines the type of tinnitus: pressure within the internal meatus generates pulsatile tinnitus whereas pressure more medially in the cerebello-pontine angle generates conventional tinnitus (Nowé et al., 2004). There is, however, considerable variation in the findings of the various relevant studies and this remains a controversial topic. A study by De Ridder et al. (2005) found a strong correlation between pulsatile tinnitus and intrameatal vascular loops. By contrast, McDermott et al. (2003) found evidence of a highly significant link between intrameatal loops and hearing loss but no association with tinnitus. It has also been observed that such loops are an incidental finding in some individuals without any tinnitus (Gultekin et al., 2008). Surgical microvascular decompression techniques have been devised to separate the nerves and vessels (Brookes, 1996; Jannetta, 1998; De Ridder and Møller, 2011). Post-operative improvement of tinnitus is reported to be more likely in persons with shorter duration tinnitus (3–5 years) (De Ridder and Møller, 2011). Initial reports of improved tinnitus varied from 40% (Brookes, 1996) to 77% (Møller et al., 1993), but the present indication is that in 30% of patients the tinnitus abates and in a further 30% it is reduced (De Ridder and Møller, 2011). However, the number of patients studied is small, studies have not used controls (though this might be ethically difficult to organise) and the surgery is potentially life threatening. For these reasons it is probably wise to regard vascular loops as a hypothetical cause of tinnitus and await a more robust evidence base. Behavioural techniques to manage tinnitus should be attempted prior to any surgery.

Superior semicircular canal dehiscence

First described by Minor et al. (1998), superior semicircular canal dehiscence is a condition in which the bone overlying the superior semicircular canal is deficient, leaving the membranous labyrinth exposed, touching the dura of the middle cranial fossa. Symptoms associated with this condition include aural fullness, awareness of one's voice and other somatosounds such as the movement of the eyes or joints. Patients may be aware of their heartbeat or the sound of their footsteps as they walk. Dizziness and balance disorders are common, especially in response to loud sounds – the Tullio phenomenon. Changes in middle ear or intracranial pressure can also trigger dizziness. Pulsatile tinnitus is common but other types of tinnitus have also been reported (Nam et al., 2010b). The aetiology of the condition is unknown but it has been suggested that affected patients have congenitally thin bone over the superior semicircular canal. It is unusual, however, for the condition to present in childhood – the most common age at presentation is in the fourth decade of life, with men outnumbering women. Diagnosis is often difficult as some of the symptoms may resemble other conditions such as otosclerosis, Ménière's disease, benign paroxysmal positional vertigo, Eustachian tube dysfunction, patulous Eustachian tube or vestibular failure. Pure tone audiometry may show an air–bone gap even though the air conduction thresholds are within the normal range. This apparent conductive hearing loss is thought to be due to the dehiscence creating a third window into the inner ear (Merchant and Rosowski, 2008). Vestibular evoked myogenic potentials (VEMPs) may show reduced thresholds for this reflex. The main investigation is high-resolution computed tomography of the temporal bone to visualise any dehiscence. Several surgical procedures have been suggested for the management of superior semicircular dehiscence. The dehiscent bone can be exposed via a middle fossa craniotomy and the defect can then be repaired by resurfacing the superior aspect of the temporal bone. Alternatively, the defect can be plugged, compressing the affected superior semicircular canal. Plugging can also be achieved via a trans-mastoid approach. All these surgical treatments carry appreciable risks and many patients with the condition have preferred to live with their symptoms. Dehiscence of the lateral and posterior semicircular canals can also occur, usually associated with cholesteatoma or high-riding jugular bulbs, respectively (Chien et al., 2011).

Myoclonus and allied conditions

Middle ear myoclonus

The muscles attached to the ossicles can cause an unusual form of tinnitus in which there is rhythmical contraction of the stapedius and/or tensor tympani muscles. Typically patients describe a clicking or buzzing sound but other descriptions are not uncommon and for some people the condition produces a somatic symptom, often described as a fluttering sensation, rather than a sound. This form of tinnitus is most commonly called middle ear myoclonus but other titles including intratympanic myoclonus, stapedial myoclonus, tensor tympani myoclonus and tensor tympani syndrome are seen. It may be subjective or objective and is usually unilateral. Middle ear myoclonus is usually said to be a rare condition but there are no relevant prevalence and incidence studies and anecdotally it seems not uncommon to encounter patients who experience brief episodes of this type of tinnitus, often in conjunction with other nonrhythmical tinnitus. The underlying pathophysiology is unknown, but a small number of cases have been reported after facial nerve palsy (Bento et al., 1998; Liu et al., 2011) and a case of congenital middle ear myoclonus has been described (Howsam et al., 2005). There is no evidence to suggest that middle ear myoclonus is a manifestation of a wider neurological condition.

The diagnosis is usually obtained by taking a careful clinical history. Close examination of the eardrum using an operating microscope set at high magnification may supply confirmation. Long time base tympanometry is also helpful as it may demonstrate a sawtooth wave (Bhimrao et al., 2012).

It is usually impossible to determine whether it is the stapedius or the tensor tympani muscle that is generating the symptom, though it has been suggested that stapedial myoclonus produces buzzing whereas tensor tympani myoclonus generates clicking (Watanabe et al., 1974). When considering middle ear myoclonus as a diagnosis it is important to differentiate it from other forms of tinnitus, particularly palatal myoclonus, but also patulous Eustachian tube syndrome, vascular pulsatile tinnitus and temporomandibular joint crepitus. Although there is no strong evidence base, it would seem sensible to investigate unilateral middle ear myoclonus in the same way that other unilateral cases of tinnitus are investigated, with MRI scanning of the trigeminal, facial and vestibulocochlear nerves and adjacent brainstem.

Treatments that have been tried are divided into drug treatments, supportive interventions and surgery. Drugs that have been used include piracetam (Ha, 2007), carbamazepine (Rajah, 1992), orphenadrine (Ha, 2007; Abdul-Baqi, 2004) and benzodiazepines (Badia et al., 1994). Most of these drugs have proved helpful to some extent, but with very small patient numbers and no randomised controlled trials it is difficult to draw any real conclusions. Botulinum toxin has been successfully used in a patient whose middle ear myoclonus was associated with ipsilateral blepharospasm, injecting the drug into the orbicularis oculi muscle (Badia et al., 1994). A recent animal study has been conducted on guinea pigs to establish whether it is safe to administer botulinum toxin intratympanically (Zehlicke et al., 2008); no ototoxic effects were detected. There is one case report of botulinum toxin being used intratympanically in a human patient to good effect (Liu et al., 2011). Supportive treatments that have been tried have included relaxation therapy (Klockhoff et al., 1971), psychotherapy (Cohen and Perez, 2003) and patient-administered zygomatic pressure (Chan and Palaniappan, 2010). Sound therapy has been recommended for the treatment of middle ear myoclonus (East and Hazell, 1987). There are several reports regarding the use of surgery for the treatment of middle ear myoclonus, by performing a tympanotomy and then dividing either or both of the stapedius and tensor tympani tendons (see Bhimrao et al., 2012, for a review). Studies have shown that surgical tenotomy is generally helpful, though, as with drug treatments, patient numbers are too small to reach confident conclusions. Although division of the middle ear muscle tendons might be expected to cause hyperacusis by depriving the ear of its normal protective reflex there are no reports of this occurring.

Palatal tremor (palatal myoclonus)

The muscles of the soft palate, some of which are also attached to the Eustachian tube, can produce a form of tinnitus called palatal tremor or palatal myoclonus by involuntary rhythmical contraction. In this rare type of tinnitus the patient hears a clicking sound with a frequency of 1 to 2 clicks per second, which may also be audible to others. The palatal contractions may be unilateral or bilateral. Palatal myoclonus has been divided into two types: symptomatic palatal myoclonus and essential palatal myoclonus (Pearce, 2008). Symptomatic palatal myoclonus is associated with lesions in the Guillain–Mollaret triangle, which is an area of the brain stem bounded by the inferior olive, the red nucleus and the contralateral dentate nucleus within the cerebellum (Pearce, 2008). This form of palatal myoclonus is unusual among movement disorders in that it often persists during sleep and cannot be suppressed by voluntary muscular action. Causative pathologies in the brainstem include cerebrovascular lesions, tumours, trauma, demyelination, infection and degenerative diseases. Symptomatic palatal myoclonus is most common in late middle age. Essential palatal myoclonus is clinically similar but no brainstem pathology can be identified. It tends to happen in younger people, between 30 and 40 years, and is more likely to stop in response to voluntary muscular action. Its aetiology is unknown. Clicking is generally associated with essential rather than symptomatic palatal tremor (Zadikoff, 2006) and it is therefore essential palatal tremor that is more likely to be seen in a tinnitus clinic setting. Palatal myoclonus may be accompanied by involuntary eye movements, usually a pendular nystagmus, in which case the condition is called oculopalatal myoclonus.

Diagnosis of palatal myoclonus is by observation of the palate. Sometimes mouth opening abolishes the phenomenon. In this case use of a fibre-optic endoscope inserted through the nose may be helpful in obtaining a diagnosis as the soft palate can then be visualised from above with the mouth closed. Because of the association of the condition with brainstem pathology patients should have a high-resolution magnetic resonance scan of this region. A neurological opinion is also recommended. Various systemic drug treatments have been tried, most noticeably antispasmodic and anticonvulsant medications, with mixed results. When patients with palatal myoclonus have clicking, local injection of botulinum toxin to paralyse the tensor veli palatini muscles gives relief, albeit temporarily (Saeed and Brookes, 1993; Penney et al., 2006). Radiofrequency ablation offers the possibility of a permanent cure (Aydin et al., 2006).

Tonic tensor tympani syndrome

Various workers in the tinnitus field feel that as well as being involved in middle ear myoclonus, the tensor tympani muscle can produce a range of auditory and vestibular symptoms by being held in a persistent state of contraction. This tonic tensor tympani syndrome was first described by Klockhoff et al. (1971). Symptoms include pain or full-ness in the ear, distortion of hearing, tinnitus, numbness or a burning sensation around the ear, unsteadiness or dizziness. It has been suggested that tonic tensor tympani syndrome is the mechanism underlying Acoustic Shock Syndrome (Westcott, 2006) and that it may also be involved in some cases of hyperacusis. Although some facets of tonic tensor tym-pani syndrome fit with clinical observation, the condition remains speculative and as yet there is little hard scientific evidence to support its existence.

Patulous Eustachian tube

The Eustachian tube spends most of its time closed, opening to equalise the pressure in the middle ear with that in the environment only during swallowing or yawning. There is a rare condition in which the Eustachian tube is abnormally open. During breathing a venturi effect sucks the eardrum medially, giving the patient a sensation of aural fullness, autophony and a flapping sensation. This condition, called patulous Eustachian tube syndrome, often starts after sudden weight loss and has been reported in patients undergo-ing bariatric surgery (Alhammadi et al., 2009; Muñoz et al., 2010) and in association with anorexia (Karwautz et al., 1999). Patulous Eustachian tube syndrome has also been reported following radiotherapy for nasopharyngeal carcinoma (Chen et al., 1999; Young et al., 1997) and in patients suffering from amyotrophic lateral sclerosis (Takasaki et al., 2008; Schellenberg et al., 2010). There may be an associated sensorineural hearing loss. Almost all case reports have been in adults but the condition is very occasionally seen in children (Wolraich and Zur, 2010).

Diagnosis is chiefly from the history but careful examination of the tympanic membrane while the patient breathes in and out can show the movement. Long-time base tympanometry during respiration can also be used to demonstrate the movement (see Figure 5.4).

Treatment is not straightforward. Unfortunately, many of the symptoms are similar to those of otitis media with effusion and the condition is often mistaken for Eustachian tube dysfunction or, in other words, an abnormally *closed* Eustachian tube, and not infrequently the first treatment is to insert a ventilation tube (grommet). Many clinicians feel that insertion of a ventilation tube in the presence of a patulous Eustachian tube is a mistake, but others feel that this is not the case and report good results from their usage (Chen and Luxford, 1990). Various materials such as Teflon (Pulec, 1967), autologous cartilage (Kong et al., 2010; Poe, 2007), autologous fat (Doherty and Slattery, 2003) and calcium

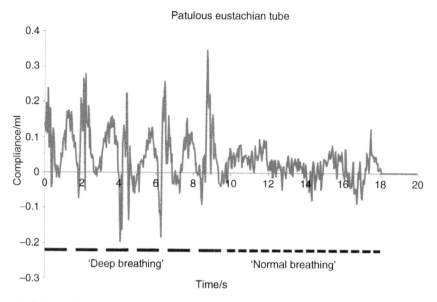

Figure 5.4   Long time base tympanometry in patulous Eustachian tube.

hydroxylapatite (Wolraich and Zur, 2010) have been injected around the opening of the tube in the nasopharynx to try to close it sufficiently to stop the symptom, but not so much that the tube becomes completely blocked. Robinson and Hazell (1989) reported use of controlled diathermy of the medial end of the tube to achieve the same result. Lasers have been used to reshape the curvature of the medial end of the Eustachian tube (Yañez et al., 2011) and one group reported ligating the tube to good effect (Takano et al., 2007). Plugs can be inserted into the lateral end of the Eustachian tube using a transtympanic approach (Sato et al., 2005; Ikeda et al., 2011). Another way to try and reduce the symptoms of patulous Eustachian tube syndrome is to apply small weights to the tympanic membrane to limit its mobility; one group reported a series of patients who were treated with small pieces of Blu-Tack (Bartlett et al., 2010). Other measures have included instructing people with the condition to stop sniffing (Ikeda et al., 2011). Most of the studies on therapeutic interventions for patulous Eustachian tube syndrome have been on very small patient populations and have not used adequate controls. It is therefore not possible to recommend any treatment above the others.

Spontaneous otoacoustic emissions

Most spontaneous otoacoustic emissions are inaudible except with the use of sophisticated instruments. The role of such small-amplitude spontaneous otoacoustic emissions in the genesis of tinnitus is discussed in Chapter 4. However, a very small number of spontaneous otoacoustic emissions are loud enough to be clearly heard by others (Schloth and Zwicker, 1983; Fritsch et al., 2001). Occurring chiefly in children, these large spontaneous otoacoustic emissions have been reported as a cause of objective tinnitus. However, in many cases, although onlookers may be aware of the sound, the patient is often unaware of it. It is therefore a moot point as to whether this should be regarded as tinnitus. Hearing is usually unaffected. Management is generally a thorough explanation of cochlear and particularly outer hair cell function. The patient and relatives should be strongly reassured that there is no serious underlying pathology and that these audible spontaneous otoacoustic emissions tend to fade with time. Low-dose aspirin has been shown to be effective in abolishing the sound in some cases (Fritsch et al., 2001). However, aspirin should not be given to patients under the age of 16 years as there is a risk of precipitating Reye's syndrome.

Temporomandibular disorder and tinnitus

Temporomandibular disorder, also known as 'temporomandibular pain dysfunction disorder' or 'craniofacial disorder' is defined as symptoms arising from the temporomandibular joints, muscles of mastication and associated structures (McNeill, 1993). Like tinnitus, temporomandibular disorder is common: prevalence is reported as up to 20% of the population. Symptoms and signs of temporomandibular disorder include pain and tenderness around the temporomandibular joints and muscles of mastication, headaches, clicking and crepitus of the temporomandibular joints, locking of the temporomandibular joints, abnormal bite and altered sensation in the face. In addition, temporomandibular disorder can be associated with tinnitus, vertigo, otalgia and altered hearing perception (Chan and Reade, 1994). With two such common conditions as temporomandibular disorder and tinnitus, it is inevitable that some patients could have both conditions, but some reports have suggested that such simultaneous occurrence of tinnitus and temporomandibular disorder is just coincidence (Brookes et al., 1980). However, other workers have suggested that there is evidence of a higher than expected prevalence of tinnitus in temporomandibular disorder patients and vice versa (Rubinstein et al., 1990; Rubinstein, 1993). The presence of temporomandibular disorder has been reported as a predictive factor in the subsequent development of tinnitus (Bernhardt et al., 2011).

This association of aural symptoms with dysfunction of the temporomandibular joints was first described by Costen in 1934, and the combination of temporomandibular disorder and tinnitus is still sometimes referred to as Costen's syndrome. The pathophysiological processes that link temporomandibular disorder to tinnitus remain obscure, but several theories have been proposed. These include a common embryological origin of temporomandibular joints and aural structures, a shared sensory nerve supply, muscles of mastication acting on the Eustachian tube and ligaments that are common to both the malleus and the temporomandibular joints (Ash and Pinto, 1991; Chen and Reade, 1994). Additionally, the hypothesis of Levine (1999) regarding the influence of somatic systems upon auditory gain and tinnitus may be implicated. Stomatognatic (dental and jaw) treatment has been studied with relevance to tinnitus, mostly by dentists with a particular interest in tinnitus (Rubinstein and Carlsson, 1987). Nonsurgical treatment of temporomandibular disorder includes analgesics and anti-inflammatory drugs, anxiolytics and antidepressants. Bite-raising orthodontic splints are helpful in preventing excessive muscle contraction and bruxism. Adoption of a soft diet also helps to reduce strain on the tempo-romandibular joints. Relaxation therapy and stress management techniques have been used to good effect in temporomandibular disorder (Turk et al., 1996).

Surgery is appropriate only when conservative measures have failed. The two commonly used surgical techniques are temporomandibular joint arthroscopy (Steigerwald et al., 1996) and arthrotomy. Both techniques aim to repair damaged structures within the temporomandibular joints. Arthroscopy employs a small endoscope to access the joint, whereas arthrotomy formally opens the joint. Arthrotomy allows more extensive work to be undertaken but is a more invasive procedure and the post-operative recovery period is longer. There have been several studies that have shown that treatment of temporomandibular disorder improves associated tinnitus (Gelb and Bernstein, 1983; Erlandsson et al., 1991; Tullberg and Ernberg, 2006). Wright and Bifano (1997) reviewed the relevant literature and concluded that between 46% and 96% of patients with temporomandibular disorder and tinnitus had reduction of the tinnitus when the temporomandibular disorder was treated with splints, although there were methodological flaws in most of the studies. The mechanism by which treating temporomandibular disorder results in reduction of any associated tinnitus remains obscure, though Campbell (1993) suggested that large doses of nonsteroidal anti-inflammatory drugs are often used to alleviate the symptoms of temporomandibular disorder and these might in fact exacerbate tinnitus. Successful treatment of the underlying condition would allow reduction or cessation of nonsteroidal anti-inflammatory drug intake with consequent relief of tinnitus.

Unilateral sudden sensorineural hearing loss

A sudden sensorineural hearing loss is considered to be an otological emergency (Arts, 1998; Hughes, 1998) and to necessitate urgent treatment. Little attention has been paid, however, to the consequence to the patient of a sudden sensorineural hearing loss in terms of a tinnitus handicap. The perceived hearing handicap of patients with unilateral hearing loss has been considered (Newman et al., 1997a). A series of 43 patients with unilaterally normal hearing completed the Hearing Handicap Inventory for Adults (Newman et al., 1990). It was noted that almost three-quarters (73%) reported a mild or greater hearing handicap, which was indicative of 'communication and psychosocial problems', despite the normal contralateral ear. The patients were recruited from otolaryngology outpatients, but it was not recorded for how long they had experienced the unilateral hearing loss, nor if the loss had been gradual or sudden. It might be expected that the sudden and possibly traumatic onset of a unilateral hearing loss might involve more handicap than a loss of insidious onset. A study by Chiossoine-Kerdel et al. (2000) investigated the tinnitus handicap associated with sudden sensorineural hearing loss in a group of patients using the Hearing Handicap Inventory for Adults and the Tinnitus Handicap Inventory (THI) (Newman et al., 1996) as outcome measures. Tinnitus was reported by 14 of the 21 patients who responded to the postal questionnaires from a total of 38 patients identified as having undergone a sudden sensorineural hearing loss in the years 1988–1997. The median total THI score for those with tinnitus was 20 (interquartile range 52), and in four patients of the 14 with tinnitus (28.6 %) the tinnitus handicap

Table 5.2 Investigations for sudden sensorineural hearing loss.*

Haematology
  Full blood count
  Erythrocyte sedimentation rate
  Clotting screen

Biochemistry
  Blood sugar
  Urea and electrolytes
  Cholesterol/triglycerides
  Thyroid function test
  Liver function tests

Clinical immunology
  Autoantibodies
  Immunoglobulins (IgG, IgM, IgA)
  Rheumatoid factors (latex agglutination, Rose Waaler)
  Cryoglobulins
  Circulating immunocomplexes
  Complement profile (C1150, C3, C4, Clq)

Microbiology/serology
  Viral antibodies, including Epstein–Barr virus and cytomegalovirus
  Syphilis serology
  Toxoplasma serology
  Rickettsia serology

Audiology
  Daily pure tone audiometry (AC/BC)
  Electronystagmography and calorics
  Brainstem evoked response audiometry

Radiology
  Magnetic resonance imaging scan of internal auditory canals and brain

---

*Not all of these investigations are appropriate to every patient with sudden sensorineural hearing loss and the tests should be tailored to meet the individual patient's requirements.

was moderate or severe. The onset of tinnitus was coincident with sudden sensorineural hearing loss in eight patients (57% of the 14 with tinnitus) and occurred within 48 hours in the remaining six (43%). In 18 patients (86% of the 21 patients) a significant hearing handicap was demonstrated by the Hearing Handicap Inventory for Adults score. The management of sudden sensorineural hearing loss remains controversial. The condition should be thoroughly investigated in an attempt to identify specific treatable pathology (Table 5.2). Many different treatment regimes have been tried including systemic steroids, intratympanic steroids, hyperbaric oxygen, antiviral drugs, vasodilators and other vasoactive drugs. Several of these treatment modalities have been the subject of Cochrane systematic reviews. A review of hyperbaric oxygen therapy (Bennett et al., 2007) commented that the published trials were generally of poor quality but there was some evidence that this therapy helped tinnitus outcome. Wei et al. (2006) investigated the use of systemic steroids and found no evidence with regard to tinnitus outcome. A review of vasodilators and vasoactive drugs (Agarwal and Pothier, 2009) identified three potential studies and one of these had used tinnitus as an outcome measure (Ogawa et al., 2002), finding that tinnitus outcome was better in a group treated with prostaglandin E1 compared to a placebo group. The early support and rehabilitation of both the hearing loss and tinnitus, using hearing therapy and amplification as appropriate, may well be of significant benefit.

Summary

There are several well-defined diseases that have tinnitus as part of the symptom complex. There are also various drugs that are known to induce tinnitus. The mechanisms by which tinnitus is generated in these situations have been well investigated and in most cases are much better understood than in the more commonly encountered nonsyndromic tinnitus. From first principles it would be expected that a good understanding of the pathophysiology should lead to enhanced treatment options and a greater chance of controlling or curing the symptom. However, in practice, the results of treating such conditions are often rather disappointing with regard to tinnitus control. This supports the neurophysiological and psychological models of tinnitus, both of which suggest that although peripheral otological disease may trigger tinnitus, central auditory processes and related systems of reaction and emotion are more important in the distress and long-term effects of the symptom.

Chapter 6

Objective correlates of tinnitus

The search for an objective measure of tinnitus perception has been a challenge in the tinnitus field for many years. In our first edition of this book we were amazed by the rapid progress in studies on the neural mechanisms behind tinnitus and this has continued apace. In this chapter we review knowledge regarding spontaneous reaction time and auditory response audiometry, and also consider findings in the field of brain imaging techniques. While there is yet no simple solution as to what causes tinnitus and there are still many uncertainties, some robust understanding of tinnitus is emerging.

Reaction time

A few studies have investigated how tinnitus patients respond to sounds in terms of reaction time. Measures of reaction time are not performed without subjects' active participation, but the results can give us some indication as to how the brain processes the tinnitus signal. Goodwin and Johnson (1980b) found that tinnitus patients ($n=9$) responded faster to tones that matched their tinnitus frequency compared with sounds of a nontinnitus frequency at which hearing was normal. A significant intergroup difference in reaction times for the tinnitus frequency was also seen when the patients were compared with a control group, with the tinnitus subjects exhibiting more rapid reaction. Nieschalk et al. (1998) partly replicated these findings in a study with 15 tinnitus patients and 15 normal-hearing control subjects. Patients were faster at the tinnitus frequencies and also at the 1000 Hz frequency. In addition, the tinnitus group displayed shorter reaction times at sensation levels near threshold, but no differences for sound stimuli in the suprathreshold region. It is not easy to explain this effect and another study found the opposite result (Attias et al., 1996a), with slower reaction times. Nieschalk et al. (1998) considered their findings to be indicative of cochlear dysfunction and went on to suggest that the cochlea could be dysfunctional even when audiometric thresholds are broadly

Tinnitus: A Multidisciplinary Approach, Second Edition. David Baguley, Gerhard Andersson, Don McFerran and Laurence McKenna.
© 2013 David Baguley, Gerhard Andersson, Don McFerran and Laurence McKenna.
Published 2013 by Blackwell Publishing Ltd.

normal (which was the case in their study). However, these authors also pointed out the importance of central processing in tinnitus. Nieschalk et al. (1998) excluded patients with signs of mood disorder from their study. Such mood disorders are common among tinnitus clinic patients (Zöger et al., 2001) and might be expected to influence reaction time. It is therefore difficult to extrapolate the findings of this study to a wider tinnitus group. Stevens et al. (2007) studied a group of 11 tinnitus patients and also had a control group. When analysing reaction time data on a Stroop task (a task in which the subject is asked to name the colour of the ink that words are printed in when the word is a different colour name: one example would be the word green written in blue colour), word reading and category naming tasks they found some indications that tinnitus patients were slower to respond for the Stroop task and for the more difficult category naming task.

Evoked response audiometry

Evoked response audiometry is a set of techniques in which electrical potentials from the brainstem or cerebral cortex are measured by means of electrodes attached to the scalp. The ears are stimulated with sound stimuli (usually clicks or tone pips) and a summating average of the responses is performed by a computer to reflect evoked auditory activity in the brain (Pratt, 2003). In tinnitus research two types of responses to auditory stimuli have been studied.

The first type consists of the short latency responses occurring within 10 milliseconds (ms) after the onset of the stimulus. This auditory brainstem response (ABR) consists of five major waveforms, which are thought to reflect electrical activity in auditory pathways at various levels of the brainstem. The second type consists of responses that occur 50–400 ms after stimulus onset and are assumed to reflect cognitive activity, such as auditory attention.

Auditory brainstem responses

There are several studies in which ABRs in tinnitus patients have been compared with similar measurements in control subjects who do not have tinnitus. Some studies have given inconclusive results (Barnea et al., 1990; McKee and Stephens, 1992; Attias et al., 1996a), but others have indicated that both early and late ABR waves are affected in tinnitus (Maurizi et al., 1985; Ikner and Hassen, 1990; Rosenhall and Axelsson, 1995). Rosenhall and Axelsson (1995) found delayed latencies for all ABR waves and interpreted these results as indicating brainstem dysfunction rather than impaired hearing. Gerken et al. (2001) studied ABRs and middle latency responses and found that only ABR wave VII was affected in repeated-measures analysis: wave VII is not routinely measured in clinical applications of ABR. In a case control study Kehrle et al. (2008) found a prolongation of latencies of waves I, II and V compared to the control group. In addition, the interpeak III–V interval was enlarged compared to the control group. In a later study, Singh et al. (2011) compared 25 normal hearing tinnitus patients with a control group and found differences in terms of wave I latency prolongation, shortening of wave V and I–III and I–V interpeak latency.

Based on a finding that tinnitus subjects demonstrated a lower amplitude ABR wave I than normal subjects (with wave V being of normal amplitude), Schaette and McAlpine (2011) proposed that a reduction in cochlear output is associated with tinnitus. They further argue that this 'hidden hearing loss' is then normalised by homeostatic mechanisms in the auditory brainstem. Further elaboration and development of these ideas is anticipated.

One remaining problem with this research is that different studies have used very different sample groups, rendering comparison difficult. In addition, there have been no efforts to control for possible psychological factors such as attention and anxiety, and while the ABR is thought to be independent of attention and anxiety this would be of interest.

Cortical evoked potentials

Cortical evoked potentials, in the form of either auditory evoked electrical responses or their magnetic field equivalents (e.g. M100), have been studied in relation to tinnitus, and are of particular interest as they reflect higher order processing of auditory stimuli. Hoke et al. (1989) found a lack of clear P200 responses and increased amplitude of N100 responses in a group of tinnitus patients. A case study corroborated these findings and showed that evoked potentials were normalised during remission of tinnitus (Pantev et al., 1989). However, these promising findings were not replicated in two subsequent studies (Jacobson et al., 1991; Colding-Jørgensen et al., 1992). More recently, sophisticated measurement strategies have been utilised and selective attention has been manipulated, showing more promising results (Attias et al., 1996a; Jacobson et al., 1996; Hoke et al., 1998; Norena et al., 1999). There are issues with the populations that have been used in these studies; for example, it can be argued that male army personnel, studied by Attias and co-workers, represent a distinct group from the mixed gender samples used in other studies.

In a study by Kadner et al. (2002) auditory-evoked potentials were recorded from eight tinnitus patients and 12 control subjects. Tone pips of 1000 Hz and 2000 Hz, as well as a tone matched to the frequency of the tinnitus (commonly around 4000 Hz), were presented at different intensities. Results showed a steeper response in the tinnitus group to the tinnitus frequency tone and the authors hypothesised that the findings derived from lateral inhibition arising from neural activity in the 4000 Hz region. In another study by Walpurger et al. (2003) a fresh approach was taken when Hallam's habituation model was tested in a study with 10 tinnitus complainers and 12 noncomplainers. Diminution of the N1 and P2 amplitudes of the evoked potentials were taken to measure habituation for consecutive trials (e.g. four tests in one session). The results supported the habituation theory, with less distinct habituation in the group with more severe tinnitus (as determined by their score on the Tinnitus Questionnaire). Delb et al. (2008) studied event-related potentials to attended and unattended tones in a sample of

41 tinnitus patients and 10 controls. They found differences between patients with low versus high distress (again as determined by their score on the Tinnitus Questionnaire) in that the low-distress group exhibited reduction in N100 amplitude and phase locking (comparing the attended with unattended conditions) whereas the high-distress group did not. They interpreted the findings as a sign that attention in high tinnitus-related distress patients is more often captured by their tinnitus compared with the low-distress patients. Overall, the low-distress group resembled the nontinnitus group in terms of their responses.

Santos et al. (2010) focused on noise-induced hearing loss in a study with 60 subjects exposed to occupational noise of which 30 had tinnitus: the groups were not matched. Results regarding evoked potientals showed increased N1 and P300 latencies in the tinnitus group.

In a study using magnetic source imaging, a magnetic encephalography technique that measures cortical responses by changes in magnetic fields rather than electrical responses, Mühlnickel et al. (1998) found evidence of cortical reorganisation in response to auditory stimulation in a group of 10 tinnitus patients compared with 15 control subjects. Weisz et al. (2005) studied map reorganization by collecting data while tinnitus patients were exposed to lesion edge frequencies that had been hypothesised to be linked with tinnitus. Patients ($N = 14$) with high-frequency hearing loss and normal hearing controls ($N = 11$) were included in the study. The results did not support the theory even if lesion edge activation was associated with right hemisphere map distortion. Diesch et al. (2010) also used magnetic encephalography to investigate responses to amplitude modulated tones in 18 tinnitus patients and 18 controls. Both groups included musicians. The tinnitus group showed a facilitation effect when multiple tones were presented whereas the controls rather showed an inhibition effect. They interpreted the finding as an indication that lateral inhibition is reduced in tinnitus.

Ashton et al. (2007) used a method called quantitative EEG power spectral mapping, which is a method that can measure regional brain activity and EEG abnormalities. In their study with 8 tinnitus patients and 25 controls they identified high-frequency activity in the gamma range (>40–80 Hz) in auditory cortex for the tinnitus patients but not the controls. Lorenz et al. (2010) studied 26 tinnitus patients and found that the negative association between alpha and gamma activity as measured by MEG was steeper (compared with 26 controls without tinnitus). They interpreted this as a sign that tinnitus patients show low alpha and high gamma activity.

Positron emission tomography and related methods

With the advent of modern brain imaging methods it has been possible to study deep brain functioning *in vivo* (Johnsrude et al., 2002) and tinnitus is no exception. Tinnitus has been investigated using single photon emission computed tomography (SPECT), positron emission tomography (PET) and functional magnetic resonance imaging (fMRI). The results are summarised in Table 6.1. For ease of interpretation, Brodmann's areas (BAs) are depicted in Figure 6.1.

Table 6.1 Overview of brain imaging studies of tinnitus.

Study	Manipulations or study group(s)	Main results
SPECT		
Shulman et al. (1995)	Blood flow at rest compared with normative data; 2 patients	Significant regional abnormalities bilaterally in temporal, frontal, parietal and hippocampal amygdala regions
Sataloff et al. (1996)	Blood flow at rest compared with normative data; 12 patients	Abnormal findings in 11 patients
Staffen et al. (1999)	Lidocaine minus rest; single case	Lateralisation between right and left auditory cortex decreased during lidocaine infusion
Gardner et al. (2002)	Depressed patients with ($n = 27$) or without ($n = 18$) tinnitus	Differences in right frontal lobe. In many patients activation of primary or secondary auditory cortex
PET		
Arnold et al. (1996)	Ears plugged at rest; 11 patients, 14 control subjects; one patient with fluctuating tinnitus	Increased activity in primary auditory cortex (BA 41). Correspondence between complaints and PET
Lockwood et al. (1998)	Oral facial movement or tone stimulation; 4 tinnitus patients and 6 control subjects	Activation in auditory cortex (BA 41). More widespread activation in patients and activation of hippocampus
Mirz et al. (1999a)	Masking versus rest; lidocaine versus rest; 12 patients	Altered activity in middle frontal and middle temporal gyri and lateral and mesial posterior sites (BAs 41, 42, 21 and 8). Activation of right precuneus (BA 7) in lidocaine condition
Giraud et al. (1999)	Gaze-evoked tinnitus; 4 patients	Activity in temporoparietal association auditory cortex, but not in primary auditory cortex. BAs 42, 21, 22, 7 and 8 activated
Andersson et al. (2000b)	Lidocaine versus rest; 1 patient	Increased rCBF in the left parietotemporal auditory cortex, including the primary and secondary auditory cortex with a focus in the parietal cortex (BAs 39, 41, 42, 21 and 22). Activations were also found in right frontal paralimbic areas (BAs 47, 49 and 15)
Lockwood et al. (2001)	Gaze-evoked tinnitus; 8 tinnitus patients and 7 control subjects	Evidence for neural activity related to tinnitus seen in auditory lateral pontine tegmentum or auditory cortex

(*Continued*)

Table 6.1   (cont'd).

Study	Manipulations or study group(s)	Main results
Mirz et al. (2002)	Five cochlear implant patients with tinnitus. Tinnitus reduced by implant	Activation of primary and secondary auditory cortex, limbic system and the precuneus (BA 7)
Reyes et al. (2002)	Lidocaine versus placebo; 10 tinnitus patients, 7 control subjects	Evidence for neural activity related to tinnitus seen in auditory lateral pontine tegmentum or auditory cortex. Less response to lidocaine than usually observed
Andersson et al. (2006)	Eight tinnitus patients. Silent counting backwards in steps of seven	Reduced activity in auditory cortex bilaterally
fMRI		
Cacace et al. (1996)	Gaze-evoked tinnitus ($n = 2$) and one case with cutaneous-evoked tinnitus	Abnormal foci of activity in the upper brainstem and frontal cortex
Cacace et al. (1999)	Cutaneous-evoked tinnitus; 2 patients	Activation of temporoparietal junction
Mirz et al. (1999b)	Masking versus rest; 8 patients	Activation of superior and middle temporal gyri, BAs 21, 22, 37, 39 (associative auditory cortex); BAs 7, 40 (parietal lobes); BAs 8–10, 44–45 (inferior frontal gyri); BAs 6, 9, 31, 32 (medial frontal and cingulated gyrus)
Melcher et al. (2000)	White noise stimulation; 4 lateralised patients, 3 nonlateralised compared with 6 controls	Binaural noise produced abnormally low activation of the inferior colliculus in lateralised tinnitus

BA = Brodmann's area.

SPECT is a technique that can be regarded as a predecessor of PET. Abraham Schulman and his colleagues found that the brain activity in two tinnitus patients was significantly different from normative data (Schulman, 1995). Sataloff et al. (1996) studied blood flow at rest in 12 patients, and when these data were compared with normative data as many as 11 patients were found to have abnormal findings. In a case study using lidocaine to temporarily abolish tinnitus, Staffen et al. (1999) compared differences in blood flow using SPECT between at rest and with tinnitus abolished by means of lidocaine. These workers found that the lateralisation between the left and right auditory cortex decreased following lidocaine infusion. Gardner et al. (2002) used SPECT in a study of 45 patients with lifetime depression, of whom 27 had severe tinnitus. Decreased blood flow was found in the right frontal lobes (BA 45), left parietal lobes (BA 39) and left visual association cortices (BA 18) in the tinnitus group compared with the depressed

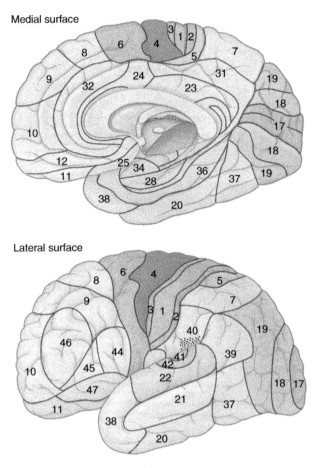

Medial surface

Lateral surface

Figure 6.1 Brodmann's cytoarchitectural map of cortical areas of the brain. Primary auditory cortex: BA 41, 42. Auditory association cortex: 22. (Reproduced from Clinical Neuroanatomy and related neuroscience, FitzGerald and Folan-Curran (2002) by permission of Elsevier.)

patients without tinnitus. These workers also found that the proportion of tinnitus patients with pronounced rCBF (a measure of cortical blood flow) alterations in the auditory cortex was increased compared with both a normal comparison sample and the depressed patients without tinnitus. It would have been interesting to know to what extent depressed versus nondepressed tinnitus patients differed in terms of cortical activity, but such a control group was not included.

PET is a more advanced technique that uses radio isotopes to obtain cross-sectional images of the body and to highlight areas of increased metabolic activity. Commonly, the brain imaging application of PET consists of tracing blood flow by labelling isotopes of oxygen and other elements (Johnsrude et al., 2002). The use of PET in tinnitus research was popular for a while, but was hampered by the costs and the need for intravenous injections of the tracer substance. Hence there have not been many new studies using this technique since the first edition of this book. Some studies have been directly related to transcranial magnetic stimulation and are not covered in this chapter (e.g. Langguth et al., 2006; Plewnia et al., 2007).

Arnold et al. (1996) used PET to study 11 tinnitus patients at rest and compared the findings with a control group. The results showed an increase of cortical activity in primary auditory cortex in the tinnitus group. Interestingly, in one of the tinnitus subjects, tinnitus was weaker than usual at the time of the testing and the patient was therefore called in for a second session in which tinnitus was back at its usual level. These subjective reports of tinnitus were found to correspond to the PET data, with increased cortical activity in auditory cortex. Lockwood et al. (1998) studied four patients who had tinnitus that they could modify by means of oral facial movements (jaw clenching). This is an interesting phenomenon that seems quite common among tinnitus patients in some studies (Pinchoff et al., 1998). This was a complex study, but the main finding was increased activity in the auditory cortex and some evidence for the involvement of the hippocampus (a structure active in emotional processing) was also observed. Lockwood and colleagues also included a control group. Using auditory stimulation, their results showed that tinnitus patients displayed more widespread cortical activation than control subjects. Mirz et al. (1999a) studied tinnitus suppression with PET using both lidocaine and masking by means of narrowband noise. In total their 12 subjects each underwent eight scans. In the lidocaine part of the study there were two nonresponders. Results were analysed using a subtraction approach. These authors found a decrease in right middle frontal gyrus and middle temporal gyri (BA 21) activity following lidocaine administration. Interestingly, the right precuneus was also activated. In a masking versus baseline condition, the results showed that all 12 subjects masked their tinnitus and a decrease in primary auditory cortex activity was found, extending into associate areas. This study has been questioned because of a suspected lack of statistical significance (Reyes et al., 2002; Cacace, 2003). Giraud et al. (1999) studied four patients with gaze-evoked tinnitus that had developed after unilateral vestibular schwannoma surgery. Changes in eye gaze resulted in activation of temporoparietal association auditory cortex (BAs 42, 21 and 22), but not in the primary auditory cortex. The precuneus (BA 7) was also activated with increased tinnitus. Andersson et al. (2000b) reported a case in which lidocaine was used effectively to inhibit tinnitus. The brain activity associated with tinnitus included the left primary, secondary and integrative auditory brain areas (Figure 6.2), as well as right paralimbic areas, which are thought to be involved in processing negative feelings. Increased activity in association with tinnitus was also found in the left parietal cortex (precuneus, BA 7). Lockwood et al. (2001) also used PET to study gaze-evoked tinnitus in eight patients and included a control group consisting of seven age- and gender-matched subjects. Results showed activation of auditory lateral pontine tegmentum or auditory cortex. More detailed tables of their data with Brodmann areas revealed that activation of secondary auditory cortex structures were evident, as was found by Giraud et al. (1999). In their lidocaine study, Reyes et al. (2002) studied 10 subjects and, surprisingly, found that only five patients had a decrease in their tinnitus, whereas four patients reported an increase. One patient had no change. Importantly, given the well-known placebo effect, these authors included a lidocaine placebo

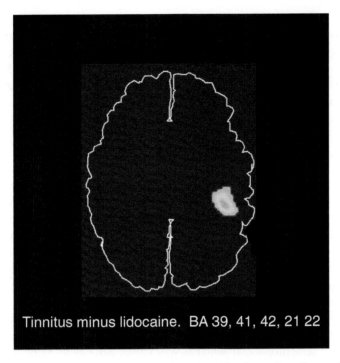

Tinnitus minus lidocaine. BA 39, 41, 42, 21 22

Figure 6.2 PET images of tinnitus-related brain activity. The figure describes activation in the tinnitus–lidocaine contrast (Andersson et al., 2000b). Increased activity is found in the primary and secondary auditory cortex.

condition. The results showed that increase of tinnitus was associated with activity in the secondary auditory cortex of the right hemisphere (BA 21). It would have been interesting to see the activation caused by the placebo minus baseline condition, but these data were not reported.

In an innovative study, Mirz et al. (2002) reported an experiment in which five cochlear implant patients with tinnitus were studied. All had in common the experience that tinnitus was totally suppressed by turning on the implant. Subtraction analyses showed that primary and secondary auditory cortex structures were activated during tinnitus, but also the parahippocampal gyrus (BA 35) on the right side and the precuneus on the right side.

Andersson and co-workers (2006) studied eight patients with tinnitus and found that silent backwards counting (serial sevens test) lead to a decrease in neural activity in the auditory cortex (BAs 41, 42 and 22), as well as a perceived decrease of tinnitus loudness and annoyance. The reduced cortical activity can be seen as a replication of what has been found in previous studies on normal subjects (Ghatan et al., 1996, 1998). It is worth noting that primary auditory cortex was more clearly involved than in the previous studies on normal subjects. Unfortunately, a control group of subjects without tinnitus was not included in the study. Osaki et al. (2005) studied three cochlear implant patients with tinnitus and found that the right cerebellum was activated during tinnitus perception and that the right anterior middle and superior temporal gyri

(BAs 21 and 38) were activated during residual inhibition. The study also included six normal hearing controls without tinnitus. Schecklmann et al. (2011) studied a large sample of 91 patients with PET. They found that tinnitus distress correlated positively with activation of left and right posterior inferior temporal gyrus (BA 45) as well as the left and right posterior parahippocampal–hippocampal interface (BA 36). They also found that tinnitus duration and distress were associated with areas involved in attentional and emotional processing.

fMRI

fMRI is a specialised form of MRI scanning that measures blood flow in tissues. Increased blood flow is used to imply increased activity within the tissue. Unlike PET scanning, this does not require the use of potentially hazardous radioactive isotopes in tinnitus research. However, fMRI scanning produces noise up to 130 dB, which limits its usefulness in auditory research, even if there are some possibilities of reducing the sound and scanning during less noisy periods (Hall et al., 1999). Although subjects undergoing fMRI scans can wear noise attenuating devices, some patients with tinnitus and hyperacusis are deterred by the noise. Cacace et al. (1996) used fMRI in two patients with gaze-evoked tinnitus and found signs of abnormal activity in the upper brainstem and in the frontal cortex. In a later study of two patients with cutaneous-evoked tinnitus (Cacace, 1999), activation of the temporoparietal junction was found. Mirz et al. (1999b) presented a study in which eight patients were investigated with fMRI at rest and while they were having their tinnitus masked. The results showed activation of associative auditory cortex (BAs 21, 22, 37 and 39), the parietal lobes (BAs 7 and 40), inferior frontal gyri and medial frontal and cingulate gyri (BAs 6, 9 and 31–32). Melcher et al. (2000) managed to use a quieter fMRI method by focusing on a restricted area of the brain. Using a complex design, four patients with lateralised tinnitus were compared with three with nonlateralised tinnitus and six control subjects, of whom several also had tinnitus; the use of such a control group is somewhat perplexing. As in the study by Mirz et al. (1999b), a masking approach was used. The main finding was that binaural noise produced abnormally low activation of the inferior colliculus in patients with lateralised tinnitus. The inferior colliculus has been suggested to be of significance in tinnitus (Gerken, 1996), given its role in lateral inhibition.

Smits et al. (2007) included 42 tinnitus patients and 10 controls and presented music while scanning with fMRI using a silent gap procedure to reduce the effect of the scanner noise. Results showed activations linked with the side of tinnitus in lateralised tinnitus. Bilateral tinnitus led to bilateral activation, whereas for the controls activation was lateralised in the left primary auditory cortex. In a study with 10 patients with unilateral tinnitus Lanting et al. (2008) found that responses to sound in the inferior colliculus were elevated compared to controls ($N = 12$). This finding does not concur with that of Melcher et al. (2000), though this may relate to methodological issues.

Melcher et al. (2009) completed another study with 12 persons with tinnitus and 20 controls without tinnitus who were exposed to acoustic stimulation. In this study they found increased activation in inferior colliculus in persons with tinnitus.

Lanting et al. (2010) studied 13 patients with tinnitus who could modulate their tinnitus by jaw protrusions and also added a control group ($n = 20$). They found that jaw protrusions led to increased activity in the cochlear nucleus and inferior colliculus compared to the controls. They also investigated responses to sound but found no group differences. In a study on brain activation during pitch matching Wunderlich et al. (2010) included six tinnitus patients and six controls. They found a more pronounced activation in tinnitus patients in the caudate nucleus, the cingulate cortex, the right hemisphere BA 8 and the superior frontal gyrus (BA 23).

Leaver et al. (2011) used fMRI in a study on 11 tinnitus patients and 11 controls. Participants were presented with band-passed white noise at tinnitus frequency and 0.5, 1 or 2 octaves above and below that frequency. They also collected data on voxel-based morphometry to assess anatomical anomalies. In tinnitus patients activity was found in nucleus accumbens, which was more pronounced at the tinnitus frequencies. They further found that tinnitus-related anomalies were intercorrelated with limbic regions and between limbic and primary auditory areas. They interpreted their findings as indicating an interaction between auditory and limbic brain areas. The same authors have further outlined a model for the understanding of the limbic–auditory link in tinnitus (Rauschecker et al., 2010).

Husain et al. (2011a) studied auditory perception and cognitive processing in a sample of eight tinnitus patients and two controls groups consisting of persons with hearing loss ($n = 7$) or normal hearing ($n = 11$). The subjects were instructed to listen passively and to do an auditory discrimination task. When groups were compared they found a decreased activation in the parietal and frontal lobes in the tinnitus group compared to the hearing loss group and decreased response in the frontal lobes relative to the normal hearing group.

Two independent reviews of the brain imaging literature on tinnitus have been published (Lanting et al., 2009; Adjamian et al., 2009). Lanting et al. (2009) concluded that tinnitus in humans may correspond to enhanced neural activity across several central auditory centres of the brain. However, they also found evidence suggesting that nonauditory areas are involved including frontal areas, the limbic system and possibly the cerebellum. In line with much tinnitus research where nontinnitus control groups have been included they pointed out the need to control for degree of hearing loss in control samples. Adjamian et al. (2009) also reviewed literature with slightly more focus on the pros and cons of different imaging techniques. They were more hesitant to draw any firm conclusions as they found the data somewhat inconsistent. This is very much in line with our updated review here, in which the data in Table 6.1 show some consistency but also much heterogeneity. For example, the evidence for the role of the limbic system in tinnitus is far from conclusive even if there are strong theoretical reasons to assume that emotions play a central role in tinnitus distress.

Studies on anatomical differences associated with tinnitus

A series of studies have investigated neuroanatomical changes in association with tinnitus. This is a different approach than the activation studies reviewed above. Schneider et al. (2009) used magnetic resonance imaging (MRI) in a sample of 61 tinnitus patients and 45 controls and found that patients had a significantly smaller volume of the medial partition of the Heschl's gyrus in both hemispheres. However, there was also a correlation between this volume and degree of hearing loss and it is not clear if volume change is a cause or a consequence of tinnitus and hearing loss.

Landgrebe et al. (2009) used MRI to study 28 tinnitus patients with normal hearing and also had a matched control group. Analysing voxel-based morphometry (VBM), they found that grey matter decreases in the right inferior colliculus and left hippocampus in the tinnitus group. In a study using diffusion tension imaging (DTI), Crippa et al. (2010) studied 10 tinnitus patients and 15 controls. With a focus on regions of interest (ROIs) they found an increased patency of the white matter tract between the auditory cortex and the amygdala in the tinnitus patients when compared to the controls. Husain et al. (2011b) used a combined VBM and DTI approach with the same sample as in Husain et al. (2011a). Overall their results showed that hearing loss rather than tinnitus has the greatest effect on grey and white matter alterations. In line with the activation-based literature the results on anatomical differences in tinnitus are far from consistent and the studies by Husain et al. highlight the importance of controlling for level of hearing loss.

Measures of neural activity associated with tinnitus

As described in Chapter 4, research into mechanisms of tinnitus has involved subjecting animals to agents that induce tinnitus in humans (specifically noise and salicylate) and recording changes in neural activity that might represent tinnitus. These recording techniques have not been widely applied to humans, however. Martin (1995) described spectral average recordings from the cochlear nerve of 14 human adult patients undergoing cerebellopontine angle surgery. In 12 patients with tinnitus, a prominent peak in the spectral average near 200 Hz was reported. Patuzzi et al. (2004) recorded the spectrum of neural noise from the round window of guinea pig cochleae and concluded that the activity recorded derived from the whole of the basilar membrane, so it would not be possible to distinguish the activity from any specific area (such as that which might be responsible for the ignition of a tinnitus percept).

Integrating the findings and future directions

Findings from brain imaging studies attest that tinnitus can be measured objectively. The findings are not consistent, but it is clear that tinnitus affects brain areas related to hearing and processing of sounds, but also that some involvement of the brain's emotional and attentional systems might be involved (e.g. amygdala). It is interesting to note that it is often the case that secondary rather than primary auditory cortex has been activated in several imaging studies. Of note, Mirz et al. (1999c) found that an interrupted stream of tones activated the secondary auditory associative cortex, whereas a tone predictably activated the primary cortex. Tinnitus has often been explained in terms of increased firing rates (Rauschecker, 1999; Lanting et al., 2009; Adjamian et al., 2009), but data from imaging studies suggest the opposite of a slower firing rate, at least in some regions of the brain, potentially leading the brain to interpret intermittent streams of neural information as a tone.

A study by Mirz et al. (2000) utilised PET and studied 12 healthy subjects to whom they presented 'tinnitus sounds' derived from actual tinnitus matching data. The results showed that the tinnitus sounds led to activation of primary (BA 41) and right associative auditory cortex (BAs 21 and 22) and limbic structures such as the amygdala or parahippocampal gyrus and hippocampus. To our knowledge there is a lack of studies on simulated tinnitus that could shed some light on how the brain perceives tinnitus.

Various imaging studies have found that the precuneus (BA 7) is activated in tinnitus patients, suggesting that it is an important area in the perception of tinnitus. Interestingly, Blood et al. (1999) found that the degree of dissonance in musical passages correlated with increased activity in BA 7 on the right side. This area has also been related to attentional mechanisms and to auditory hallucinations (Shergill et al., 2000). Moreover, increased activity in the precuneus has been found in association with cognitive tasks (Ghatan et al., 1998; Zatorre and Binder, 2000).

Imaging tinnitus is an emergent field and several important research issues remain to be investigated. The modulation of an emotional state is a possible area for further work, given that both the neurophysiological and the psychological models emphasise this aspect of tinnitus experience. Another possible area to explore is the outcome of habituation-based treatments to try to ascertain objective evidence of their efficacy – or otherwise. Thus far it is mainly the effects of low-frequency repetitive magnetic stimulation that has been studied using brain imaging techniques (Eichhammer et al., 2007, for example), and there are no studies on the effects of psychological tinnitus treatments on brain functioning, which have been conducted in other fields such as anxiety disorders (Furmark et al., 2002). Most imaging studies on tinnitus fail to account for possible co-morbid psychiatric conditions, which are likely to influence the findings in particular in emotional regions of the brain. A notable exception is the study by Gardner et al. (2002), in which patients with concurrent tinnitus and depression were included. In future imaging studies it would be interesting to investigate the differences between distressed versus nondistressed tinnitus patients (e.g. Delb et al., 2008), as it is possible that cortical activation, in particular cortical reorganisation, might differ in relation to levels of distress.

Moreover, more studies could focus on selective attention to tinnitus; to our knowledge only one study has investigated cognitive distraction (Andersson et al., 2006) and that study did not include a control group. Husain et al. (2011b) did indeed study the effects of a discrimination task, but that is within the auditory domain, and it may be important to distinguish differences between auditory and nonauditory cognitive tasks.

Despite encouraging work concerning the neuroimaging of tinnitus, some workers have sounded notes of caution. Imaging techniques may not be sensitive enough to capture the relevant brain mechanisms involved in tinnitus (Adjamian et al., 2009) and the results are scattered. Further, the main results to date indicate activity in the auditory cortex and in areas involved in emotional experience; in a patient group complaining of the perception of a sound that evokes distress, these findings are to be expected. Despite this slight scepticism, this field is one to watch for future developments.

Summary

Researchers and clinicians have long suspected that tinnitus involves certain specific areas of the brain, in particular those that subserve the perception and promotion of the experience (Minton, 1923). There are indications that tinnitus patients' reaction times differ from control subjects without tinnitus: tinnitus patients seem to display a faster reaction time to sounds.

Additional data have been collected by use of evoked response audiometry. In a few studies the results have not been conclusive, but other studies have indicated that early as well as later latency waves are affected in tinnitus. It is possible that sample characteristics of the studies, such as differences of the test populations, may explain these contradictory findings. Imaging techniques have produced some interesting results, with the overall message that auditory areas of the brain show increased activity in tinnitus patients. There are some inconsistencies in the data from imaging studies but, despite this, it remains an exciting and productive area of tinnitus research.

Chapter 7

Consequences and moderating factors

Although tinnitus is one of the most common physical symptoms to affect humanity it continues to pose particular challenges to clinicians and researchers alike. In large measure this is because the effects of tinnitus are so variable and the impact of tinnitus ranges from little or nothing to profound and life changing. Tinnitus has been associated, to varying degrees in different individuals, with changes in thinking, stress arousal, mood, sleep and behaviour and with auditory interference. These changes in turn may lead to other behavioural and psychological consequences. Many tinnitus patients suppose that tinnitus has an impact through a linear process that starts with the psychophysical characteristics of the tinnitus percept. Although, intuitively, it might be expected that particularly loud tinnitus or tinnitus of a certain frequency might lead to a greater impact, this does not seem to be the case (House, 1981; Meikle and Taylor-Walsh, 1984; Kuk et al., 1990; Dineen et al., 1997a). The exception seems to be in people's subjective judgements of the complexity of the tinnitus sounds. People who experience more complex sounds report greater problems (Dineen et al., 1997a), but the cause and effect relationship is by no means clear. It has also been said that tinnitus that is present all the time has a greater impact on quality of life than tinnitus that is intermittent (Davis, 1995). Notwithstanding these observations, the variability in the tinnitus experience cannot easily be attributed to differences in the perceptual characteristics of the symptom. The process is better understood as one in which the impact of tinnitus reflects the influence of other moderating and mediating processes that, in turn, influence the perception of tinnitus; thus it is a system involving feedback loops rather than a simple linear one. For the most part, the moderating and mediating variables are psychological in nature and are almost certainly underpinned by physiological processes. A useful starting point in seeking to understand the tinnitus experience is with the tinnitus patient's thinking processes.

Tinnitus: A Multidisciplinary Approach, Second Edition. David Baguley, Gerhard Andersson, Don McFerran and Laurence McKenna.
© 2013 David Baguley, Gerhard Andersson, Don McFerran and Laurence McKenna.
Published 2013 by Blackwell Publishing Ltd.

Tinnitus and thinking

Two aspects of thinking need to be considered: the content of a person's thoughts and the person's ability to attend to or concentrate on things.

The thought content of tinnitus patients

When a person experiences tinnitus, either for the first time or when there is a variation in it he or she will think about what is happening. The exact content of these thoughts will vary from individual to individual. Some people will have calm, neutral thoughts about tinnitus but some will have anxious or depressed thoughts. Questionnaire studies have identified common themes in the thoughts of tinnitus patients. Their thoughts have been found to reflect despair, persecution, hopelessness, loss of enjoyment, a desire for peace and quiet, and beliefs that others do not understand what they are going through (Wilson and Henry, 1998). Other common themes that have been identified are: resentment about persistence of tinnitus, a wish to escape it and worries about health and sanity (Hallam et al., 1988; Kuk et al., 1990; Wilson et al., 1991). In the first instance the person's thinking can be seen as having been provoked by tinnitus. The thought content of the tinnitus patient, however, plays a more important role as a mediator of the tinnitus experience. The variation in response to tinnitus starts at this point. Several studies have found evidence of the importance of an appraisal process in tinnitus-related distress (e.g. Erlandsson and Hallberg, 2000; Langenbach et al., 2005; Rienhoff et al., 2002). It can reasonably be supposed that thoughts that include a theme of threat or loss will lead to an increase in sympathetic autonomic nervous system arousal (stress arousal) with a number of ensuing consequences.

The efficiency of tinnitus patients' thoughts

It has been suggested that people complaining of tinnitus are more preoccupied in their thinking about tinnitus than people with tinnitus who do not complain about it (Hallam et al., 1984). Many tinnitus sufferers certainly complain that they are constantly focused on tinnitus and as a consequence have difficulties in concentrating on other things (Tyler and Baker, 1983; Sanchez and Stephens, 1997). As with sleep problems, there is some evidence that these difficulties are associated with more complex tinnitus involving several sounds (Hallberg and Erlandsson, 1993). Traditionally, these concentration problems have been assumed to be an aspect of the emotional distress associated with tinnitus. Factor analytic studies of tinnitus complaint (Hiller and Goebel, 1992; Hallam, 1996a) did not reveal a specific 'concentration' factor, but rather suggested that these cognitive difficulties form part of an emotional distress or an intrusiveness factor. This may, however, be a reflection of the fact that the questionnaires used in such studies do not include enough questions about attention or concentration problems.

There has been a small series of studies on this hitherto neglected aspect of tinnitus complaint. Initial studies (McKenna et al., 1996; McKenna, 1997; McKenna and Hallam, 1999) compared people complaining of tinnitus with people complaining of hearing loss without tinnitus on clinical tests of cognitive functioning and on a self-report measure of cognitive function, the Cognitive Failures Questionnaire (Broadbent et al., 1982). These studies found that while the tinnitus group reported more difficulties in cognitive functioning there was only weak objective evidence of poorer cognitive performance. It appeared that the effects of tinnitus on cognitive functioning were disguised in these studies because hearing loss also seemed to have an effect on cognitive functioning. Interestingly, the difficulties in cognitive functioning that were apparent in the tinnitus groups could not be easily explained by higher anxiety levels. In a more elaborate study Andersson et al. (2000a) compared the performance of tinnitus subjects with that of hearing-impaired control subjects and normal subjects, on a number of Stroop tests (tests of executive functioning). Tinnitus subjects performed more poorly on all of the tests administered. Again, the poorer performance of the tinnitus subjects could not be accounted for by differences in emotional state and, as with the earlier studies, it was not possible to rule out some effect from hearing loss. Hallam et al. (2004) administered a number of computer-presented tests of cognitive function. The tests used in this study differed from those used in previous studies by these researchers in that they were experimentally based rather than tests in general clinical use. The tests assessed cognitive performance under single- and dual-task (carrying out the task while doing something else) conditions. In this study a group of tinnitus subjects was compared with a hearing-impaired group and also with a nonclinical control group. As in earlier studies, the tinnitus group reported more everyday cognitive failures than the control groups. The tinnitus group performed more poorly on only one objective test (the variable fore-period reaction task) under dual-task conditions. Andersson et al. (2003a) investigated autobiographical memories in 19 tinnitus patients and 19 control subjects without tinnitus. Participants were given a test of autobiographical memory and the Controlled Word Association test, along with self-report measures of depression, anxiety and tinnitus distress. Compared with control subjects, tinnitus patients had difficulty retrieving specific memories and took longer to recall things. Additionally, tinnitus patients had fewer specific memories to positive cue words. This is a finding commonly observed among depressed patients (Williams et al., 1997). Rossiter et al. (2006) found that performance on tasks requiring voluntary, conscious, effortful and strategic control was impaired in the tinnitus sample compared to healthy controls. For example, they found a reduced reading span on a test of auditory verbal working memory and slower reaction times together with lower accuracy in high demanding visual divided-attention tasks.

In a welcome addition to the literature, Pierce et al. (2012) applied a standardised battery of tests of cognitive function on a group of 14 patients with troublesome tinnitus compared with an age, gender and education matched normative population: no attempt was made to match for hearing. The effect of depression was minimised as none of the patient group had a significant Beck Depression Inventory score, but there was no control for anxiety. Additionally, an exclusion criteria was that the patients should not be taking psychoactive medication, which made for a good experimental design as such drugs can have an effect upon cognitive function; however, it renders the group less representative of the clinical tinnitus population. In the tinnitus group deficits were found in learning, learning rates, immediate recall of heard words and in the use of a serial order encoding strategy. The authors set aside the thought that these deficits might be attributed to hearing difficulty, but did not evidence that: rather they proposed that tinnitus leads to a weakness in associative memory processes. Further work controlling for anxiety and hearing abilities is needed in this area.

The results of these studies suggest that tinnitus patients do experience some inefficiency in cognitive processing that cannot be completely accounted for in terms of emotional disturbance. The exact nature of the difficulties experienced is still unclear. There is evidence that tinnitus has a greater impact on people's ability to perform more complex tasks but there is also some evidence that it can interfere with the performance of mundane tasks more than with high-priority tasks. Clearly, this is an area where more research is needed and until that is completed the mechanisms underpinning this effect must be a matter of speculation. It has been suggested that this impact on cognitive functioning may be due to the depletion or disruption of the attentional resources as a result of attending to tinnitus or/and tinnitus-related negative thoughts or possibly increased somatic and self-focused attention (Newman et al., 1997b). Stevens et al. (2007) suggest that the impact on cognitive performance is likely to be attributed to a general depletion of resources, rather than only controlled processes, where tinnitus is thought of as a competing stimulus/schema that is responsible for attracting attention away from the task. Pierce et al. (2012) proposed that their data regarding cognitive function in tinnitus support this hypothesis.

It has been observed that an auditory stimulus that changes in pitch has the capacity to adversely affect cognitive processing (Jones and Macken, 1993). It has been suggested that a similar process happens with tinnitus, in that changes in tinnitus perception due to changes in environmental noise levels may disrupt a person's cognitive functioning. This in turn triggers an orienting reaction to the tinnitus and an emotional response to it (Andersson et al., 2002b). As such, this impact of tinnitus on cognitive functioning may provoke further responses and a greater overall perception of tinnitus.

Psychological state

Tinnitus and anxiety and depression

Although many people with tinnitus manage the symptom without distress, it is widely accepted that a high proportion of those seeking help for tinnitus do suffer from emotional disorder, particularly anxiety and depression. These disorders involve a number of elements, most notably changes in mood and behaviour as well as the types of changes in thinking and arousal referred to above. As yet a detailed breakdown of the component parts of emotional disorders in tinnitus patients is not available. Rather, tinnitus patients have been studied in terms of more global categories such as 'anxiety' and 'depression', which include judgements about mood, behaviour, thinking and arousal. The experiences involved in such disorders may represent a 'next step' after the changes in thinking referred to above. For many people, however, changes in mood, behaviour and thinking are experienced as running in parallel alongside an increase in arousal (referred to below). They can certainly be understood as aspects of the same process.

The link between tinnitus and emotional disorder has been investigated in several studies (Wood et al., 1983; Stephens and Hallam, 1985; Harrop-Griffiths et al., 1987;

Simpson et al., 1988; Kirsch et al., 1989; Collet et al., 1990; Halford and Anderson, 1991; McKenna et al., 1991; Scott and Lindberg, 2000). Most studies in this area have used questionnaire measures such as the General Health Questionnaire (Goldberg, 1978) or the Beck Depression Inventory (Beck et al., 1996) to assess psychological problems and have tended to find a higher prevalence of psychological disorder among tinnitus patients than among the general population. For example, McKenna et al. (1991) reported that 45% of those whose main complaint was tinnitus showed signs of significant psychological disturbance. Some researchers, however, have assessed tinnitus patients' psychological state using formal psychiatric diagnostic methods (American Psychiatric Association, 2000). For example, Simpson et al. (1988) found that a high proportion (63%) of tinnitus sufferers could be classified as psychiatrically disturbed or as having had a mood disorder (46%) as assessed by the Structured Interview for the Diagnostic and Statistical Manual of Mental Disorders (DSM-III-R) (First et al., 1997). The structured interview was also employed in a study by Sullivan et al. (1988). These researchers also found that a high proportion (78%) of their sample of tinnitus patients had experienced one or more episodes of major depression in their lifetimes compared with the experiences of a control group (21%). Sullivan et al. (1988) also found that 60% of tinnitus patients had a major depression at the time of interview compared with 7% of the control group. Hiller and Goebel (1992) found that 26 of 27 tinnitus patients fulfilled the DSM-III-R criteria for at least one lifetime diagnosis. Russo et al. (1994) used the DSM-IV to estimate the prevalence of psychiatric disorder among 88 tinnitus patients. No specific figures were provided for separate diagnoses, but it was reported that the average number of current and past diagnoses were 0.7 and 0.6, respectively. Zöger et al. (2001) studied a group of 82 tinnitus patients using DSM-IV diagnostic criteria. Their results showed that 62% of the patients had signs of lifetime depressive illness and that 39% had an ongoing depression. Current anxiety disorders (one or more) were found in 45% of patients, but of these a majority had co-morbid depression (69%). A high prevalence of psychiatric disorder (77% of cases) was also found among tinnitus patients in an Italian audiology clinic (Marciano et al., 2003). Similarly, Reynolds et al. (2004) found a high prevalence of psychiatric disorder among their tinnitus patients. Having excluded patients with an existing psychiatric diagnosis, Belli et al. (2008) found that 27% of tinnitus patients met formal psychiatric diagnostic criteria; anxiety and somatoform disorders predominated. Again having excluded patients with an existing psychosis, Goebel and Floetzinger (2008) found that 69% of a series of tinnitus patients could be classified as suffering from a psychiatric condition as assessed using the International Statistical Classification of Diseases and Related Health Problems (ICD-10). They noted significantly more psychiatric disorder in tinnitus patients who also suffered from hyperacusis than among those who did not. The Internet has been used to generate probable psychiatric diagnoses (Andersson et al., 2004a). In that study, the World Health Organization Composite International Diagnostic Interview – Short Form (CIDI-SF) (Kessler et al., 1998) was administered in a computerised Internet-based version to a self-selected sample of tinnitus patients ($n=48$). Using the cutoff for 'probable case' (12-month prevalence), 69% of the tinnitus patients fulfilled the criteria for depression. It must be remembered, however, that most studies on the emotional consequences of tinnitus have been conducted on highly selected samples of patients with severe tinnitus distress (Briner et al., 1990). Using larger samples Kirsch et al. (1989) and Wilson et al. (1991) revealed mean scores on self-report measures of emotional state within the range of mild mood disturbance.

Ooms et al. (2011) noted that there is an overlap between items in standard questionnaires used for tinnitus and for anxiety. Specifically, they considered the Tinnitus Handicap Inventory (THI) (Newman et al., 1996) and the State and Trait Anxiety Inventory (STAI) (Spielberger et al., 1970), finding an overlap in 10 THI items with the STAI. Taking this into account, they investigated anxiety in a group of 71 patients, finding greater than average cognitive anxiety (characterised by worry and negative self-talk) in 60% and clinically relevant somatic anxiety (characterised by rapid heart rate and shortness of breath) in 41%.

Some studies have suggested a link between problematic tinnitus and scores on depression scales (Wilson et al., 1991; Goebel and Floetzinger, 2008), whereas others have highlighted the importance of anxiety (McKenna et al., 1996; McKenna and Hallam, 1999; Ooms et al., 2011). Erlandsson (1990) theorised that there were two types of psychological reactions to tinnitus: one characterised by anxiety and one by depression, but these thoughts have not yet been validated empirically. As with hearing impairment, psychoacoustic measures (e.g. matching of tinnitus loudness) have not been found to be good predictors of distress (Hinchcliffe and King, 1992). Clinical experience suggests that tinnitus distress is associated with autonomic arousal, either in the form of anxiety or agitated depression, and possibly anger. Which emotion is dominant will depend on what types of beliefs the individual holds about the tinnitus. If the focus of the beliefs is about something that has been lost then depression is likely to be dominant. If it is about the possibility of future threat, or loss, then anxiety is likely to prevail. If the focus is about basic rules or assumptions being broken (e.g. 'it's not fair') then anger is likely to be uppermost.

Tinnitus and suicide

There is a popular idea that tinnitus acts as a trigger for suicide. Periodically, reports appear in the media of people with tinnitus committing suicide, and some tinnitus patients have second- or third-hand accounts of tinnitus-related suicides. There is, however, very little published scientific literature on this subject. Initial observations suggested that the incidence of suicide among patients attending a tinnitus clinic was high (Lewis et al., 1992). In a subsequent study, however, it was found that only 1.6% of people who attempted suicide had tinnitus (Lewis and Stephens, 1995), suggesting that the prevalence of tinnitus among that group of people was much less than among the general population (Axelsson and Ringdahl, 1989; Davis, 1995). None of the tinnitus cases identified in that study stated that tinnitus had played a role in their attempted suicide. These studies involved very small numbers and have several caveats associated with them; as a result, it is difficult to arrive at firm conclusions on the basis of their observations. Considered together, however, they do not lend strong support to the idea that tinnitus is associated with a high risk of suicide.

The characteristics of people with tinnitus who commit suicide have been reported in a small number of studies. It was reported by Lewis et al. (1992) that left-sided tinnitus was overly represented in their case series. In a later study, Lewis et al. (1994) obtained information from clinics around the world on a total of 28 people with tinnitus who had committed suicide in the preceding year. No particular tinnitus parameter, or associated audiological symptom, was overly represented in their suicide series. Stronger associations have been noted between psychological and demographic factors and suicide. People with tinnitus who commit suicide have the same sort of psychological profiles as the wider population of suicide victims (Lewis et al., 1992, 1994; Frankenburg and Hegarty, 1994; Johnston and Walker, 1996). The profile is one of a history of psychiatric problems, poor current psychiatric state, being male, elderly, socially isolated, with poor social support and living in an urban environment. It can be argued that the cases described were at high risk of suicide anyway and that tinnitus is not particularly important in a suicide context. Indeed, having reviewed the literature, Jacobson and McCaslin (2001) state: 'it is not tinnitus per se that results in suicide but concomitant psychiatric conditions that amplify the effects of tinnitus on the individual patient'. In a discussion of the topic, Jacobson and McCaslin (2001) went on to assert that tinnitus does not increase the risk of suicide in depressed patients. This seems a rather sweeping assertion. It is worth noting that Lewis et al. (1994) reported that 40% of their suicide cases had killed themselves within one year of the onset of tinnitus and approximately half had done so within two years.

The expression of suicidal ideas is not uncommon among patients attending tinnitus clinics, although these are usually passive thoughts. It is also worth remembering that the psychological factors thought to be paramount in suicide, such as hopelessness, depression and anger, are often complained of by patients attending tinnitus clinics. It seems reasonable to contend that if tinnitus feeds into these psychological processes then it will add to the risk of suicide. It can be concluded that for most people tinnitus does not significantly increase the risk of suicide, but that among vulnerable patients, tinnitus (in particular of recent onset) can act as an additional stressor, in the same way as, say, unemployment, thereby increasing the risk of suicide. Professionals involved in the care of tinnitus patients should be alert to the expression of suicidal ideas in their patients. They should not be shy of enquiring further about suicidal ideas if necessary; an enquiry will not put suicidal ideas into a patient's head. If suicidal ideas are encountered, the tinnitus professional should seek immediate expert guidance, preferably from a psychologist or psychiatrist, on the management of the patient. None of this should alarm the tinnitus professional; it should be remembered that the vast majority of people with tinnitus do not suffer from significant psychological problems, let alone are at risk for suicide, in spite of the high prevalence of depression in clinical tinnitus patients.

Psychological state as a trigger for tinnitus

An assumption in much of the research in this field is that the psychological disorders that tinnitus patients complain of are a result of their tinnitus. It is, however, possible to argue for a more complex relationship between tinnitus and a person's psychological condition. In a review of tinnitus literature Henry et al. (2005c) stated that the trigger for the adverse effects of tinnitus can be 'emotional stress, psychological factors, bereavement, unemployment, ... or mental illness' (p. 1205). They did not cite empirical evidence for the suggestion, but strands of evidence for this widely held clinical opinion do exist. Some of these strands suggest that for a proportion of people the tinnitus and psychological problems occur together and, for some, the tinnitus precedes the psychological problems (Stouffer and Tyler, 1992; Schmidtt et al., 2000). Other evidence indicates that the psychiatric disorder precedes the onset of tinnitus; Goebel and Floetzinger (2008) found that in 64% of those tinnitus patients who could be classified as suffering from a psychiatric disorder, that disorder preceded the onset of tinnitus. Similarly, in a study of a consecutive series of tinnitus patients seen in a routine neuro-otology clinic, Andersson et al. (2012) noted for 23.5% of patients, tinnitus preceded the mood disorder and for 20.5% of patients the onset of tinnitus and depression was simultaneous. For 56% of the patients, however, the mood disorder preceded the tinnitus onset. Many tinnitus patients, however, relate the onset of tinnitus to noise exposure rather than stress (Meric et al., 1998), while others cannot relate the onset of tinnitus to any specific event (George and Kemp, 1991; Meric et al., 1998). The evidence on this point is therefore varied but it supports the idea that, for a substantial proportion of people, tinnitus either follows or coincides with a period of stress.

There is also the question of whether other stresses or a poor psychological state aggravate existing tinnitus. Most tinnitus sufferers acknowledge that stress does aggravate tinnitus, at least insofar as making it more difficult for them to cope with their symptoms. In addition to influencing tinnitus through heightening autonomic nervous system arousal it is likely that the demands of other stresses dilute a person's ability to cope with tinnitus. There is some research evidence supporting the view that stress acts as an aggravating factor for tinnitus. In a study of tinnitus in air traffic controllers it was found that a high workload probably contributed to the problem (Vogt and Kastner, 2002). It was also noted, however, that difficult shift work patterns acted as a risk factor; it is possible that the disruption of the daily biorhythm played an important role in this respect. Andersson et al. (2012) noted that patients with an ongoing psychological mood disorder had significantly higher scores on measures of tinnitus complaint. An interaction between tinnitus distress and poor psychological state was pointed out by Sullivan et al. (1988). They noted that those tinnitus patients who were depressed had more psychological and somatic complaints than tinnitus patients who were not depressed. Those tinnitus patients who were not depressed did not have more problems than the control group, strongly suggesting that tinnitus patients' problems were more closely related to the depression than to the tinnitus. The interaction between tinnitus and psychological state has also been highlighted by Fagelson (2007), who pointed to a relationship between tinnitus and Post Traumatic Stress Disorder, which has been confirmed empirically (Hinton et al., 2006). Overall, it seems likely that once a person begins to suffer with tinnitus a vicious cycle of events becomes established; tinnitus provokes distress and the stress exacerbates the experience of tinnitus.

It is possible that a psychologically more vulnerable person will be unable to tolerate even 'mild' tinnitus and even a very 'tough' person may suffer a lot when tinnitus is perceived as very loud. In other words, there is a diathesis–stress interaction taking place in which the diathesis is the vulnerability to distress, and tinnitus level is the stress. This idea was investigated by Andersson and McKenna (1998), who studied the relationship between depression and minimum masking levels for tinnitus. They found one group of patients with low depression and average minimum masking levels. Another group had high depression and low minimum masking levels, as predicted, but they also found a group of more depressed patients who had severe tinnitus as measured by minimum masking levels. They suggested that the lower minimum masking levels in depressed people implied that their problems were mediated by them focusing on internal sensations. The results are in keeping with a diathesis–stress model.

Personality and coping style

One possible answer to why some people suffer more than others is that long-term psychological characteristics affect the way a person reacts to tinnitus. A person's personality characteristics and coping style is relevant in this context.

Personality is usually assessed by use of questionnaire measures, such as the Minnesota Multiphasic Personality Inventory (MMPI) (Hathaway and McKinley, 1940) or the Eysenck Personality Questionnaire (EPQ) (Eysenck and Eysenck, 1975). Most studies that have used such questionnaires have found that, as a group, tinnitus patients have normal personality profiles (Reich and Johnson, 1984; Collet et al., 1990; Meric et al., 1998; Vallianatou et al., 2001). Some studies, however, have found an association between tinnitus severity and psychological distress and personality characteristics such as hysteria and hypochondriasis (Bayay et al., 2002) and lower levels of extraversion (Rizzardo et al., 1998). Reich and Johnson (1984) found elevated MMPI schizophrenia subscale scores in tinnitus subjects with normal hearing. Meric et al. (1998) reported that almost half of their tinnitus subjects had at least one MMPI scale score beyond the normal limits. In most cases the abnormal scale was hysteria. Correlations between scores on the MMPI scales and scores on the Tinnitus Handicap Questionnaire (THQ) and the Tinnitus Reaction Questionnaire (TRQ) were also found by Meric et al. (1998). The strongest correlations were with the MMPI depression scale. More of their subjects with abnormal MMPI profiles had high scores on the THQ and TRQ than did those with normal MMPI profiles. Contrary to these findings, it was noted by Vallianatou et al. (2001) that there was no significant relationship between personality scores and subjective rating of tinnitus intensity. It should, however, be noted that the majority of subjects in this study cannot be regarded as representative of the most problematic of tinnitus cases. A significant correlation between the neuroticism scale of the EPQ and Tinnitus Handicap Inventory (THI) scores was noted by Zachariae et al. (2000). Unfortunately, these researchers did not state the actual EPQ scores so it is not clear whether their subjects had abnormal personality profiles or not. Using psychometric tests and psychiatric diagnostic methods, Erlandsson and Persson (2006) assessed a group of tinnitus patients. In addition to the presence of significant emotional distress, 50% of a subgroup of patients were diagnosed as suffering from a personality disorder. Erlandsson (2000) puts this in context by stating that 10–13% of the general population suffers from personality disorders. Phobic personality disorder and phobic tendencies were the most common diagnosis. Borderline personality disorder was confirmed in three male patients and obsessive compulsive disorder in one female. The majority of patients were found to have two or more disorders. Patients who were diagnosed as personality-disordered did not show a change in their distress profile at subsequent review.

Although these studies seek to assess stable personality characteristics it is possible that such measures are influenced, in some part, by the experience of tinnitus distress. The finding of Langguth et al. (2007) that the personality trait 'agreeableness' had a negative correlation with the THI score (so the less agreeable the personality, the more severe the tinnitus) is perhaps an example. This possibility was found to be less likely in a study by Langenbach et al. (2005). These researchers examined the psychosocial and personality profile of people within weeks (mean time of 11 days) of the onset of tinnitus. They reported that the presence of anxiety and dissatisfaction with life at this time predicted later tinnitus distress while factors such as localisation of tinnitus and other concomitant physical symptoms did not. They argued that as the psychological factors being measured were present very close to the onset of tinnitus stable traits were likely to have been present prior to the onset of tinnitus. The cause and effect issue is further informed by the work of Bartels et al. (2010). These researchers examined the relationship between Type D personality and tinnitus distress and quality of life. Type D personality is characterised by high levels of negative emotion (a generally sad and gloomy view of life) and social inhibition that means the person does not tell others about their emotions. The concept of Type D personality therefore refers not only to negative emotions but also to how the person typically deals with those emotions. The concept has been found to be associated with higher morbidity and mortality in other conditions independently of the disease severity. Bartels et al. (2010) reported that tinnitus patients with Type D personality had greater psychological distress and poorer health-related quality of life than non-Type D patients. Using structural equation modelling they found that the impact of Type D personality on tinnitus severity was in part mediated by the presence of anxiety and depression (i.e. possible reactions to tinnitus). The greater tinnitus distress and poorer quality of life was also, however, in part directly predicted by Type D personality.

It was noted by Scott and Lindberg (2000) that tinnitus patients not only reported a poor psychological state (i.e. problems such as anxiety and depression) but also had greater long-term psychological problems (such as a more unhelpful dispositional style, anger and response to stress) when compared with people with tinnitus but not seeking help for it, and when compared when a normal control group. High levels of trait anxiety (i.e. a general disposition to anxiety rather than a reaction to a particular stress) among tinnitus sufferers were noted by Halford and Anderson (1991) and by McKenna (1997). An association between the subjective severity of tinnitus and the degree of trait anxiety was noted by Halford and Anderson (1991). Looking at the issue from another point of view, Andersson (1996) found that a disposition towards optimism, as assessed by the Life Orientation Scale (Scheier and Carver, 1985), was negatively related to tinnitus complaints or, in other words, the greater the optimism the lower the tinnitus complaint.

The relationship between perceived tinnitus severity and patterns of coping style was investigated by Hallberg et al. (1992). These researchers reported that men with severe tinnitus more often engaged in 'escape coping' (e.g. wishful thinking, taking drugs or alcohol to feel better) than did men with equal hearing status but milder tinnitus or no tinnitus. These authors assessed general strategies for coping with stress rather than specific strategies for coping with tinnitus. The relationship between specific coping strategies that people used when dealing with tinnitus and the severity of tinnitus was assessed by Budd and Pugh (1996a), who used a questionnaire and factor analysis method that revealed three tinnitus coping styles. These were labelled 'maladaptive coping', 'effective coping' and 'passive coping'. The maladaptive coping style was characterised by catastrophic thinking about tinnitus and by ineffective attempts to avoid it by means such as daydreaming of life without it, by praying that it would go away and also by avoiding social situations because of it. Budd and Pugh (1996a) reported that sufferers who scored highly on the 'maladaptive coping' scale reported higher levels of tinnitus severity and more anxiety and depression than did sufferers who had a low score on this subscale. The passive coping style was characterised by the use of sound to mask tinnitus, by the use of relaxation techniques to cope with stress and by consulting professionals to 'offload' the difficulties of tinnitus. There was no indication that people who scored highly on this scale accepted tinnitus, and high scores were associated with increased tinnitus severity and emotional distress. The style labelled 'effective coping' was characterised by an acceptance of tinnitus and the use of a broad range of coping strategies, such as positive self-talk, attention switching and distraction through increased activity. Curiously, this style was not associated with less severe tinnitus and there was only a small association between it and better emotional adjustment. The authors suggest that this may be because the key feature in adaptation to tinnitus is the avoidance of maladaptive coping strategies rather than the use of so-called effective ones. They point out that tinnitus distress might provoke the use of strategies such as catastrophic thinking rather than the distress being caused by such strategies. They suggest that avoiding such unhelpful strategies may allow habituation to take place. It is noticeable, however, that several of the items that make up the effective coping subscale are essentially forms of distraction from tinnitus and represent avoidance behaviour, which might be expected to retard adjustment.

A sense of personal control has been found to be an important factor when facing tinnitus and hearing impairment. The concept of 'locus of control' refers to the tendency a person has to explain events as caused by internal (within the person's responsibility) or external (outside the person's responsibility) factors. Clearly, the sense of personal control that a person has is likely to have some bearing on his or her ability to cope. Locus of control has been described as one of the most important factors for health-related behaviour (Lazarus and Folkman, 1984). Personal control has also been found to be an important predictor of tinnitus discomfort and adaptation in a study by Scott et al. (1990). A significant relationship between locus of control, tinnitus severity and emotional distress in tinnitus sufferers was also found by Budd and Pugh (1995). In a study of the psychological profile of tinnitus patients, Attias et al. (1995) found that patients who sought help for tinnitus had a greater external locus of control than those who did not seek help for tinnitus. This suggests that the treatment of tinnitus patients should be aimed at facilitating coping strategies using the concept of locus of control.

Collectively, these findings strongly suggest that people with anxious personality characteristics or employ unhelpful coping strategies are at greater risk of experiencing tinnitus distressing. The professional should, however, be cautious about adopting stereotypical views of people who suffer from tinnitus as 'emotionally weak'. Anxious personality characteristics often have a positive side to them. Andersson et al. (2005a) found that people with perfectionist styles are more likely to find their experience of tinnitus distressing. It is quite likely that perfectionism leads to considerable success in other areas of life and people who suffer with tinnitus do not always present with obvious long-term emotional vulnerabilities. It does, however, make sense that people who typically take an anxious view of life in general, or who usually use avoidant coping strategies, or who become anxious when they cannot solve problems or make things perfect, will react in the same way to tinnitus. Such styles are likely to influence the types of thinking that the person adopts about tinnitus and these thinking patterns are likely to encourage the development of an anxious or depressed state. Elevated levels of arousal are likely to be a central element of this experience.

Arousal level

An important component of a distressed psychological state is an elevated level of arousal. This is all the more likely to be present if the person's long-term predisposition is towards anxiety or depression. A number of studies, using a variety of measures, have pointed to heightened arousal levels in tinnitus patients. Neuroimaging studies have identified various regions of hyperactivity in the auditory pathway of tinnitus patients (see Chapter 6). There is also evidence of increased activity in cortical regions outside the auditory cortex; these areas include the prefrontal and temperoparietal areas. Imaging studies have also revealed hyperactivity in limbic areas in tinnitus patients (again implying a high level of arousal in tinnitus patients. Walpurger et al. (2003) reported that tinnitus patients habituate more slowly, as measured by ERP, than controls, the contention here being that slowed habituation reflects higher central nervous system arousal.

There has been some research into the levels of stress hormones in tinnitus patients. People with more 'severe' tinnitus have been found to have chronically higher basal cortisol levels (reflecting hypothalamic activity) than people with less 'severe' tinnitus and control subjects (Hébert et al., 2004). Elevated cortisol levels were more closely linked to State anxiety levels than to Trait anxiety, suggesting that they were a response to the situation (tinnitus) rather than that the situation reflected constitutional disposition. Hébert and Lupin (2007) have also observed blunted cortisol responses in tinnitus patients presented with stress. They suggest that this points to tinnitus acting as a chronic stress, which results in diminished efficiency in the stress hormone system. Their conclusions took account of patients' depression. Weber et al. (2002a) reported a reduction in endocrine and immunological variables following relaxation training, suggesting that greater tinnitus distress is associated with higher levels of biological markers of distress. It must be assumed that the increased arousal observed in these studies was provoked by emotional stresses, particularly that arising from a negative interpretation of tinnitus. Indeed, Sahley and Nodar (2001) consider the possibility of a model of tinnitus based on increased auditory neuronal excitability.

Studies have also pointed to increased peripheral arousal in tinnitus patients as measured by heart rate and muscle tension. For example, Datzov et al. (1999) reported patterns of heart rate variability in tinnitus patients that reflected high levels of sympathetic autonomic nervous system activity. Electromyography provides another indicator of stress levels. Tinnitus patients often report a higher level of muscle tension (in face, jaw and shoulders) (Weise et al., 2008a; Rief et al., 2004). Rief et al. (2005) reported reductions in muscle activity following psychophysiological treatment for tinnitus, implying that tinnitus distress is related to higher arousal levels. Following a similar line of argument, Sanchez et al. (2002) demonstrated the importance of muscle contraction in tinnitus modulation.

There are a small number of findings that do not give clear support to the notion of increased arousal in tinnitus patients. Examining peripheral indicators of arousal, Carlsson and Erlandsson (1991) found no difference in physiological arousal markers of habituation between tinnitus patients and nonpatients. Heinecke et al. (2008) reported a mixed picture, higher subjective reports of strain among tinnitus patients subjected to laboratory stress than among controls but no differences in EMG or skin conductance measures. Notwithstanding these observations it is generally accepted that increased arousal is a characteristic of tinnitus patients.

Increased arousal as a trigger for tinnitus

As is the case with cognition and emotional state, it is likely that increased arousal is not only an effect of tinnitus but also plays a role as a moderator of tinnitus perception. It has even been suggested that increased arousal may be a causal mechanism in the onset of tinnitus (Schmitt et al., 2000; Sahley and Nodar, 2001). Rauschecker et al. (2010) argued that tinnitus information is usually blocked at a limbic system level through a gating mechanism. They suggested that tinnitus is consciously perceived when this gating system is compromised. Their suggestion therefore is that increased limbic system activity is not only a reaction to tinnitus but may actually have a causal role in the perception of tinnitus. It is certainly accepted that increased arousal leads to increased selective attention. The effect of this is to make whatever is being attended to more prominent compared to competing stimuli. This is as likely to be true for tinnitus as for anything else. Selective attention will be discussed further below.

Selective attention

As arousal levels increase attention becomes more selective. It is suggested that this process involves both automatic (Kahneman, 1973) and conscious processes. Clinical experience indicates that tinnitus patients monitor for events such as: perceived increases in tinnitus intensity or changes in quality; environmental noises that change the signal-to-noise status of tinnitus; environmental noises (clock, car engine, sound generator) against which to compare tinnitus. Commonly, people who are troubled by tinnitus also monitor themselves for other bodily or cognitive sensations suggestive of poor functioning, e.g. tiredness, concentration problems. If threatening tinnitus cues are detected a further source of worry is established. The finding of Hallam et al. (1984) that tinnitus patients are more persistently aware of their noises than noncomplainers (although the two groups did not differ on psychoacoustical measures of tinnitus) can be taken as evidence of a selective attention effect.

There is also a body of research evidence that points to the importance of selective attention in the tinnitus process. Andersson et al. (2000a) employed an Emotional Stroop Test using clinically derived tinnitus words (e.g. Tone, Buzz) and neutral words to investigate attentional bias in tinnitus patients. They did not find a classic Stroop effect although the tinnitus group was slower overall than a control group, regardless of stimulus condition. They speculated that the presence of tinnitus itself may have interfered with the

Stroop effect in the way that the presence of a feared object can lead to fear arousal and a reduction of the emotional Stroop effect (Mathews and Sebastian, 1993). In a subsequent study, Andersson et al. (2005b) administered an emotional (tinnitus) Stroop test, via the Internet. Their findings support an attentional bias in tinnitus patients. They speculate that the difference between the two studies may arise from different methodologies and/or from the possibility that the electronic version of the test assesses attentional bias at a later stage in the information processing system. Andersson et al. (2003a) investigated autobiographical memories in tinnitus patients using a modified version of the Autobiographical Memory Test (AMT) (Williams and Broadbent, 1986). They report that, compared to control subjects, tinnitus patients had difficulty retrieving specific memories and showed longer retrieval latencies. Additionally, tinnitus patients had fewer specific memories to positive cue words. While AMT scores were associated with depression (BDI) scores the differences between controls and patients remained significant for positive words after controlling for depression scores. Although the study has a number of limitations (e.g. small sample size) the results of this study are supportive of the idea of selective information processing in tinnitus patients. Knobel and Sanchez (2008) reported that directed attention plays a role in the perception of tinnitus.

As mentioned in Chapter 6, a number of studies have examined tinnitus patients' reaction times to sound stimuli. Goodwin and Johnson (1980a) found that tinnitus patients show faster reaction times to sound presented at the same frequency as their tinnitus than to other sounds and that they respond more quickly to sounds at the tinnitus frequency than do control subjects. Nieschalk et al. (1998) also report that tinnitus patients have faster reaction times to noises at the tinnitus frequency than control subjects. Cuny et al. (2004) investigated the ability of patients with unilateral tinnitus and control subjects to categorise sounds in one ear while other sounds were presented to the other ear using an 'odd ball' paradigm. They report classic attention capture by deviant stimuli. They also report that tinnitus patients were able to categorise sounds more accurately when they were presented to the tinnitus ear. They conclude that tinnitus patients find it more difficult to direct attention to other information when that information is presented to the tinnitus ear and suggest that this is evidence of an automatic selective attention process in tinnitus patients. Attias et al. (1996a), however, have found slower reaction times among tinnitus patients.

A number of studies have investigated electrophysiological indices, particularly event-related brain potentials (ERP), of automatic selective auditory attention in tinnitus patients. In some studies the results have not been conclusive (Barnea et al., 1990; McKee and Stephens, 1992), but other studies have provided evidence in support of the selective attention hypothesis in tinnitus patients (Ikner and Hassen, 1990; Rosenhall and Axelsson, 1995; Jacobson et al., 1996; Nieschalk et al., 1998). The neuro-imaging studies reviewed elsewhere in this book (Chapter 6) also suggest that there is an increased amount of cerebral substrate devoted to processing sounds in the range of the tinnitus frequency.

Selective attention can be regarded as the result of thinking about tinnitus in threatening terms and of the ensuing increase in arousal (for experimental studies on selective attention see Chapter 6). The effect of selective attention must be to increase the perception of tinnitus. If this increases the perceived threat of tinnitus then a maintenance cycle will be established. It is possible, however, that the effect goes beyond this and that a distortion of perception occurs. This possibility is referred to by Fowler (1943) when he suggests that tinnitus patients 'experience an exaggerated sensation as to both its loudness and its timbre, and it is then overestimated and sensed as a most disagreeable or unbearable noise' (p. 396). Just as monitoring and selective attention have been found to result in a distortion of insomnia patients' perception of their sleep loss (Harvey and Schmidt, 2000) so it is possible that selective attention leads people who suffer with tinnitus to experience a distortion in their perception of their noises. Patients' comparisons of their tinnitus to jet engines, steam trains, whistling kettles, etc., need to be reconciled with the results of matching and masking studies, which suggest that tinnitus is matched to low levels of external sound. It may be that matching and masking studies simply provide an inadequate measuring system. It is possible, however, that the differences can be accounted for by a distortion in perception resulting from selective attention. This idea, however, remains speculative.

The tinnitus experience is therefore one that is best understood in terms of a number of feedback loops and interacting systems rather than a linear one. Current theorising in psychology suggests that once tinnitus (or a change in tinnitus) is detected the person thinks about this; if the interpretation is a threatening one then increased arousal, changes in mood and alterations in behaviour ensue. These processes focus attention on tinnitus and may provoke further threatening interpretations, so creating a vicious cycle of events. It is likely that these processes occur, to a greater or lesser extent, in all those who experience tinnitus as distressing. Once established this cycle of events can, but does not necessarily, give rise to a number of other consequences. There is also a question of whether this loop is influenced by other processes.

Sleep

One of the most important aspects of tinnitus complaint is sleep disturbance. Open-ended questionnaire studies indicate that sleep disturbance is the most common, or second most common, aspect of tinnitus complaint (Tyler and Baker, 1983; Sanchez and Stephens, 1997). As many as 71% of tinnitus patients report sleep problems (Andersson et al., 1999). In a survey of tinnitus sufferers in New Zealand, George and Kemp (1991) found that all of their subjects indicated that tinnitus affected their sleep. On the basis of the UK National Study of Hearing, Davis (1995) reported that 5% of the population describe tinnitus that disturbs their sleep. Sleep problems may also be prevalent among children complaining of tinnitus. In a study of children's experiences of tinnitus, Kentish et al. (2000) reported that 80% of children referred for help with tinnitus complained of sleep problems, these problems usually being the reason that led parents to request help for their child. In an epidemiological study ($n = 10\,216$) on sleep problems in older adults with tinnitus, it was found that poor sleep was reported by 14.4% of the men and by 27.9% of the women with tinnitus (Asplund, 2003). It is clear from these reports that many people who suffer with tinnitus also suffer with sleep disturbance. Importantly, however, it is also clear that not everyone who is troubled by tinnitus suffers from poor sleep.

Insomnia is not, an inevitable effect of tinnitus. Interestingly, in a study on patients seen at a sleep laboratory unit, only 10 of 1500 patients reported tinnitus, and of those only two were annoyed (Alster et al., 1993). It is also noteworthy that Eysel-Gosepath and Selivanova (2005) reported that a high proportion of their tinnitus patients had other causes, such as obstructive sleep apnea or periodic leg movements, for their sleep disturbance. A similar observation was made by Cronlein et al. (2007).

In addition to being very common, there is evidence that troubled sleep is among the most significant complaints for tinnitus sufferers. Sleep disturbance was the largest single factor in the factor analysis of tinnitus complaint undertaken by Hallam et al. (1988), and Jakes et al. (1985) reported that difficulty sleeping was the main complaint in 50% of severe tinnitus sufferers. There is also evidence that sleep problems are associated with more distressing tinnitus. Scott et al. (1990) reported that the most important predictors of greater tinnitus discomfort and decreased tolerance of the symptom were depression and insomnia. Langenbach et al. (2005) reported that insomnia occurring at the onset of tinnitus predicted greater distress later on. Other researchers have reported that sleep problems are associated with more annoying and more severe tinnitus (Axelsson anad Ringdahl, 1989; Hallam, 1996b; Dineen et al., 1997a; Folmer and Griest, 2000), although the cause and effect relationship is difficult to work out. It is possible that sleep loss results from more complex or distressing tinnitus but it is equally possible that sleep loss results in the person having a greater opportunity to focus on and find complexity within tinnitus. This possibility is supported by the observations of Cronlein et al. (2007). These researchers compared tinnitus patients who had poor sleep with a control group of insomniacs without tinnitus across a number of objective and subjective sleep measures. They found no significant differences between the groups on any objective measures but the subjective estimate of time taken to fall asleep was longer among the tinnitus patients. Cronlein et al. (2007) suggested that tinnitus may provide some patients with evidence of their lack of sleep and so provoke worry about lack of sleep.

In spite of the importance of insomnia in tinnitus complaint, it has received relatively little attention in the tinnitus research literature. It is usually referred to as just one of a number of aspects of tinnitus complaint, or outcome factors, and it has not been clearly defined in most cases. Therefore, little is known about the exact nature of the relationship between tinnitus and insomnia. Although many tinnitus sufferers believe that tinnitus prevents them from sleeping or wakes them up in the night, it seems unlikely that tinnitus is actually a specific sleep antagonist. Sleep disturbance is not a universal aspect of tinnitus complaint. Indeed, anecdotal clinical reports suggest that many tinnitus sufferers sleep very well. Clinical reports also suggest that the pattern of awakenings among tinnitus sufferers complaining of insomnia corresponds with the usual awakenings that are part of a normal night's sleep. These observations point to the influence of some mediating factors. It has been suggested by McKenna and Daniel (2006) that a cognitive behavioural model of insomnia can be applied in the tinnitus context and that it is anxiety associated with tinnitus, rather than tinnitus per se, that leads to insomnia. The ensuing anxiety about poor sleep adds to the problem by feeding into the vicious cycles described above. They suggested that the pre-sleep period (at the start or in the middle of the night), with its few other distractions and low levels of ambient noise, offers an opportunity to focus on tinnitus. This leads to unhelpful thoughts about tinnitus and to changes in behaviour, such as delaying going to bed when tinnitus is more intrusive, and checking their tinnitus, which in turn leads to increased arousal and distress. This anxiety leads to poor sleep that, in turn, leads to further anxiety, so maintaining the insomnia and the awareness of tinnitus. The use of alcohol to either reduce anxiety or as a hypnotic can have the effect of disrupting the usual sleep cycle and can lead to depression symptoms. While McKenna and Daniel (2006) emphasised anxiety as a key factor in this process these authors recognised that the anxiety may be an aspect of depression in many cases. They suggested a cognitive behavioural treatment approach.

Family relationships

The influence of family relationships in the experience of tinnitus has received only a small amount of research interest. The possibility that a person's distress might have an impact on family relationships seems obvious; it is, however, also possible that those relationships influence the experience of tinnitus. People who are distressed by tinnitus do a number of things that communicate their distress to others. These behaviours can come under the control of reinforcements of one kind or another from other people, in particular the patient's spouse. Thus, conceivably, a spouse who provides attention and sympathy (i.e. responds solicitously) to a patient's tinnitus behaviour may unwittingly reinforce and maintain it. Alternatively, it is possible that a spouse who ignores or punishes the tinnitus behaviour may have the effect of reducing the behaviour and so improving the patient's overall level of functioning. This process was investigated by Sullivan et al. (1994), who examined coping, depression and marital support as correlates of tinnitus disability, where disability was defined as interference with activity at work, at home and in the patient's social life. Contrary to the prediction of a conditioning model, these researchers found that punitive responses from the spouse did not have a helpful effect on the patient. They concluded that, for tinnitus patients, criticism results in demoralisation rather than activation. This was particularly true when the patient experienced greater levels of depression, and Sullivan et al. (1994) suggested that in such circumstances criticism may lead to poor habituation to tinnitus. They also reported that poor marital cohesion was associated with greater disability. This study, however, focused on only one aspect of disability, namely the ability to function in very specific areas of life. Further work was done by Pugh et al. (2004), who investigated the effect of spouses' responses to patients' 'tinnitus behaviour' on the perceived severity of tinnitus and on the level of emotional distress experienced. These workers concluded that solicitous responses on the part of spouses had a detrimental effect on the experience of chronic tinnitus and enquiries about tinnitus tended to increase expressions of distress. They also found that punishing responses by spouses were correlated with maladaptive coping and tinnitus severity. It seems that, rather than reducing tinnitus behaviours, punitive responses from spouses amounted to a removal of social support. The relationship between punitive responses and tinnitus severity appeared to be mediated by emotional distress. Interestingly, however, Pugh et al. (2004) noted that there was a direct relationship between solicitous responses and tinnitus severity as well as one mediated by emotional distress. This suggests that the influence of rewards and punishments needs to be built into any model of tinnitus distress. These researchers also found that dissatisfaction within the marriage was associated with greater anxiety and depression.

The role of family support was also investigated by Granqvist et al. (2001), who investigated the relationship between attachment patterns and tinnitus-related problems. Attachment theory originally focused on infants' ties to their mothers but has subsequently gone on to be applied in many other settings, including seeking to understand people's experiences of illness. There are two broad types of attachment patterns, referred to as 'secure' or 'insecure' (the latter being divided into avoidant or ambivalent). These researchers reported that avoidant attachment was linked to tinnitus-related problems and that avoidant and ambivalent attachment was related to punitive family responses. Furthermore, avoidance predicted tinnitus-related problems over and above the effects of family support. Contrary to expectations, however, secure attachment patterns were not related to fewer tinnitus problems. Granqvist et al. (2001) speculated that people who have an avoidant attachment style, and who presumably perceive other people as unlikely to be able to support them, may use unhelpful coping strategies such as emotion-focused and avoidant strategies instead of problem-focused ones when dealing with tinnitus. An avoidant attachment style might also influence how a person relates to others and how others, in turn, relate to them, and hence might increase the likelihood of punitive responses from the family. Alternatively, it is possible that people high in insecurity do actually have fewer supportive family members because they choose partners who are similar to themselves.

Work

Few studies have investigated the effects of tinnitus on people's ability to work. There is the potential for tinnitus to interfere with people's ability to perform certain tasks that require precision hearing, such as the performance of classical music. As a consequence, some people with tinnitus conceal the fact that they have it. It is interesting to note that in such circumstances people often carry on working in the supposedly compromised profession. Despite the concentration problems associated with tinnitus, in practice few people are unable to work because of tinnitus itself (Andersson, 2000a). Indeed, Vallianatou et al. (2001) noted that the patients in their study group did not report that tinnitus had a detrimental effect on their ability to work. Most of their patients, however, had tinnitus of long duration and were reasonably well adjusted to it. It is also noteworthy that some people with tinnitus who are in high-profile jobs still manage to perform their duties with no apparent difficulty. In spite of these observations, some people who suffer with tinnitus do have difficulty carrying on their everyday lives, including their jobs. It seems most likely that the difficulties that such people experience can be attributed to the psychological problems associated with tinnitus (i.e. anxiety and depression) rather than the tinnitus itself.

Gender

Gender differences in tinnitus have been reported in several studies. Women have been found to report more complex tinnitus sounds (Meikle and Griest, 1989). Although more complex tinnitus tends to be associated with more problems, it is less clear whether there are gender differences in how problematic tinnitus is. On the one hand, George and Kemp (1991) found that men reported more tinnitus-related problems than did women. On the other hand, Dineen et al. (1997a) found that women reported a greater reaction to tinnitus than did men. In a study with 146 tinnitus patients, using the Anxiety Sensitivity Index (Reiss et al., 1986), anxiety sensitivity correlated significantly with tinnitus distress ($r=0.60$). Interestingly, the association was significantly stronger for female participants ($r=0.74$ versus $r=0.53$ for the males), who also scored higher on the anxiety sensitivity index (Andersson and Vretblad, 2000). In another previously mentioned study Andersson et al. (2005a) investigated the relationship between perfectionism and tinnitus distress. In addition, associations between perfectionism and sleep problems, and anxiety or depression were investigated. Gender-differentiated multiple regression analyses showed that anxiety and depressive states were related to tinnitus distress for both genders. However, for the males the perfectionism subscale Personal Standards was related to tinnitus distress, whereas in females it was the Organization subscale that was most predictive of tinnitus distress. Other studies have found no gender differences in problems related to tinnitus (Hallberg and Erlandsson, 1993). As the evidence is contradictory it is currently unwarranted to suggest that men and women with tinnitus should be managed differently.

Other somatic symptoms

The presence of other somatic symptoms may increase the burden that tinnitus patients have to bear. For example, George and Kemp (1991) found that people who experienced dizziness in addition to tinnitus reported more problematic tinnitus. In contrast to this, however, it was reported by Dineen et al. (1997a) that tinnitus subjects who experienced headaches, back pain, neck pain or balance problems reported their tinnitus to be no louder, no more annoying and no more difficult to cope with than subjects who did not have these symptoms. They did, however, find that subjects who suffered from jaw pain reported tinnitus as more annoying and more difficult to cope with, but not louder. Notwithstanding the findings of Dineen et al. (1997a), it seems intuitively obvious that if a person has more than one problem he or she will have greater levels of distress. Indeed, McKenna et al. (1991) found greater psychological problems in neuro-otology patients complaining of more than one symptom. Although there may be greater overall distress, however, it is not necessarily the case that more symptoms will result in more problematic tinnitus. It is often the case that other symptoms, in particular dizziness, diminish the significance of tinnitus. Nonetheless, it would seem to make sense that coexisting symptoms should be tackled where possible as part of the management of the tinnitus patient.

Hearing impairment

In the population at large, the degree of hearing loss is one of the things most closely correlated with tinnitus (Davis, 1995). The possibility that hearing loss has some mediating influence on tinnitus must therefore be considered. The evidence about this is mixed, however. Some work has suggested that hearing loss predicts greater tinnitus distress and the idea that hearing loss will affect tinnitus is a central tenet of the neurophysiological model of tinnitus (Jastreboff, 1990). Several studies have found that the characteristics of associated hearing loss are not correlated with self-reported assessment of tinnitus (Newman et al., 1996; Meric et al., 1998; Zachariae et al., 2000; Vallianatou et al., 2001). Similarily, Scott and Lindberg (2000) found that anxiety, depression and reaction to stress in tinnitus patients remained high even when hearing impairment had been suitably rehabilitated. In other words, these problems are not related to hearing loss. Nonetheless, it seems sensible to try to alleviate a hearing loss through the use of hearing aids where one is present. Intuitively, it seems likely that if there is some external auditory input it will help to offset the internal tinnitus. The clinician needs to be aware, however, that this seemingly sensible approach has not always been successful (Andersson et al., 2011; Melin et al., 1987).

Smoking, alcohol and caffeine

Many tinnitus sufferers believe that smoking, drinking alcohol or excessive intake of drinks such as tea and coffee will influence their tinnitus. Many sufferers believe that these substances will worsen their tinnitus and are careful to abstain. Others take the view that a glass of wine or beer, or a cigarette, has a beneficial effect. The evidence linking tinnitus with any of these substances is at best equivocal. There is a suggestion that the incidence of hearing loss is greater in smokers than in nonsmokers (Zelman, 1973), but a direct relationship between tinnitus and smoking still needs to be established. Similarly, no relationship between caffeine and tinnitus has been established. In a double-blind crossover study St Claire et al. (2010) found no relationship between the withdrawal or introduction of caffeine and the experience of tinnitus. Nicotine and caffeine are, however, stimulants and, in theory, they might increase arousal and increase tinnitus detection through that mechanism. Alternatively, increased arousal may lead to greater anxiety levels and so reduce coping ability. This is, however, a theoretical point and anecdotal evidence suggests that few patients who cut out smoking and drinking coffee show dramatic improvements in their tinnitus.

The link between alcohol and tinnitus has received moderate research attention (McFadden, 1982; Kemp and George, 1992; Pugh et al., 1995; Stephens, 1999; Vallianatou et al., 2001) but the picture to emerge from studies is unclear. Most tinnitus sufferers report that modest alcohol consumption makes no difference to their tinnitus, but some report a temporary improvement while others report a temporary worsening. It was found by Stephens (1999) that a worsening of tinnitus after drinking alcohol was particularly noted by people who drank less alcohol; however, higher intake was found to worsen tinnitus in another study (Goodey, 1981). The consumption of alcohol was found to be a risk factor for tinnitus in a study of the epidemiology of hearing problems in Italy (Quaranta et al., 1996).

There are obvious general health benefits to stopping smoking and avoiding excessive alcohol intake but there is a risk that removing pleasures from life also reduces the rewards that might help to maintain a sense of wellbeing and therefore the ability to cope with tinnitus.

Environment

It has been noted clinically that a change in environment can alleviate tinnitus distress. For example, some patients report an improvement in their overall wellbeing when they go on holiday. Unfortunately, many very distressed patients do not attempt to change their environment for fear that their ability to cope will be destabilised. This idea is never put to the test and such patients' distress persists perhaps partly as a consequence of this. Interestingly, Vallianatou et al. (2001) suggested that the agreeable environment of a Greek island may be responsible for the greater wellbeing of people with tinnitus who live there. Many distressed tinnitus patients who take their holidays in that part of the world would agree. A holiday, however, involves many changes, including a change in physical environment, change in stress levels, altered ambient noise levels (e.g. cicadas on a Greek island), increased alcohol intake, etc., and so it is difficult to know what the key elements involved are. Unfortunately, the reported benefits, or otherwise, of changing an environment are entirely anecdotal.

Summary

The consequences of tinnitus are many and varied. For some people tinnitus is of little consequence; for others it is life changing. There is also a variety of factors that influence the tinnitus experience. Understanding this variability is one of the greatest challenges in tinnitus therapy and research. Intuitively it would seem reasonable to suppose that variability in the psychophysical measures of tinnitus would be associated with variability in suffering. Historically, however, it has been argued that the evidence does not support this contention (House, 1981; Meikle and Taylor-Walsh, 1984; Kuk et al., 1990; Dineen et al., 1997a) and there seems little ground for rejecting this argument. The way forward with this challenge is to understand the experience of tinnitus in terms of a series of events that contains a number of possible feedback loops rather than as a simple linear process. Once tinnitus has been detected variability starts with the way the signal is interpreted. Very negative thoughts about it give rise to emotional distress and to increased stress arousal. Feedback loops may become influential at this stage, with deteriorating mood and increasing arousal leading to changes in thinking. Increased arousal leads to selective attention and monitoring of tinnitus. This process leads to greater tinnitus detection and helps to confirm some overly negative thoughts about tinnitus. The person is therefore led back through the above process and distress is maintained. The relevance of the component parts of this process is supported by a growing body of research from several disciplines. The importance of factors outside this system, such as gender, the presence of other symptoms, including hearing loss, diet and environment, seems even more variable. This may be because these factors do not have a direct effect on tinnitus but rather influence one or other of the elements within the system.

Chapter 8

Psychological models of tinnitus

Introduction

Several psychological theories have been proposed for explaining why tinnitus becomes a distressing experience. Among the earliest were psychodynamic theories (Schneer, 1956; Weinshel, 1955), but since there was no proper research to underpin these theories they have been largely forgotten and play no major role in our current understanding of tinnitus. Briefly the early psychodynamic theories postulated that unconscious conflicts were the reasons behind tinnitus distress. The notion that psychological disturbances could influence the perception of tinnitus did feature in an early discussion of tinnitus (Fowler, 1948) and is still highly relevant (see Chapter 7), but psychodynamic theory has not been part of that literature.

There is not one single psychological theory that dominates the field but rather a range of different theories and empirical observations. However, the behavioural and cognitive theories have dominated the literature.

Behavioural theories

Behavioural psychology has been around for a long time (Watson, 1913) and is still widely used in research and theories on anxiety, fear and a range of other phenomena (Sundell and Sundell, 1999). Briefly, the first form of behavioural psychology focuses on *respondent conditioning* (also called classical conditioning), which has a major role in the neurophysiological model outlined by Jastreboff and Hazell (2004) (see Chapter 9).

A second form of behavioural psychology is *operant psychology* (Baum, 1994), which has rarely been mentioned in the tinnitus literature, but which is the basic theory in behaviour therapy and in behavioural analysis. One exception in the field of tinnitus is early work by Scott and Lindberg who based their studies on operant psychology (Lindberg, 1989; Scott, 1989). Briefly, operant psychology holds that behaviour is determined by its consequences

Tinnitus: A Multidisciplinary Approach, Second Edition. David Baguley, Gerhard Andersson, Don McFerran and Laurence McKenna.
© 2013 David Baguley, Gerhard Andersson, Don McFerran and Laurence McKenna.
Published 2013 by Blackwell Publishing Ltd.

and therefore it is important to consider the consequences of 'tinnitus behaviour' – in other words, what the person with tinnitus does and how the consequences maintain the behaviour. As is often the case there is much more written in the field of chronic pain than in the tinnitus field. Operant psychology has been a central theory in the pain literature for many years (Fordyce et al., 1982) and still informs pain management.

An early form of basic behavioural theory was presented in 1984 by Richard Hallam and colleagues. These workers observed that most cases of tinnitus are associated with 'some neurophysiological disturbance in the auditory system at any point between periphery and cortex' (Hallam et al., 1984, p. 33). However, they also noted that some cases of tinnitus occur without aural pathology, citing the findings of Heller and Bergman (1953), in which people who stated that they had no hearing impairment and no previous tinnitus reported hearing tinnitus-like noises when placed in a soundproof environment. Hallam et al. (1984) went on to suggest that psychological processes were involved in tinnitus and, as well as psychological factors affecting tinnitus, the converse could also happen. This suggestion of both psychosomatic and somatopsychic interactions echoed the findings of previous work by Tyler and Baker (1983), and indeed work by Fowler (1948), in which clear psychosomatic links were proposed. Hallam et al. (1984) suggested that efficient central neural processing requires selective inhibition of sensory input and that this process may be impaired when the attentional system is required to process excessive levels of input, in particular during states of high central nervous system and autonomic nervous system arousal. They further suggested that tinnitus does not receive continuous conscious attention and can be modified by factors such as masking, distraction and changes in arousal, including circadian rhythm. Hallam (1987) further elaborated on the role of self-attentiveness in the development of tinnitus distress. Hallam et al. (1984) observed that the majority of people who experience tinnitus do not complain about the symptom and suggested that the normal situation is for people to habituate to their tinnitus. Work by Tyler and Baker (1983) supported this hypothesis by showing that the range and intensity of tinnitus-related problems decreased with time and that there was also no correlation between perceived loudness of the tinnitus and the degree of distress. Habituation has been defined as 'a decrease in response to a benign stimulus when that stimulus is presented repeatedly' (Kandel et al., 2000) and is described in work by Pavlov and by Sherrington (see Kandel et al., 2000, for a review). Using Horvath's (1980) rules of habituation, Hallam and colleagues (1984) postulated that tinnitus should rapidly lose its novelty and habituation should occur, but that in certain situations this process could be expected not to occur. Such situations include high levels of autonomic nervous system arousal, sudden onset of tinnitus, particularly intense aversive or unpredictable tinnitus or if the tinnitus develops emotional significance through a learning process (Groves and Thompson, 1970). Habituation could also be affected if the neural pathways involved in habituation were damaged. Conversely, tinnitus awareness could be attributed to dishabituation of a previously tolerated signal because of psychological change. In this model it was further proposed that an orienting response to tinnitus could interrupt normal behaviour, thereby increasing arousal and consequently reducing habituation. This would produce a pathophysiological positive feedback loop, resulting in persistence of the symptom. This proposal is supported by the observation that tinnitus distress tends to increase in quiet environments where the signal (tinnitus) to noise (background sound) ratio is greater. Extending this theory, Hallam et al. (1984) suggested that anything that alters the signal-to-noise ratio may affect tinnitus perception and that distress will increase as awareness of the tinnitus interferes with normal central neural activity. This model can be used to develop treatment strategies. Firstly, reducing levels of autonomic system arousal would be expected to be beneficial. This is generally achieved by relaxation therapy. Secondly, changing the emotional meaning of tinnitus should reduce the distress. This can be achieved by formal cognitive therapy, but also by vouchsafing information about the mechanisms of tinnitus and associated distress.

Unfortunately, surprisingly little research has followed the important theoretical contribution of Hallam et al. (1984). Hallam and colleagues concentrated on cognitive habituation processes that described habituation of reaction, whereas most research studies have considered psychophysiological measures of habituation, such as skin conductance and event-related potentials (see Chapter 6). Carlsson and Erlandsson (1991), for example, studied 14 patients of whom seven were complainers and seven noncomplainers, measuring skin conductance and heart rate changes in response to a series of tinnitus-like sounds. No differences in habituation were observed, but in fact some signs of opposite mechanisms (e.g. sensitisation) were found in the complainer group. Complainers compared with noncomplainers increased their heart rate. For many reasons this small-scale study cannot be regarded as a fair test of the habituation model. Walpurger et al. (2003) (see Chapter 6) tested Hallam's habituation model and found some support for a lack of habituation to tone pips by use of auditory evoked potentials. Other previous experiments on evoked potentials have also been interpreted as showing evidence of habituation failure (Attias et al., 1993a). When it comes to psychological habituation (e.g. caring less about it) the evidence is mixed, as older adults with longstanding tinnitus may have more instead of less severe annoyance. It is also unclear if psychological and physiological habituation are related (Heinecke et al., 2008, for example, did not find an association).

A fourth kind of behavioural psychology can be considered. It might not be classical conditioning that takes place but rather 'evaluative conditioning' (De Houwer et al., 2001). Evaluative conditioning refers to changes in the liking of a stimulus because the stimulus has been paired with other, positive or negative, stimuli. In evaluative conditioning studies, a neutral stimulus is paired with an affective stimulus and changes in the valence of the neutral stimulus are measured. Interestingly, unlike most forms of Pavlovian conditioning, evaluative conditioning is highly resistant to extinction. There is yet no research to support this theory.

Cognitive theories

Cognitive psychology is arguably the most widely spread and popular branch of psychology and underpins most current research in clinical psychology and indeed cognitive neuroscience as well. The concept of cognition is extremely broad but covers such diverse activities as sensation, perception, language, thinking, reasoning, problem solving, memory, consciousness, and attention. Andersson and McKenna (2006) proposed a model for how tinnitus and cognition may interact. They suggested that cognition can influence tinnitus at three different levels (see Figure 8.1). Firstly, they argued that tinnitus is likely to disrupt

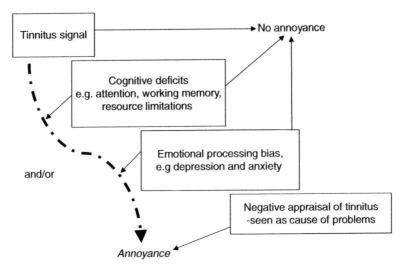

Figure 8.1   A cognitive model of tinnitus.

cognitive functioning, and there are some indications that tinnitus patients have impaired capacity to perform certain cognitive tasks. Secondly, they cited evidence that tinnitus patients show cognitive bias in the way they handle information. Such an information processing style suggests either depressive functioning, or anxious vigilance, or both. Finally, they mentioned that self-report measures of tinnitus distress all require conscious recollection of how tinnitus is perceived and the consequences of tinnitus. Such reports necessitate cognitive capacity. Thus cognition may make a difference at three different levels, but most research has dealt with the third level with patients reporting their level of distress and cognitions on self-report inventories.

With regards to the first level, there is some limited evidence suggesting that tinnitus patients perform worse on neuropsychological tests than do people without tinnitus over and beyond the effects of hearing impairment. Moreover, there is no clear theoretical framework for why impaired cognitive function might lead to more tinnitus distress. Indeed, as suggested by Andersson and McKenna, it may be that cognitive function can protect against the intrusiveness of tinnitus, but there is yet not much support for the notion that cognitive problems make tinnitus worse or the other way around that tinnitus would impair cognitive function (even if that might be the case).

When it comes to the second level, there are more studies even if they are far from conclusive. Research on information processing holds that people process information is certain ways and that psychological disturbance may result if information is interpreted in a biased manner. For example, cognitive theory of depression suggests that depressed persons have a negative view of themselves, the world and their future (Beck et al., 1979). Depressed individuals tend to remember negative information better than positive information and memory bias is a typical feature of depression. It can also come in the form of cognitive avoidance of memories, which consistently have been found to be less specific in depressed individuals (Williams et al., 2007). In anxiety other cognitive processes are involved even if interpretation plays a central role here as well. Anxiety tends to be associated with selective attention and it is often found that patients with anxiety disorder selectively attend to information related to their concern (e.g. threat stimuli in specific phobia). How does this relate to tinnitus? Several authors have proposed cognitive models of tinnitus (Henry and Wilson, 2001; McKenna and Andersson, 2008). A more elaborate cognitive model of tinnitus has yet to be fully developed, but the data thus far suggest that people with tinnitus show more signs of 'depressed' information processing rather than selective attention to threat. This is possibly due to the fact that many tinnitus patients after a while realise that their tinnitus will not make them mad or soon become much louder, but of course there are people with tinnitus who 'catastrophise' and fear their tinnitus. However, the evidence regarding catastrophising in tinnitus only derives from nonexperimental correlational research (Cima et al., 2011; Hesser and Andersson, 2009). In cognitive theories on related conditions like chronic pain catastrophising and maladaptive misinterpretations play a central role (Vlaeyen and Linton, 2000). Avoidance in tinnitus may involve avoidance of situations that are perceived to make tinnitus worse and situations that are viewed as dangerous in terms of loud sounds causing more hearing loss. However, catastrophising more relates to the third level of appraisal in the model presented in Figure 8.1. There may be some 'automatic' character to the avoidance, and interpretation and indeed selective attention is involved in tinnitus distress. Several authors have proposed that attentional factors may play a crucial role in moderating the adverse effects of tinnitus. For example, Jastreboff (1990), in his seminal paper, wrote: 'The psychological components related to the evaluation of tinnitus and the type of emotion it evokes are of particular importance, and the procedures which affect this evaluation are likely to be effective in tinnitus alleviation.' Jacobson et al. (1996) found that tinnitus patients showed evidence of early selective auditory attention by means of an experimental paradigm in which participants were asked to attend and respond to an occasional target stimulus presented in one ear while ignoring information (including the target stimulus) presented in the opposite ear. Selective attention in terms of interpretation bias has been less well researched and the few studies that exist do not indicate that tinnitus patients have a bias related to words describing their tinnitus (e.g. Andersson et al., 2000a).

At the third level of the cognition–tinnitus link we place appraisal theories usually described under the name of coping theories. Coping was mentioned in Chapter 6. Coping theory holds that people handle stressful events by first appraising if it is a threat or not and then if it is something that the person can handle (Folkman and Lazarus, 1988). Depending on the outcomes of this process the person can choose between either problem-focused or emotion-focused coping. Coping theory is important in health psychology and has indeed informed tinnitus research as well (e.g. Budd and Pugh, 1996a, 1996b). However, this leads us to a more recent development in the literature, namely acceptance.

Acceptance-based theory

Acceptance has been put forward as an important psychological construct that may mediate between the sound and the annoyance caused by it (Andersson and Westin, 2008; Schutte et al., 2009; Tyler et al., 2006). Acceptance is a difficult concept to convey in clinical settings as it may lead to the impression of giving up. However, in the current conceptualisation it refers to a process of actively taking in an event, to fully experience bodily sensations, thoughts, memories and feelings and in a specific situation, without having to follow or change them (Hayes, 2003). Acceptance is conceptualised not as an end in itself but as a means by which more useful behaviour can occur even in the presence of negative experiences (Hayes, 2003). On a theoretical level acceptance is closely related to its opposite psychological process – *experiential avoidance*. This is defined as the avoidance of internal sensations, thoughts, etc., and is regarded as an underlying process behind psychological distress (Hayes et al., 1996). The literature on acceptance of tinnitus is emerging, but involved the development of new instruments (Westin et al., 2008a), experimental studies (Hesser et al., 2009; Westin et al., 2008b), mechanisms of change in treatment (Hesser et al., 2009) and treatment studies (Zetterqvist Westin et al., 2011). Acceptance-based theory has a direct link to new theories about language (Hayes et al., 2001) and is not a disease-specific theory.

Emotion-based theory

Surprisingly, few researchers have commented on the role of emotion regulation in tinnitus, which is a central feature of our current understanding of anxiety and depression (Gross, 2002). Emotion does, however, play a central role in both the neurophysiological and psychological models of tinnitus and it has even been suggested that emotional centres in the brain play a causal role in the perception of tinnitus (Rauschecker et al., 2010). Most theories regard emotional reactions more as a consequence of tinnitus and do not regard emotion per se as a cause of tinnitus. Memory is closely linked with emotion and De Ridder and Vanneste (2011) convincingly argued that memory mechanisms play a role in tinnitus, for example by means of reinforcing the distress.

Cognitive-affective links: the changing state theory

While some psychological theories provide plausible explanations about how tinnitus becomes more distressing by means of how it is interpreted and the role of habituation there is still surprisingly little written about the tinnitus signal itself and how it becomes a distressing experience. Noble and Tyler (2007) argued that tinnitus is not a neutral stimulus and that classical conditioning theory as outlined by Jastreboff is less plausible since tinnitus hardly can be regarded as being without emotional significance (an argument made by McKenna, 2004, as well). Andersson (2002a) presented a model that took account of the potentially disturbing aspects of tinnitus sound on cognitive functioning by suggesting that working memory is affected by tinnitus (Andersson et al., 2002a). Working memory is the memory system that holds perceptual input while interpretation of it is worked out (Baddeley, 1986). In this context is has been important to investigate the role of background sounds in relation to tinnitus. It is well known that tinnitus often can be covered (masked) by environmental sounds and that it can in some circumstances be totally masked. However, consideration of masking is complicated by the fact that tinnitus does not 'behave' as an acoustic sound and that it might resurface if one attempts to mask it (Penner et al., 1981).

Andersson (2002a) proposed that the 'changing-state' character of the tinnitus signal may increase tinnitus distress. This had been suggested already in the habituation model by Hallam. In brief, experimental literature on the changing-state effect has found that not only speech but also tones that vary in pitch and segmentation disrupt cognitive performance. Although irrelevant sounds can be habituated to, even a brief hiatus has the capacity to restore the disruption (Banbury et al., 2001). Habituation is not likely to occur if the disturbing sound varies in complexity. Even if tinnitus were a stable neural signal (which neuroscience research implies is not the case), it might be a stimulus of changing-state character because of the influence of environmental sounds masking the tinnitus in an unpredictable manner. In a review Banbury et al. (2001) outlined the conditions during which cognition is disrupted by irrelevant sounds. They pointed out that both the properties of the sound and of the cognitive task are crucial. Interestingly, loudness of the disrupting sound is not important (as in tinnitus) and neither is the meaning of the sound (e.g. speech disrupts cognition even when in another language). However, there is one caveat: if the degree of change in the auditory stimulus becomes very marked, the degree of disruption can also diminish. This would account for the clinical observation that tinnitus with large variations in sound quality and presence does not appear to be more annoying than tinnitus that is experienced as stable. The brain-imaging literature on tinnitus suggests that tinnitus in many ways is processed as a complex auditory stimulus, involving the secondary associative auditory cortex and areas related to attention (see Chapter 6). The cognitive disruption might serve as a starting point for later conditioned emotional reactions to tinnitus. It is thought that tinnitus has an interfering effect on cognitive function and that this effect is noted by the person who starts to attend to the tinnitus. Focus on tinnitus leads to less attention to other conflicting sounds (or camouflaging sounds), which might then be perceived as an increase in loudness (or contrast). Fundamental to all such hypotheses is the possibility of emotional responses to tinnitus. This might occur at all points, including when tinnitus first appears, when it is found to disrupt cognitive function and when fluctuations are experienced. Unfortunately, there has not been much research into the possibility that the tinnitus sound itself is generating the distress via cognitive interference. Indeed, it may be that simulated tinnitus is necessary to test the changing state theory.

Moderators and mediators

Andersson and Westin (2008) presented a conceptualisation of tinnitus which involved a distinction between moderators and mediators of distress. A moderator variable is one that influences the strength of a relationship between two other variables (Baron and Kenny, 1986). In their paper they proposed that several variables might act as moderators of tinnitus distress. Degree of hearing loss, arousal, insomnia, characteristics of tinnitus, noise sensitivity, serotonin functioning and a range of psychological factors such as personality and perceived control were discussed as potential moderators. They then moved on to mediator variables. A mediator variable is one that explains the relationship between the two other variables, and must by definition be caused by a predictor, and then mediate between the predictor and the dependent variable. Potential mediators were stress levels (caused by tinnitus), classical conditioning (as in the neurophysiological model),

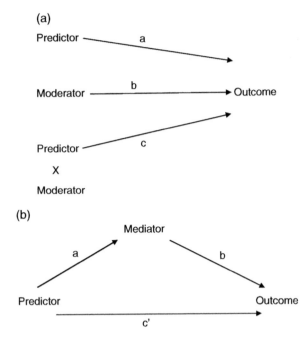

Figure 8.2 (a) Example of a moderator model. In a tinnitus example the predictor could be tinnitus, the outcome tinnitus distress and the moderator the level of hearing loss. (b) Example of a mediator model. In a tinnitus example, with the tinnitus presence as the predictor and tinnitus distress the outcome, attention with negative connotations could act as a mediator.

selective attention towards tinnitus and psychological acceptance of tinnitus (versus experiential avoidance). While the moderator–mediator distinction is not a theory in itself, it can inform our understanding of tinnitus as there has been some confusion regarding what is an effect of tinnitus and what is actually causing tinnitus to become distressing. A graphical presentation of moderator and mediator associations is presented in Figure 8.2.

Summary

Among the psychological theories about tinnitus, Hallam's habituation model remains the most widely known. In this chapter we described behavioural theories, cognitive theories and also commented on the distinction between moderators and mediators of tinnitus distress. Clearly, tinnitus can only be fully understood from a biopsychosocial approach and all theories need to consider biological underpinnings, psychological mechanisms and also the social aspects of tinnitus. Overall, the literature on the psychology of tinnitus is scattered and there is a surprising lack of scientific progress when it comes to theoretical advancements. One example of this is the lack of research on emotion regulation in tinnitus.

Chapter 9

The Jastreboff neurophysiological model

Having reviewed potential physiological mechanisms of tinnitus, Jastreboff (1990) presented a neurophysiological model of tinnitus. This was based on the tenet that, in addition to the classical auditory system pathways, other central neural pathways are involved in the emergence and maintenance of tinnitus. In particular, the limbic system, sympathetic autonomic nervous system and reticular formation are pivotal to the hypothesis. Jastreboff proposed that signal recognition and classification circuits are involved in persistent tinnitus as neural networks that become tuned to the tinnitus signal, even when that signal is of low intensity or intermittent. Peripheral processes might indeed be involved in the generation of tinnitus-related activity, but bearing in mind the findings of Heller and Bergman (1953), it was not necessary for an auditory system dysfunction to be present for tinnitus to be perceived. This Jastreboff 'neurophysiological model' was published in diagrammatic form in 1996 and in slightly more detailed form in 1999 (Figure 9.1).

It was noted that after a short period of awareness of tinnitus-related activity, a process of habituation generally occurs so that the activity is no longer consciously perceived. However, in cases where there is some 'negative emotional reinforcement', described as fear, anxiety or tension, then limbic system and sympathetic autonomic activation cause the activity to be enhanced and perception persists. The distinction between the perception and the behavioural and emotional reaction to tinnitus was implicit, as was the potential for a feedback loop between these processes. The Jastreboff neurophysiological model suggests that, in tinnitus, the links between these elements of the central nervous system are governed by classical conditioning or associative learning (Schwartz et al., 2002). Although not described in detail by Jastreboff, these processes are based on Aristotle's third principle of contiguity. This states that if two or more experiences occur together frequently enough then eventually one occurring on its own will evoke memory of the other(s). The most famous examples of this are Pavlov's experiments (1927), in which a neutral stimulus (a bell ringing) was presented to dogs at the same time as they

Tinnitus: A Multidisciplinary Approach, Second Edition. David Baguley, Gerhard Andersson, Don McFerran and Laurence McKenna.
© 2013 David Baguley, Gerhard Andersson, Don McFerran and Laurence McKenna.
Published 2013 by Blackwell Publishing Ltd.

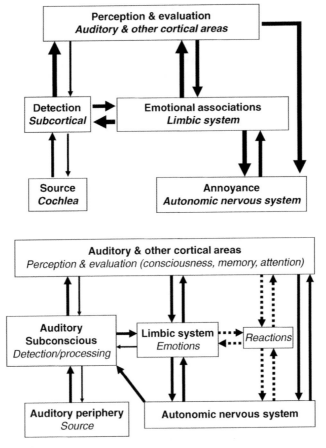

Figure 9.1   Diagrammatic representations of the Jastreboff neurophysiological model of tinnitus. Arrows denote interrelations between different functional areas.

were given another stimulus (food) which naturally produced salivation. After a while the dogs salivated when the bell was rung even if no food was present. The presentation of food was the natural or unconditioned stimulus; the bell ringing was the neutral stimulus or conditioned stimulus; the salivation without the presence of food was the conditioned reflex. Jastreboff (1999) suggested that tinnitus becomes a problem when it becomes associated with negative experiences, though he did not clearly elaborate upon what comprises the unconditioned stimulus, the conditioned stimulus and the conditioned response in that process. Although the negative experience may be a change within the auditory system, it may also be an unrelated stressful event such as bereavement, relationship difficulties or work problems. Indeed, Jastreboff (1999) suggested that in the majority of cases of tinnitus the emergence is not related to auditory system change. Negative information or beliefs about tinnitus can supply negative reinforcement, which, via the limbic system, stimulates the sympathetic arm of the autonomic nervous system, releasing catecholamines and producing a fight or flight response. Because this autonomic response is unpleasant, it in turn acts as further negative reinforcement.

There are several points within the auditory, reactive and emotional systems where feedback can occur. One of the main feedback pathways occurs in the lower part of the model (Figure 9.1) between the auditory subconscious, the limbic system and the autonomic nervous system. This lower loop operates at a pre-conscious level. An upper feedback loop also involves the limbic system and the autonomic nervous system, but in addition incorporates higher cortical centres and hence operates at a conscious level. Jastreboff (1999) suggested that the lower loop is dominant in most people who have severe tinnitus. The neurophysiological model hypothesis also suggests that once the central feedback loops have become established the auditory periphery becomes relatively unimportant. There is evidence to support this as section of the auditory nerve fails to control severe established tinnitus in up to 50% of cases (see Chapter 13).

Jastreboff et al. (1996) used this neurophysiological model to develop a treatment strategy called tinnitus retraining therapy (see Chapter 14), but has subsequently agreed that tinnitus retraining therapy is not the only treatment that is congruent with the neurophysiological model. The model itself has been criticised for being oversimplistic (Andersson, 2002a), but this is perhaps to miss the point: within that simplicity lies the ease of communication to patients and indeed to nonspecialist clinicians.

The assertions made in the Jastreboff neurophysiological model are also not as well supported as sometimes claimed. For example, it is not clear that tinnitus can be likened to a tone to which the patient is classically conditioned. Further, the role of the limbic system in tinnitus distress might seem hard to contest, but imaging research has not been fully consistent with this theory (Chapter 6). Indeed, from a learning psychology point of view, there is much left to explain within the neurophysiological model, such as the temporal properties and actual instances when aversive reactions have become conditioned (McKenna, 2004). Personal attributes such as experience and personality are marginalised in the Jastreboff neurophysiological model, and this does not fit well with observations in the clinic.

Given that tinnitus is not viewed as an unconditioned stimulus for unconditioned aversive reactions (which it might very well be, for example, as a sign of becoming deaf), there is a missing link to explain, namely, how a tone without meaning (i.e. tinnitus) becomes paired with an unconditioned aversive stimulus. Here, the Jastreboff model takes a tautological approach and does not explain *why* tinnitus becomes bothersome. Indeed, it might not be classical conditioning that takes place but rather 'evaluative conditioning' (De Houwer et al., 2001) (see Chapter 8). Evaluative conditioning refers to changes in the liking of a stimulus because the stimulus has been paired with other, positive or negative, stimuli. In evaluative conditioning studies, a neutral stimulus is paired with an affective stimulus and changes in the valence of the neutral stimulus are measured. Interestingly, unlike most forms of Pavlovian conditioning, evaluative conditioning is highly resistant to extinction.

Despite the many criticisms that have been levelled against the Jastreboff neurophysiological model of tinnitus its basic principles are still used by many, perhaps the majority, of tinnitus clinicians worldwide, more than two decades after its publication. It is difficult to overemphasise the improvements in tinnitus management that developed as a result of this work.

Summary

The Jastreboff neurophysiological model of tinnitus undoubtedly represented one of the major turning points in our understanding of tinnitus and helped to provide a useful management strategy. It relegated the cochlea to a minor role in tinnitus distress and gave much greater importance to the role of the brain and autonomic nervous system. It highlighted emotional processing as the major factor in generating tinnitus distress and promoted habituation as the means of reducing that distress. In many respects these are features that are shared by psychological models of tinnitus. The neurophysiological model, however, differed from the psychological models in that it regarded the subconscious processing of auditory information as being more important than conscious evaluation of the symptom in most patients. The treatment strategy that developed from this model, tinnitus retraining therapy, is discussed in Chapter 14.

Chapter 10

How tinnitus is perceived and measured

Attempts to measure tinnitus have a long history (Henry and Meikle, 2000; Tyler, 2000). Perhaps the most influential contribution was by Edmund Prince Fowler in the 1940s (Fowler, 1942), who undertook systematic investigations, but earlier attempts were published (Wegel, 1931; Josephson, 1931). In these two early studies a serious attempt to measure tinnitus was made by means of comparisons with pure tones, a strategy that was later to be used in many studies. However, it was Fowler's work that developed many of the principles that researchers and clinicians still adhere to today. For example, it was Fowler (1942, 1944) who noted the discrepancy between the reported loudness of tinnitus and the loudness measured in the sensation level (SL). This chapter examines the sound quality of tinnitus, how localisation can be assessed, the pitch and loudness of the tinnitus sound, masking level and finally the effects of masking tinnitus. It is not easy to measure tinnitus and there are many reasons why no standard set of tests has been reached for the psycoacoustical description of tinnitus. Tyler (2000) mentioned three sources of difficulty: test–retest variability, the normal fluctuation of the tinnitus in many patients and changes in the tinnitus produced by the measurement stimulus in some patients. In addition, some patients do not have one, but several, tinnitus sounds and these sounds may have different temporal and loudness characteristics.

Sound quality

In order to know how tinnitus is perceived it is important to ask the patient, since no objective way to measure this aspect of tinnitus exists. Some tinnitus patients have tinnitus that is difficult to describe in words, but it is important to try and understand the patient's tinnitus experience by careful history taking. The audiometer can be used to try and match the patient's tinnitus. Unfortunately, this is not an easy task, and almost always fails because the sound produced by the audiometer rarely sounds the same as the tinnitus: the tinnitus sound is often too complicated to be replicated by an audiometer. Mitchell et al. (1984) and

Tinnitus: A Multidisciplinary Approach, Second Edition. David Baguley, Gerhard Andersson, Don McFerran and Laurence McKenna.
© 2013 David Baguley, Gerhard Andersson, Don McFerran and Laurence McKenna.
Published 2013 by Blackwell Publishing Ltd.

Penner (1993) studied whether the tinnitus sound could be simulated using a synthesiser, but, even with this sophisticated technology, failed to solve the problem. However, interestingly, Penner (1996) found that there was no real difference between how tinnitus patients and people without tinnitus rated a set of 'tinnitus sounds' in terms of annoyance. These tinnitus sounds had been derived from computer simulation. One conclusion from the study was that tinnitus sounds are perceived as annoying by most people. In a study reported by Wahlström and Axelsson (1996), 50 normal hearing subjects from an audiology department were asked to describe a set of sounds (pure tones at 250 Hz, 4 kHz and 8 kHz) that were presented via an audiometer at a comfortable sound level for 5 seconds. The same stimulus material was presented to 50 tinnitus patients. Results showed that tinnitus patients perceived the tones as less clear, compared with the normal hearing subjects.

Despite the difficulties in generating tinnitus sounds that exactly match the sensation of tinnitus, there are several reports of how the sounds are described from the patients' own words. Stouffer and Tyler (1990) studied over 500 tinnitus patients and found that the most common description was ringing (37%), in second place came whirling (11%), third crickets (9%) and fourth hissing (8%). The remaining descriptions included a large range of different sounds. In a study of 1800 tinnitus patients, Meikle and Taylor–Walsh (1984) found that 30% of their patients described their tinnitus as ringing. This is a common observation both in clinical practice and in research, with the addition that patients often report a combination of sounds that can sound very different and distinct: for example, a buzzing sound in one ear and a tone in the other ear. In some research there is a brief characterisation of tinnitus as either tonal, buzzing or a combination of the two. Douek (1981) proposed that tinnitus could be categorised from the patients own description into (a) low tones, (b) high whistles, (c) humming machines, (d) multiple sounds and (e) complex sounds.

Tinnitus patients describe their tinnitus in many diverse ways. Sometimes the patient will find a metaphor for the sound. It is useful for the clinician to ask the patient if the tinnitus sounds like anything they have heard previously. Some examples written by patients from the Tinnitus Clinic in Uppsala, Sweden, are listed in Table 10.1.

Table 10.1   Examples of descriptions of tinnitus sounds by patients (Andersson, 2000b).

- A soft ringing sound
- Like crickets playing (sometimes over 100)
- Metallic sound, like from a decoration from a Christmas tree plus some other sounds
- Tonal buzzing or 'fluorescent tube'
- A high tone with wind in the background
- Buzzing, like someone flushing water
- A loud cutting tone surrounded by buzzing in colour
- Scream
- Rushing
- Loud bagpipe
- A high-pitched tone heard all the time
- Just as when the television broadcasting ends (buzzing sound)
- Buzzing
- Like a signal and scream; persistent most of the time, but sometimes pulsating and jumpy during movement
- Buzzing, like a midge or mosquito

Clearly there are many commonly used metaphors for tinnitus, but it is usually the case that tinnitus is not described as something dramatic and interesting. More commonly, mechanical and rather boring sounds are likened to tinnitus. In fact, often the patient can only come up with 'ringing sound' as a metaphor for tinnitus. Surprisingly, little systematic research has been devoted to the perception of the tinnitus sound. None of the commonly used tinnitus questionnaires address the different aspects of the perceived sound quality of the tinnitus. This is definitely an area that deserves further research as there are useful clinical implications for some patients. In some cases, a more meaningful metaphor for tinnitus (e.g. diamond drill with a craftsman sitting in a room working) can be used as a way of helping to attain habituation.

Pitch

Pitch matching is undertaken with the objective of trying to generate a sound that matches the tinnitus pitch that later can be used to estimate tinnitus loudness. This is only relevant in tonal tinnitus and this may not be the most common experience of tinnitus. Descriptions dating back to the 1930s have described ways to do this (Wegel, 1931; Josephson, 1931) and further studies have been published subsequently (Henry and Meikle, 2000; Tyler and Stouffer, 1989). Measuring tinnitus pitch is somewhat arduous both for the clinician and the patient, and Vernon (1987a) notes that many patients have 'octave confusion', by which he means that the selected pitch turns out to be an octave above or below the tinnitus pitch. Moore (2012) indicated that this octave confusion can be minimised by training patients to make pitch matches. Tinnitus may not be easy to match to a single tone, but according to Tyler and Babin (1993) most patients can at least compare their tinnitus with a tone or a tone that is part of the whole tinnitus perception.

Using synthesisers to find a tinnitus tone closer to the tinnitus may not be practical in clinical settings. However, it is possible that computerised assessment of tinnitus (pitch and loudness) will facilitate this (Henry et al., 1999, 2006a; Mitchell et al., 1984). There are two approaches in use at the time of writing, the first being an automated software program developed by Dr James Henry within the USA Veterans Administration. This approach releases the audiologist from a tedious task, but it remains arduous for the patient. The software is reported to assess test–retest variability in real-time and so allows the clinician to assess the reliability of the data. Another approach is taken by Dr Larry Roberts of McMaster University in Canada, who has developed subject-driven computer tools to assess the psychoacoustic characteristics of the tinnitus (e.g. pitch, spectrum, loudness) and residual inhibition. These tools are being commercialised. Thus, in addition to clinician administered tinnitus matching, there could be a role for self-generated matching. However, most clinics have access to nothing more sophisticated than a traditional audiometer – this can still supply useful information. Summarising data from several studies it is common to match tinnitus to a tone at 4000 Hz. The majority of patients describe a pitch that exceeds 3000 Hz. For many patients tinnitus pitch corresponds to the start of the measured hearing loss on their audiogram. This is of theoretical importance given the discordant damage hypothesis put forward by Jastreboff (1990). A study by Sereda et al. (2011), however, investigated 67 people with chronic bilateral tinnitus and did not find any relationship between the tinnitus pitch and the edge frequency. The tinnitus pitch generally fell within the area of hearing loss. In a subset of subjects with a narrow tinnitus bandwidth, pitch was associated with the audiometric edge. On the other hand, Moore and Vinay (2010) trained their subjects to provide more accurate pitch matches. After the training, pitch matchings were generally lower and there was a strong correlation between matchings and edge frequency of the audiogram. Overall, the literature is not consistent, with some studies finding an association between pitch and edge frequency and others not (e.g. Pan et al., 2009).

Obtaining measures of pitch can be done in different ways. Tyler and Conrad-Armes (1983a) compared three ways of assessing pitch and came to the conclusion that it was best to measure pitch from the ear with tinnitus. Others, however, have instead recommended that the contralateral ear should be used for pitch estimates (Henry and Meikle, 2000). In most cases it does not appear to be of major importance if the tinnitus ear or the contralateral ear is used. The process becomes more complicated with bilateral asymmetrical tinnitus. However, there is a consensus that one ear at a time should be tested rather than presenting simultaneous binaural stimuli.

The diagnostic value of tinnitus pitch has been discussed (Douek and Reid, 1968; Tyler and Conrad-Armes, 1983a). For example, in noise-induced hearing loss tinnitus is often high-pitched (Henry and Meikle, 2000) and in the early stages of Ménière's disease tinnitus is reportedly low-pitched (Douek and Reid, 1968; Vernon and Johnson, 1980). However, to use tinnitus pitch as a diagnostic tool is of questionable value. From a diagnostic point of view it is also important to look at test–retest reliability of pitch estimates, and in this respect the results are far from encouraging (Henry et al., 1999).

Loudness

Many patients want to get some kind of estimate of the loudness of their tinnitus, which they can use to inform other people of their condition. However, an early observation by Fowler (1942) was the lack of correspondence between the patient's view and the obtained loudness estimates. Loudness of tinnitus can be measured in many ways, but most commonly the patient is instructed to say when a tone or a broadband noise reaches the same level as the tinnitus – typically a tone at 1000 Hz is used (Vernon, 1987a) or some other frequency where hearing is normal, though the matching frequency may also be used.

One early research finding was that tinnitus, for most patients, matches to sound of low intensities relative to the threshold of hearing (Fowler, 1942; Reed, 1960; Tyler and Stouffer, 1989). In practical terms, if tinnitus is matched to a tone of 40 dB hearing level (HL) and the patient has a hearing threshold of 35 dB HL for that frequency, the level of tinnitus in terms of sensation level (SL) becomes only 5 dB (40 minus 35 dB), which corresponds to a very low intensity sound. However, describing tinnitus in terms of sensation level may be inappropriate (Penner and Klafter, 1992), as it is grounded in the concept that tinnitus is just like any other sound or tone. Andersson (2003) reviewed the literature on the differences between expressing tinnitus loudness in HL versus SL and found that the association with annoyance was stronger for HL. Hence, one alternative would be to describe tinnitus in dB HL. However, this inevitably makes the level of hearing loss part of the definition of loudness and it is known from epidemiological studies that hearing impairment is significantly associated with both the presence and annoyance of tinnitus. One alternative is to match tinnitus against a tone for which the patient has normal hearing (Penner, 1986; Goodwin and Johnson, 1980b), which may result in a more reliable estimate of loudness (Risey et al., 1989).

From a clinical point of view it is often unhelpful to talk about tinnitus in terms of SL as it implies that the patient is imagining that the tinnitus is loud when it is really not. The title of one of Fowler's papers 'The "illusion of loudness" of tinnitus', clearly suggests this (Fowler, 1942). Largely because of these practical and theoretical objections, loudness estimates have gone out of fashion in the management of tinnitus.

There are alternative and more complex ways of measuring tinnitus loudness (Hinchcliffe and Chambers, 1983; Matsuhira et al., 1992; Ward and Baumann, 2009), for example, by considering the effect of recruitment (nonlinear loudness growth). Tyler and Conrad-Armes (1983b) derived a formula for calculating tinnitus loudness correcting for recruitment, which indicates the loudness in sones (a psychoacoustical measure of loudness growth in an individual) (Tyler, 2000). Later research has tended to ignore recruitment as a possible reason for the discrepancy between measured loudness and the experienced annoyance. Even if these alternative ways of getting loudness estimates have their advantages, they are rarely used in clinical practice because of time constraints and lack of clinical relevance. Another alternative is to use self-reported loudness (Hiller and Goebel, 2007), but that approach is close to self-reported annoyance and probably not a true representation of how loud tinnitus is when measured using audiometric procedures.

Estimates of the loudness of tinnitus can vary when subjects are retested (Burns, 1984; Penner, 1983b), in a similar way to measurements of tinnitus pitch, and as with pitch computer-based testing may improve that, though this variability reflects an inherently poor test–retest reliability or may show that the tinnitus actually changes. Changes in loudness often occur within short time periods and these variations may be a contributing factor to the tinnitus distress experienced by the patient. Tinnitus seems more problematic if the patient cannot predict or control the loudness.

Another perspective upon the discrepancy between the descriptions by patients of their experiences of intense tinnitus and the low-level intensity match data has been provided by Cope et al. (2011). Using a group of patients with tinnitus in a deaf ear following translabyrinthine surgery for the removal of a vestibular schwannoma (VS) and a control group of general tinnitus patients, they conducted two experiments. The first calculated the matched intensity of tinnitus in sones and in phons. Sones are the standard unit of loudness in psychoacoustics, where 1 sone is equivalent to the perceived loudness of a 40 dB SPL 1000 Hz tone to a normal hearing listener. To that person a 50 dB SPL tone is twice as loud and is 2 sones. The phon is a measure of loudness level, where that level is the level (in dB SPL) of a 1000 Hz tone that is equal in loudness (for a normal hearing person) to a specific sound of interest. For the general tinnitus group, the mean matched intensity was 30.2 dB SL (standard deviation 22 dB) and when converted ranged between 20 and 50 phons (equivalent to 0.14–2 sones). For the VS tinnitus group, the mean matched intensity was 30.0 dB SL (standard deviation 22 dB) and when converted ranged between 6 and 51 phons (equivalent to 0.012–2.25 sones). Measures were repeated in threshold equalising noise (TEN) – wideband noise spectrally shaped so that for normal hearing persons it leads to an equal masked threshold for tone across a wide range of frequencies, which is used in testing of cochlear dead regions. For the general tinnitus group matching tinnitus in TEN made minimal difference to matched intensity, whereas for the VS group a significant increase in match intensity was demonstrated. This study indicates that tinnitus can be matched to a signal of moderate intensity and that the complaint of post-surgery VS patients that background noise increases the perceived intensity of their tinnitus is borne out.

It is hard to ignore the fact that one of the most important measures of tinnitus – the perceived intensity – is afflicted with a host of problems. The notion that tinnitus in most cases is a low-intensity sound is problematic as current psychoacoustical measures do not mirror how the brain handles tinnitus (e.g. the cortical representation).

Maskability

Another perspective upon the intrusiveness of tinnitus is to measure the minimal masking level, in other words the level of sound required for the tinnitus to disappear from awareness. Anecdotally, masking was discovered by Vernon in the early 1970s (Vernon, 1998), but the knowledge that external sound can mask tinnitus has probably been around for as long as there have been humans with tinnitus (see Chapter 1). Overall, the phenomena of masking has been researched extensively (Henry and Meikle, 2000), with various approaches and interesting findings revealing that tinnitus does not behave in the same way as 'natural' sounds (e.g. tones) in terms of masking characteristics.

The frequency relationship of tinnitus masking using tones was investigated in early work by Feldmann (1971). He tested 200 tinnitus patients and investigated how tones with increasing frequencies masked tinnitus and by doing this generated tinnitus masking curves. Feldmann found evidence for different types of masking curve. For the first type of masking curve entitled 'convergent', the threshold curve and the masking curve converge from low to high frequencies (see Figure 10.1). Once the tinnitus pitch is reached the curves converge and follow each other afterwards. From Feldmann's data 34% of patients show this pattern, which was said to be typical of noise-induced hearing loss. The second type, said to be very rare (3%), show the opposite pattern, entitled 'divergent', as threshold and masking curves diverge from low to high frequencies. The third type, called the 'congruence' type, was found to be common (32%) and was characterised by the fact that any tone or narrowband noise, raised above threshold, will mask the tinnitus. The fourth type, 'distance', was seen in 20% and is what many people would expect from annoying tinnitus, that is the threshold curve and masking curve are distant from each other. The fifth type is the 'resistance' type, when tinnitus is not masked by any kind of sound. In Feldmann's material as many as 11% showed this pattern. These findings and other studies (Penner, 1987; Tyler and Conrad-Armes, 1984) show that tinnitus is not masked as an ordinary tone and Henry and Meikle (2000, p. 149) concluded, 'tinnitus masking appears to be categorically different from the conventional masking of one external tone by another'.

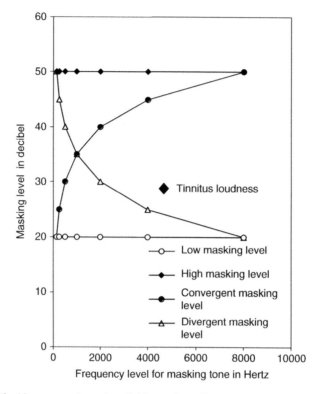

Figure 10.1   Masking curves based on Feldmann's work.

White noise or pink noise can be utilised to mask tinnitus. The question of using broadband versus narrowband noise as masking for tinnitus has been widely debated. One study by Shailer et al. (1981) found that some patients could benefit from a narrowband noise as a lower level of sound was needed to mask the tinnitus. The authors concluded that different patients might prefer different characteristics of the masking sound. Smith et al. (1991) tested this notion and asked 10 experienced tinnitus patients to test and later choose which bandwidth of masking they preferred. The authors found no convincing evidence that a certain masking sound would be preferred, but interestingly a majority of patients chose a masking sound that only partially masked their tinnitus. One potential explanation, which corresponds with reports from patients, is that a lower masking sound makes it easier to attend to environmental sound such as conversation, especially if the individual concerned has any degree of hearing loss.

An important observation by Tyler (1987) is that for many patients the laterality of the masking sound makes no difference. Even if tinnitus is perceived predominantly in the right ear, it can still be masked by a sound in the left ear. This observation suggests that tinnitus is masked at a higher level of the brain and not at the level of hair cells. This is not a new idea: Minton (1923, p. 509) suggested that tinnitus masking probably was 'a property of the auditory nerves or even of the acoustic centres of the brain itself'.

Another interesting issue regarding minimal masking level is that it has been found to respond to treatment (Jastreboff et al., 1994) and to predict long-term outcome (Andersson et al., 2001).

Effects of masking

One remarkable finding in the tinnitus literature is the fact that, for some individuals, tinnitus can disappear for a short period following masking. This phenomenon is called 'residual inhibition' and was noted by Feldmann (1971), and has since been much explored by Vernon and co-workers (Vernon and Meikle, 2000). The discovery raised much hope for a cure, but the effect is most often short lived, often just a few minutes (Terry et al., 1983), and the effect is not seen in all patients. In fact, residual inhibition is just one of several possible outcomes after masking. For example, Tyler (1987) found that, for some tinnitus patients, tinnitus instead becomes stronger after termination of masking.

An interesting finding was reported by Penner et al. (1981) who found that the minimal masking level for tinnitus was raised over repeat test conditions. In a later investigation Penner further found that increased masking level was associated with increased annoyance (Penner, 1983a). Two explanations for this phenomenon have been considered by Penner. The first is that the masking sound temporarily worsens tinnitus, thus rendering it more noticeable. The second explanation is that auditory adaptation to the masking sound occurs without any corresponding adaptation to the tinnitus sound (Penner and Bilger, 1988). Masking as a treatment tool is discussed in Chapter 11, though modern methods of tinnitus management suggest that total masking of tinnitus is unhelpful when habituation is the goal.

All of the above measurements of tinnitus have demonstrated poor test–retest reliability, but even this is not a constant observation. Some researchers have reported large variability of tinnitus measurements (Burns, 1984) and Penner (1986) suggested that the reliability of tinnitus measurements was poor because tinnitus seemed to behave as a fluctuating external stimuli. However, in other studies reliability has been more satisfactory (Mitchell et al., 1993; Nageris et al., 2010).

Summary

The perceived sound quality of tinnitus is very varied but still gives important clinical information for further counselling. Generating data on tinnitus pitch is notoriously difficult and in practical terms is often restricted to those patients who have tonal tinnitus. When pitch matching is possible, most patients have a pitch that exceeds 3000 Hz. Measurement of tinnitus loudness is also somewhat fraught and there is still considerable debate about the implications of the results of such measurements. In particular there is poor correlation between the tinnitus sensation level (SL) and annoyance. Masking of tinnitus has been studied in many ways and historically has been one of the most influential management options. Overall the measurement of tinnitus is still far from satisfactory and, in particular, the psycholological aspects of tinnitus loudness, pitch and masking have yet to be explored. There has been little progress in this area since the first edition of this book.

Chapter 11

Self-report and interview measures of tinnitus severity and impact

As stated previously, there are no objective ways to determine the severity of tinnitus. While there are indeed associations between degree of hearing loss and tinnitus annoyance, audiometric data provide little information about tinnitus distress in the individual case. In many ways, what distinguishes mild from severe tinnitus is difficult to establish, apart from variations in subjective ratings of intrusiveness and loudness. Moreover, attempts to determine the handicap caused by tinnitus using the characteristics of the tinnitus itself, such as loudness, pitch and character, have not proved particularly helpful to date. Therefore, it is necessary to carefully interview the patient to get an idea of the level of distress associated with tinnitus. This is crucial as psychological complaints are of major importance in determining the severity of tinnitus.

In line with the difficulties associated with measuring tinnitus (Chapter 10), no consensus has been reached regarding its classification, although several schemes have been proposed (e.g. Nodar, 1996; Douek, 1981; Holgers et al., 2000), which have included guidelines on how to measure severity. In addition there have been several alternative suggestions in terms of cutoff scores on questionnaire measures (e.g. McCombe et al., 2001), but it is fair to say at the outset of this chapter that there is no consensus on how severity of tinnitus should best be assessed.

Dauman and Tyler (1992) proposed a system involving several classifications (see Table 11.1 adapted from Davis and El Rafaie, 2000). They distinguished between normal and pathological tinnitus, the former being a sensation experienced sometimes by most people (Heller and Bergman, 1953) and the latter being defined by its prolonged nature (more than five minutes every week) and its association with hearing loss. They classified tinnitus regarding its severity, duration, site of origin and aetiology. Of particular interest is the classification of tinnitus severity into acceptable and unacceptable. However, exactly how unacceptable tinnitus was defined was not described, although this was probably intended to be based on an interview with the patient.

Tinnitus: A Multidisciplinary Approach, Second Edition. David Baguley, Gerhard Andersson, Don McFerran and Laurence McKenna.

Table 11.1   Dauman and Tyler's (1992) classification system of tinnitus.

Pathology	Severity	Duration	Site	Aetiology
• Normal • Pathological	• Acceptable • Unacceptable	• Temporary • Permanent	• Middle ear • Peripheral neural • Central neural	• Noise-induced • Ménière's disease • Ototoxicity • Presbyacusis • Unknown aetiology

Table 11.2   Klockhoff and Lindblom (1967) and Scott et al. (1990).

Grade I stands for when tinnitus is audible only in silent environments.
Grade II is when tinnitus is audible only in ordinary acoustic environments, but masked by loud environmental sounds; it can disturb going to sleep, but not sleep in general.
Grade III is when tinnitus is audible in all acoustic environments, disturbs going to sleep, can disturb sleep in general and is a dominating problem that affects quality of life.

Klockhoff and Lindblom (1967) devised a system for determination of tinnitus severity and distress that has been used in Sweden following slight modification by Scott et al. (1990). The grading system is presented in Table 11.2 and can be regarded as a mixture of the perceptual and experiential aspects of tinnitus. Andersson et al. (1999) reported data from a study in which a subsample of 39 patients for whom tinnitus grading had been assessed both by a clinical psychologist and an ENT physician. A significant correlation was found between the two forms of assessment ($\rho = 0.80$, $p = 0.0001$). Further, similar proportions of patients were assessed as grades I (5.1%), II (64.1%) and III (30.8%) by the physician when comparing the rating conducted by the clinical psychologist (4.2%, 57.5% and 38.3%, respectively). A set of discriminant analyses was conducted on the data set to investigate variables discriminating between tinnitus of grades II–III. This resulted in a final model that included pitch, minimal masking level (MML), tolerance in relation to onset and avoidance of situations because of tinnitus. This model correctly classified 73% of the subjects into the two levels of distress (grades II and III).

In comparison, the Dauman and Tyler (1992) system is more comprehensive, but the Klockhoff and Lindblom (1967) system does have the advantage of providing a single global rating of the severity of tinnitus and is used as such in current clinical practice. The grading system has been used in research studies and a common observation is that among patients seeking help for hearing loss (with co-morbid tinnitus) and in patients operated on for vestibular schwannoma relatively few have grade III tinnitus (6–14%) (Lindberg et al., 1984; Andersson et al., 1997). Lindberg et al. (1984) reported that 35% of their tinnitus sample of hearing aid centre clients had tinnitus of grade I and 51% had grade II. Tinnitus of grade III appears to be rare in the general population, but the relative prevalence of tinnitus of grades I and II is not known.

Table 11.3 Summary of the questions asked in a structured tinnitus interview.

1. Background data (age, etc.)
2. Hearing loss and use of hearing aid (including effects on tinnitus)
3. Tinnitus localisation
4. Tinnitus primary character including descriptors of tinnitus
5. Duration of tinnitus
6. Event(s) associated with onset of tinnitus (e.g. trauma)
7. Tinnitus grading (Klockhoff and Lindblom, 1967) (see above)
8. Variation in tinnitus loudness
9. Attention directed towards tinnitus during an ordinary day
10. Most problematic situations associated with tinnitus
11. Time of the day most problematic
12. Possibility to do something to lessen the problems with tinnitus
13. Possibility to change the loudness of tinnitus
14. Situations when tinnitus is less problematic
15. Avoidance of situations and activities because of tinnitus
16. Psychological consequences of tinnitus including irritation, depression, anxiety and concentration difficulties
17. Sleep problems (hours of sleep per night, sleep onset latency, awakenings during the night, time awake in the morning)
18. Influence of background sounds or noises on tinnitus
19. Masking of tinnitus by background sounds
20. Noise sensitivity including hyperacusis
21. Influence of stress and fatigue
22. Influence of weather
23. Medication or other causes than tinnitus and and their effects on tinnitus
24. Use of caffeine and its effects on tinnitus
25. Alcohol use and effects on tinnitus
26. Tobacco use (cigarette and snuff) and effects on tinnitus
27. Role of relatives/spouse when coping with tinnitus
28. Major or minor change of tinnitus characteristics since onset
29. Tolerance of tinnitus in relation to onset (e.g. much better or much worse)
30. Earlier or ongoing treatments for tinnitus and hearing loss (including counselling)
31. Perceived cause of tinnitus
32. Problems with headache
33. Dizziness or unsteadiness
34. Muscular tension (in face, jaws or shoulders)
35. Earlier or ongoing psychiatric consultations/treatments
36. Attitude towards tinnitus
37. Attitude towards referral to psychologist
38. Presentation of a cognitive–behavioural model of tinnitus annoyance and check for acceptance of the model and the approach to treatment (including time investment, not a cure, etc.)

Table based on Andersson (2001).

Structured interviews

There are few reports on the use of structured interviews with tinnitus patients. Most clinicians follow an interview protocol that gives a framework of topics to discuss at the first consultation but few have evaluated if the questions used are appropriate. Lindberg and Scott developed a structured interview, which was later revised (Andersson et al., 1999). The interview is conducted following audiological and medical examination. The questions are summarised in Table 11.3. Other researchers have developed similar approaches (Hiller and Goebel, 1999) and there is also an interview that has been developed for use in tinnitus retraining therapy (Henry et al., 2002c). Structured interviews need to be complemented with questionnaire data and are best regarded in relation to findings from audiological tests.

Tinnitus self-report measures

Self-report measures are increasingly used in both the management of tinnitus patients and in tinnitus research (Meikle et al., 2008). With the advent of evidence-based medicine, the use of clear and robust outcome measures is of great importance. In particular, controversies about the efficacies of treatment methods will not be resolved until those efficacies can be determined in a manner that allows direct comparison.

Visual analogue scales

Daily diaries provide an indispensable tool both in research and in practice. It is common for tinnitus to fluctuate, and on occasions patients have difficulty identifying reasons for such fluctuations. Diaries can supply the answer in many cases. Daily diaries need to be easily comprehended and unobtrusive while still providing usable data. One alternative, which is commonly used in pain management, is the Visual Analogue Scale (VAS). This is simply a straight line, the end anchors of which are labelled as the extreme boundaries of the sensation, feeling or response being measured (Wewers and Love, 1990). Sometimes ratings on VASs are collected on single occasions and not for a series of days (or hours). It is important to note that one single rating on a VAS is not very reliable and the strength of the method lies in the aggregation of several measurements (e.g. weekly average of tinnitus annoyance). While VASs have been recommended for use in tinnitus research (Axelsson et al., 1993), it is not clear how commonly they are used in clinical practice. An example of VAS is given in Figure 11.1.

A more recent way to obtain daily ratings and to capture the fluctuations in tinnitus loudness and distress was presented by Henry et al. (2012). The method is known as ecological momentary assessment and involves the real-time measurement of states, situational factors and symptoms by individuals as they go about their day-to-day activities. Henry et al. used a personal digital assistant that sent reminders to participants to complete a questionnaire dealing with tinnitus. In their sample of 24 participants they found high compliance and at most sampling points participants could hear their tinnitus. With the spread of smart phones, mobile phone data collection in ecologically valid settings will be facilitated, even if it is still uncertain whether the method will be useful for more than research purposes.

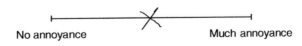

No annoyance   Much annoyance

Figure 11.1   Visual analogue scale.

Tinnitus-specific questionnaires

For clinical use a questionnaire must be brief and easy to interpret. It should also be appropriate and understandable to the patient and the results should be easy to feed back in the consulting room. It should be reliable, in that it should measure what it purports to measure (construct validity), should be in broad agreement with other measures of the same or very similar situations (convergent validity) and give the same result when applied repeatedly (test–retest validity). Further, it should be sensitive to the effects of treatment and to reliably report outcomes.

There are several instruments available, and although a comparative assessment is difficult many of the items included in the questionnaires are often rather similar (for reviews see Tyler, 1993; Noble, 2000; Meikle et al., 2007, 2008). Examples of items included in two common questionnaires are given in Table 11.4.

Similar factors tend to become evident on conducting factor analyses, reflecting the fact that a substantial overlap exists in questionnaire wording of items and content. A list of questionnaires is presented in Table 11.5.

One of the first questionnaires developed specifically for the assessment of tinnitus complaints was the Tinnitus Questionnaire (Hallam, 1996b), which exists in several versions. The questionnaire was first called the Tinnitus Effects Questionnaire, but was later shortened to Tinnitus Questionnaire. The full Tinnitus Questionnaire contains 52 items and covers sleep, emotional disturbances, audiological/perceptual difficulties and intrusiveness. In a factor analysis of an earlier 40-item version, Hallam et al. (1988) extracted three factors: sleep disturbance, emotional disturbances and audiological/perceptual disturbances. Hiller and Goebel (1992) factor-analysed the 52 item version and found a five-factor solution. In addition to Hallam's factors they added a factor called intrusiveness and one entitled somatic complaints. The intrusiveness factor was also noted in an earlier study by Jakes et al. (1985). There is also a briefer 33-item version of the TQ, for which Hallam (1989) proposed six factors: helplessness, capacity for rest and relaxation, acceptability of change, emotional effects and related beliefs, hearing speech and sounds, and the ability to ignore. This ordering of items into subscales was not, however, derived from empirical analysis. An even shorter version of the TQ (12 items) has been

Table 11.4 Examples of items in the Tinnitus Reaction Questionnaire and the Tinnitus Handicap Inventory.

Tinnitus Reaction Questionnaire (Wilson et al., 1991)
  My tinnitus has made me unhappy.
  My tinnitus has 'driven me crazy'.
  My tinnitus has lead me to avoid noisy situations.
  My tinnitus has interfered with my ability to work.

Tinnitus Handicap Inventory (Newman et al., 1996)
  Because of your tinnitus is it difficult for you to concentrate.
  Do you complain a great deal about your tinnitus?
  Do you feel that you have no control over your tinnitus?
  Does your tinnitus make you feel insecure?

Table 11.5   Overview of a selection of tinnitus self-report inventories.

Title	Number of items and factors	Psychometrics
Tinnitus Questionnaire (Hallam, 1996b)	52 items, 5 factors	$a = 0.91$ for total scale, for subscales $a = 0.76$ to $a = 0.94$
Mini TQ (Hiller and Goebel, 2004)	12 items	>90% correlation with TQ Test–retest $= 0.89$
Tinnitus Handicap Questionnaire (Kuk et al., 1990)	27 items, 3 factors	$a = 0.93$ for total scale
Tinnitus Severity Scale (Sweetow and Levy, 1990)	15 items	α not reported
Tinnitus Reaction Questionnaire (Wilson et al., 1991)	26 items, 4 factors	$a = 0.96$ and a test–retest correlation of $r = 0.88$
Subjective Tinnitus Severity Scale (Halford and Anderson, 1991a)	16 items	$a = 0.84$
Tinnitus Handicap/Support Scale (Erlandsson et al., 1992)	28 items, 3 factors	α not reported
Tinnitus Handicap Inventory (Newman et al., 1996)	25 items, 3 scales	$a = 0.93$ for total scale
THI-S (Newman et al., 2008)	12 items	Correlation with THI $= 0.9$, test–retest of 0.81
Tinnitus Functional Index (Meikle et al., 2012)	25 items, 8 factor solution	$a = 0.97$ test–retest $= 0.78$

developed (Hiller and Goebel, 2004) and is used internationally. Official translations of the mini TQ are available at www.eutinnitus.com/country-selection.php.

The Tinnitus Reaction Questionnaire (TRQ) was developed by Wilson and co-workers (1991) and has been used in several research studies and in different languages (e.g. English, German, French and Swedish). It has also been validated for Internet use (Andersson et al., 2003b). The TRQ was designed specifically to measure distress – such as tension, depression and anger – that may be related to tinnitus. The TRQ has repeatedly been found to generate good psychometric properties. A principal components analysis suggested four factors, which they labelled 'general distress', 'interference', 'severity' and 'avoidance'. Meric et al. (2000) refrained from factor analysing the French version, assuming a priori the factorial structure to be extant. However, given the high internal consistency found and on the basis of factor analyses of the Swedish version of the TRQ, it is very likely that the scale just contains one reliable factor from a statistical point of view. In other words, there is a substantial overlap in how patients respond to the items in the TRQ.

The Tinnitus Handicap Questionnaire was developed by Kuk et al. (1990), informed by their previous research on open-ended questions (see below). The questionnaire was properly analysed by means of principal components factor analysis, which resulted in three factors, with the first two being particularly noteworthy. The first reflected physical, emotional and social consequences of tinnitus and the second factor reflected hearing. The last factor was seen as mirroring the patients' views on tinnitus. Together they explained 57.6% of the variance, but as has been seen in subsequent factor analyses of other tinnitus questionnaires, the first factor explained the majority of the variance (42.6%). This suggests that a basic overarching annoyance factor is involved. This questionnaire has not been widely used in research, but was recently validated for a French population (Bouscau-Faure et al., 2003). However, Goebel and Hiller (1999) raised some concerns over test construction and composition of the scales.

The Tinnitus Severity Scale (Sweetow and Levy, 1990) is a small scale with 15 items, but was developed with the aim of covering several aspects with few items. Brevity is often advantageous in clinical settings, rendering this scale attractive in some settings. However, the published report did not include enough information to assess the suitability of the scale from a psychometric point of view.

Another questionnaire, the Subjective Tinnitus Severity Scale (Halford and Anderson, 1991a) was developed with items again reflecting the annoyance/intrusion dimension of tinnitus. In another report (Halford and Anderson, 1991b), the authors found the scale correlated with measures of anxiety and depression, a common finding in the literature.

A Swedish research group developed a Tinnitus Handicap/Support Scale (Erlandsson et al. 1992). This scale includes several important dimensions, such as social support, and seems to posses adequate psychometric properties. Unfortunately, this scale has not been translated into any other language.

The Tinnitus Handicap Inventory (THI) (Newman et al., 1996) is the most widely used scale internationally in the clinical context to assess tinnitus related self-reported handicap and to report treatment outcomes (Newman et al., 1998; McCombe et al., 2001; Rosenberg et al., 1998). Moreover, high convergent validity with other measures of tinnitus distress, specifically with the Tinnitus Questionnaire (Hallam, 1996b), have been reported (Baguley et al., 2000). The THI has been translated into Danish (Zachariae et al., 2000), Spanish (Herraiz et al., 2001), German (Kleinjung et al., 2007), Swedish (Kaldo et al., 2007), Brazilian Portuguese (Schmidt et al., 2006), Turkish (Aksoy et al., 2007b, no. 5616), Italian (Monzani et al., 2008), Chinese (Cantonese) (Kam et al., 2009), French (Ghulyan-Bedikian et al., 2010), Greek (Korres et al., 2010) and Hebrew (Oron et al., 2011). Newman et al. (1996), in the original presentation of the THI, suggested a three-component model for the THI, naming the factors Emotional, Functional and Catastrophic. However, the factor structure of the scale was not initially reported. Factor analysis of the subscales of the THI has later been reported for the Danish translation (Zachariae et al., 2000). In this study an exploratory factor analysis (incorrectly presented as a confirmatory factor analysis) demonstrated that a three-factor solution could be derived, but the factors were not identical to the ones suggested a priori by Newman et al. (1996). In a factor analysis the THI was found to contain only one factor and not the three suggested in the original paper (Baguley and Andersson, 2003). Zeman et al. (2011) considered what change in THI score could be considered clinically relevant. Change in the THI score was compared with clinician ratings of clinical improvement (utilising a Clinical Global Impression-Improvement score). This analysis indicated that the minimal clinically relevant change in the THI score was 7 points. This may better reflect the modest clinician expectations of the outcome of tinnitus therapy rather than a change that a patient would consider clinically relevant. The THI is now available in a screening form (THI-S; see Newman et al., 2008) with 12 items and a robust correlation with the original version ($r = 0.90$), but it does not claim to be sensitive to outcomes.

In an attempt to build upon the best of the existing questionnaires, Dr Mary Meikle drew together a group of experts to construct a new questionnaire: the Tinnitus Functional Index (Meikle et al., 2011). After many iterations the final version has 25 items and robust psychometric validity data. It is thought to be sensitive to outcomes and has a preliminary 13-point change criterion for clinically significant change. The TFI should be borne in mind when designing research studies and it may become a widely used tool for tinnitus assessment.

A number of targeted tinnitus questionnaires have been developed. For example, an Australian research group have devised a Tinnitus Coping Strategy Questionnaire (TCSQ) (Henry and Wilson, 1995). It contains 33 items dealing with cognitive and behavioural strategies used to cope with tinnitus. Two ratings are made for each item, one dealing with frequency of usage and the other dealing with derived benefit. The questionnaire is very much inspired by the Coping Strategy Questionnaire used in pain research (Rosenstiel and Keefe, 1983). The TCSQ is reported to have excellent psychometric properties (Chronbach's $\alpha = 0.88$), for each of the two summary scales (e.g. Frequency and Benefit). There is yet another questionnaire targeted towards coping with tinnitus, the Tinnitus Coping Style Questionnaire (Budd and Pugh, 1996a, 1996b). It includes 40 items and has been factor analysed into two stable factors called 'maladaptive' and 'effective' coping styles. Wilson and Henry (1998) have also developed a Tinnitus Cognitions Questionnaire and have used it in outcome research (e.g. Henry and Wilson, 1998). More recently, acceptance-oriented questionnaires have been developed (Schutte, 2009, no. 5625). One example is the Tinnitus Acceptance Questionnaire (TAQ), which is a measure of experiential avoidance and acceptance in relation to tinnitus (Westin et al., 2008a). The TAQ consists of 12 items and provides a total score of maximum 72 points. Higher scores indicate higher levels of tinnitus-related acceptance. The TAQ has an internal consistency of Cronbach's $\alpha = 0.89$ and a test–rest reliability of $r = 0.74$ (Westin et al., 2008a).

Smith and Fagelson (2011) aimed to measure tinnitus self-efficacy, which they referred to as 'the confidence individuals have in their capabilities to perform courses of action needed to manage their tinnitus successfully', and they produced the Self-Efficacy for Tinnitus Management Questionnaire (SETMQ). This instrument comprises 40 items (with two additional nontinnitus practice items) and patients are asked to answer by circling a percentage of certainty in their ability to perform an action, where 0% is 'cannot do this at all', 50% 'moderately certain I can do this' and 100% 'I am certain I can do this'. Examples of the actions sampled include:

- I can ignore my tinnitus when reading in a quiet place.
- I can manage feelings of fear when I hear my tinnitus.
- I can have a conversation on the telephone even when I hear my tinnitus.

The SETMQ is psychometrically robust and holds promise for use in future research and clinical application.

Open-ended approaches

Stephens and co-workers suggested an alternative approach to questionnaire assessment involving open-ended questions that are classified and quantified. It has been suggested that treatment effects may be more easily detected by open-ended questions than by structured questionnaires, such as the TQ (Sadlier and Stephens, 1995). This method could potentially be useful in the study of tinnitus, but may also result in inconsistencies. For example, using the open-ended approach, Tyler and Baker (1983) reported that 33% of the tinnitus patients had concentration problems. Sanchez and Stephens (1997, p. 211) found a slightly lower percentage of 22% reporting concentration problems in response to the request to 'make a list of the difficulties you have as a result of your tinnitus'. However, when confronted with the question in either a structured interview (Andersson et al., 1999) or in a questionnaire (Andersson et al., 2001), 70% and 78%, respectively, of tinnitus patients reported that they had concentration problems. Discrepancies between open-ended versus closed question sets, with open-ended questions yielding lower frequencies, has been observed in other studies (Schwartz, 1999). While open-ended questions are certainly valid they are not necessarily reliable.

Other useful self-report instruments

Proper multidisciplinary management of tinnitus patients often requires the assessment of related aspects, which can be even more disabling than tinnitus. One such example is the experience of hearing loss for which several questionnaires have been developed and validated (Andersson et al., 1995a; Ringdahl et al., 1998). Noble (1998) provided a comprehensive review of these measures. Self-report measures of hearing disability and handicap may provide useful information regarding hearing dysfunction. This can be of particular importance when it is possible to fit a hearing aid to improve communication, but it can also be the case that communication strategies (e.g. hearing tactics) are lacking and need to be targeted in rehabilitation.

Given the increased recognition of psychological factors when dealing with tinnitus, the use of validated measures of depression and anxiety can be useful, both when planning and evaluating the treatment. One option is the Hospital Anxiety and Depression Scale (HADS) (Zigmond and Snaith, 1983), which only includes 14 items (response scale 0–3). One advantage with the HADS is that it has been developed for use with somatic patients (Bjelland et al., 2002) and adequately captures the mood issues in tinnitus. The HADS has been used in tinnitus both in person (Zöger et al., 2004; Adoga et al., 2008) and by the Internet (Andersson et al., 2003b). Zigmond and Snaith (1983) recommended a cutoff score for 'cases' of 11 or more on each of the two subscales as being indicative of being 'cases' of either anxiety or depression. Other cutoff scores have, however, been suggested, for example eight on each of the subscales (Bjelland et al., 2002). It needs to be made clear that the HADS, and any other self-report inventory for that matter, is not a substitute for a proper psychiatric assessment, which should be requested in difficult cases. It should also be borne in mind that the HADS is a screening instrument and hence not sensitive to treatment outcomes.

Insomnia can be assessed with the Insomnia Severity Index (ISI) (Bastien et al., 2001). The ISI is a seven item questionnaire suitable for detecting changes in perceived sleep difficulties (Bastien et al., 2001). Each item is scored on 0–4 Likert-type scale and a sum is calculated. Bastien et al. (2001) reported an internal consistency of $a = 0.74$. An alternative is the Pitsburgh Sleep Quality Index (Buysse et al., 1989), which was applied to tinnitus patients by Handscomb (2006).

Tinnitus patients often report cognitive failures. The Cognitive Failures Questionnaire (CFQ) (Broadbent et al., 1982) is a self-report inventory for the assessment of common everyday errors regarding perception, memory and motor function. It contains 25 items and has adequate psychometric properties. It has also been used with tinnitus patients (McKenna, 1997).

There are several questionnaires available for the assessment of quality of life. Perhaps the most common is the Short Form 36 (SF-36) (Ware, 1993), which is available in a second version (see Hawthorne et al., 2007, for norms) and measures mobility and physical function, for which robust normative data are published. The SF-36 has also been used in studies on tinnitus (Wilson et al., 2002). Alternative instruments are the EQ-5D (EuroQol, 1990) and the Health Utilities Index (Feeny et al., 1995); these have not to our knowledge been applied specifically to tinnitus. Although quality of life measures may be useful for research, they do not add much in clinical practice. El Rafaie et al. (1999) reported data on a newly developed Quality of Family Life Questionnaire, but this questionnaire has not yet been widely used.

How tinnitus affects the family and primary relations surrounding the individual with tinnitus is not well understood. Granqvist et al. (2001) used a tinnitus-adapted version of the Family Support Scale of the West Haven-Yale Multidimensional Pain Inventory (Kerns et al., 1985) with the purpose to measure perceptions of family members´ responses to the individual with tinnitus (see also Sullivan et al., 1994). This measure is not widely used.

Discussion

Assessment of tinnitus severity and impact is very much dependent on valid and reliable self-report instruments. To date, there has been no consensus in the research nor clinical communities about which of the available instruments is the most useful. Unfortunately, this means that neither research data nor audit of clinical activities can be compared. Goebel and Hiller (1999) did a critical comparison of the nine scientifically relevant and tinnitus-specific questionnaires that were then in existence worldwide. They recommended Hallam's Tinnitus Questionnaire, and the mini-TQ is widely known in the audiological community. Instead, the TFI now represents an alternative that could serve as an initial step towards consensus across communities (Meikle et al., 2012). This remains to be seen. In addition, there are aspects not covered in the existing scales. Such aspects include common co-morbid problems such as hyperacusis, matters relating to avoidance of either noisy environments or silence and their direct effects on the experience of tinnitus. Other neglected factors include sound characteristics of tinnitus and masking properties of environmental sound.

Summary

Although several classification schemes have been used in the literature there remains a need to develop classification of tinnitus further, and in particular to assess the effects of tinnitus on general wellbeing and quality of life. In order to get an idea of the disability caused by tinnitus, reliable and valid instruments are needed. It is interesting to apply the World Health Organisation definition of 'body functions and structure; activities, participation, and contextual factors' (WHO, 2001), which was recently proposed by Langguth (2011). Noble (1998) suggested that interference with hearing functions represents the disability component of tinnitus and that the emotional, health and sleep problems reflect the handicap component. At present there are several instruments devoted to the assessment of tinnitus, but as yet there is no self-report inventory encompassing all the relevant aspects of tinnitus severity, though the TFI may prove an advance in this regard.

Chapter 12

Hyperacusis

The experience of becoming troubled by decreased sound tolerance can be catastrophic for a patient and their family, and represents a real challenge for the audiologist. Although the symptom has been described for many years (as will be demonstrated below), it is only in the last decade that protocols for diagnosis and treatment have been formulated and that an evidence base for treatment efficacy has begun to be built.

The fact that clinical recognition of disorders of sound tolerance is relatively recent is not to say that these issues have arisen in modern times. For example, the prolific Victorian author Wilkie Collins (1824–1889) uses hyperacusis as an essential element of the plot in his gripping novel *The Woman in White* (1860). Mr Fairlie is the uncle and guardian of Laura and is derelict in his duty (leading to his niece's downfall) as he is unable to tolerate spoken conversation and therefore is unable to advise her. For example, Mr Fairlie states:

> Pray excuse me but could you contrive to speak in a lower key? In the wretched state of my nerves, loud sound of any kind is indescribable torture to me. You will pardon an invalid?

Many individuals with decreased sound tolerance might well recognise aspects of their situation in this statement.

Definitions and related constructs

The terminology describing disorders of loudness perception is not consistent, due in part to the small amount of rigorous work in this area (Phillips and Carr, 1998) and in part to the observation that noise sensitivity has been described in at least four separate bodies of literature: audiology, neurology, psychiatry and in research on noise sensitivity and annoyance from a public health perspective.

The term *hyperacusis* was introduced to the medical literature by Perlman (1938), and the term was modified to 'hyperacusis dolorosa' by Mathiesen (1969). This latter term,

Tinnitus: A Multidisciplinary Approach, Second Edition. David Baguley, Gerhard Andersson, Don McFerran and Laurence McKenna.
© 2013 David Baguley, Gerhard Andersson, Don McFerran and Laurence McKenna.
Published 2013 by Blackwell Publishing Ltd.

Table 12.1 Terms used to describe decreased sound tolerance. (Adapted from Baguley and McFerran (2011)).

	Synonyms	Derivation	Dictionary definition *
Recruitment	Loudness recruitment	*French*: recruter	An abnormally large increase in the perceived loudness of a sound caused by a slight increase in its intensity
Hyperacusis	Hyperacousia Hyperacusia Hyperakusis Acoustic hyperaesthesia Auditory hyperaesthesia	*Greek*: hyper (above), akousis (hearing)	Exceptionally acute hearing, the hearing threshold being unusually low
Phonophobia		*Greek*: phone (voice or sound), phobia (fear)	Irrational fear of sounds or of speaking aloud
Misophonia		*Greek*: misos (hatred), phone (voice or sound)	Not yet in widespread usage
Dysacousis	Auditory dysesthesia dysacousia dysacusis	*Greek*: dys (bad), akousis (hearing)	A condition in which certain sounds produce discomfort
Odynacusis		*Greek*: odyne (pain), akousis (hearing)	Not yet in widespread usage
Auditory allodynia		*Latin*: auditorius (pertaining to hearing); *Greek*: allos (other), odyne (pain)	Not yet in widespread usage

*Definitions from *Dorlands Medical Dictionary*.

though redolent of the sadness of some individuals with hyperacusis, was not widely adopted. Hyperacusis has been defined as follows:

'unusual tolerance to ordinary environmental sounds' (Vernon, 1987b),

'consistently exaggerated or inappropriate responses to sounds that are neither threatening nor uncomfortably loud to a typical person' (Klein et al., 1990),

'abnormal lowered tolerance to sound' (Baguley, 2003).

Common to each of these definitions is that sound of low intensity can evoke this experience and that sounds in general (i.e. everyday sounds) are problematic rather than specific sounds.

A number of similar and related terms are in use (Table 12.1). The term *loudness recruitment* (Fowler, 1936; Moore, 1998) describes an experience commonly associated with cochlear hearing loss and OHC dysfunction in particular (Phillips and Carr, 1998). Many individuals with a cochlear hearing loss experience a rate of growth of loudness level with increasing sound level that is greater than normal (Moore, 1998). This phenomenon may be distinguished from hyperacusis if the individual experiences sound of moderate intensity as uncommonly loud (recruitment) or sound of low intensity as uncomfortably loud (hyperacusis), but the two experiences are not mutually exclusive. Loudness recruitment has not been reported to vary with mood, however, as is the case with hyperacusis. This has not yet been tested in experimental research and it is indeed very likely that the annoyance associated with loudness recruitment is linked to mood and how the symptom is perceived.

The term *phonophobia* (the literal meaning of which is fear of sound) has also been used for the experience of reduced sound tolerance and is frequently used in the neurological literature (Silberstein, 1995). In fact, increased noise sensitivity is a common finding in migraine, with at least 50% of attacks being accompanied by phonophobia (Woodhouse and Drummond, 1993). In addition, reduced uncomfortable loudness levels have been observed during migraine attacks (Woodhouse and Drummond, 1993). The suffix *phobia* describes the emotional impact of disordered loudness perception, but carries the implication that the dysfunction is strongly linked with fear and hence to be considered as a psychiatric symptom. As migrane patients experience their reduced sound tolerance as an overwhelming intensity of sound, rather than as an emotional intensity, the term hyperacusis might be a better fit than phonophobia for their auditory experiences (Baguley and McFerran, 2011).

In some contexts the suffix phobia implies that treatment might be optimally, and sometimes exclusively, the province of psychiatry. In response to this, the word *misophonia* (Jastreboff and Jastreboff, 2003) has been proposed, deriving from the Greek for 'dislike of sound'. While this is a laudable attempt at removing the implied phobic element while still retaining the emotional aspect of the experience, the word has not been uncritically adopted to date. One potential reason is the fact that this term is very close in meaning to the much more widely used concept of *noise annoyance* in epidemiological research and therefore only adds to the terminological confusion. Misophonia is described by Jastreboff and Hazell (2004) as when 'a negative reaction to sound results from an enhanced limbic and autonomic response, without abnormal enhancement of the auditory system'. They propose that phonophobia is thus a subsection of misophonia where fear is the chief component.

The terms *decreased* or *collapsed sound tolerance* are in use in the patient community, and examples can be found at the Hyperacusis Network website (www.hyperacusis.net). This network provides a rich resource for persons with sound tolerance issues, and the use of these terms underlines the extent to which people with this symptom are adversely emotionally affected.

The phenomenon of acoustic shock will be examined in Chapter 19. This can arise after exposure to abrupt unexpected sound, even if of modest intensity at times, and is more likely to be evident if the person is stressed or if the origin of the sound is careless or of ill intent. A reduction in sound tolerance is one of the defining symptoms, as are tinnitus and severe otalgia, and the extent to which this tolerance can be considered as hyperacusis is considered below.

Another area in which the symptom of noise sensitivity is mentioned is psychiatry. For example, the startle response is one of the symptoms used in the diagnosis of post-traumatic stress disorder (American Psychiatric Association, 2000). The way noise sensitivity is described in the psychiatric literature often makes it indistinguishable from what audiologists understand as hyperacusis. Noise sensitivity has been observed in association with depression, leading some workers to suggest that deficits in serotonin functioning may be implicated in both depression and hyperacusis (Marriage and Barnes, 1995). In fact, given the overlap between tinnitus and depression (see Chapter 8) it would not be surprising if at least a proportion of patients with hyperacusis would have diagnosable depression (Carman, 1973). Supporting this theory is the clinical observation that hyperacusis sometimes disappears once psychological wellbeing returns to normal.

Noise, defined as unwanted sound perceived as harmful or uncomfortable, has been studied from a public health perspective, mainly with respect to its detrimental effect on psychological wellbeing and on health (Job, 1996). Hence, noise sensitivity and noise annoyance have been the subject of extensive research (Abel, 1990; Stansfeld, 1992; Staples, 1996). In this literature it is common to distinguish *noise sensitivity* and *noise annoyance*, the first being seen as an intervening variable between exposure and individual annoyance responses (Stansfeld, 1992). This distinction has not been made in the literature on hyperacusis. In community surveys a co-morbidity between noise sensitivity and psychological problems has been observed (Stansfeld, 1992), and Weinstein (1980) argued that noise sensitivity may be a personality characteristic. Stansfeld et al. (1985) suggested that between 40% and 50% of highly noise-sensitive subjects had a recognisable psychiatric disorder. Research has found that noise sensitivity is not only related to neuroticism, but also to sensitivity to other aspects of the environment (Stansfeld, 1992). The experience of being specifically troubled by perception of low-frequency sound in the environment is discussed in Chapter 19.

Axelsson and co-workers studied the problem of hyperacusis (Axelsson et al., 1995; Anari et al., 1999) in a sample of consecutive patients referred for treatment of hyperacusis and concluded that sensitivity to sounds consists of different conditions, of which hyperacusis is one example. In the differential diagnosis of hyperacusis they proposed distinctions between hyperacusis and recruitment, distortion, psychiatric problems, noise annoyance and phonophobia. Unfortunately, this suggested categorisation has not resulted in further research. The group also noted a large co-morbidity of hyperacusis and tinnitus.

In reviewing the literature on noise sensitivity and annoyance Stansfeld (1992) argued that whereas sensitivity is related to noise level annoyance is not. From this reasoning hyperacusis would be included under the heading of noise sensitivity, representing a particularly severe form of noise sensitivity. The distinction between phonophobia and hyperacusis has also been questioned (Marriage and Barnes, 1995), but most workers believe that the term is sufficiently distinct to be retained.

Prevalence

Epidemiological data regarding hyperacusis has not been robustly determined and this is a major shortcoming in the literature. Several papers have been published as conference proceedings. Fabijanska et al. (1999) undertook a postal questionnaire epidemiological study of tinnitus in Poland, which included an unspecified question on hyperacusis. Of the 10 349 respondents, 15.2% reported hyperacusis, comprising 12.5% of the male respondents and 17.6% of the females. Regional differences were also reported. This report is interesting, but not sufficiently specific to be robust. This verdict also pertains to another conference report by Rubinstein et al. (1996) who described findings from a random sample of 1023 females from Gothenburg, Sweden (aged 38 years). In that study the point prevalence of hyperacusis was estimated at 23%. Unfortunately, no data on response rate or any detailed definition of hyperacusis was provided. In the only published peer reviewed study, Andersson et al. (2002b) investigated the prevalence of hyperacusis in the adult Swedish population: a specific definition of hyperacusis was included in their questionnaire (translated from Swedish):

> In our society we are surrounded by sounds of various kinds. Some of these sounds can be annoying or even unpleasant in character. We all differ in how vulnerable we are to these sounds. In this survey we study sensitivity to everyday sounds in the sense that they evoke adverse reactions. By this we mean, for example, reactions to conversation, chirping of birds, paper noises (rustle), the ringing sound at a pedestrian crossing, or the sound of a running water-tap. In other words, we ask about sounds of moderate loudness that most people experience daily without being annoyed. Our interest is thus not restricted to loud sounds such as drilling machines or low flying aircraft.

Two methods were utilised: firstly, an Internet study, wherein visitors to the website of a Swedish newspaper were invited to complete a web-based questionnaire, and, secondly, a postal population study. Of 1167 individuals who clicked upon the web banner, 595 responded, yielding a response rate of 51.9%. The point prevalence of hyperacusis in this group was 9%. The postal group comprised 987 individuals of whom 589 responded (a response rate of 59.7%) and a point prevalence of 8% was determined. Excluding participants who reported hearing impairment resulted in point prevalence rates of 7.7% and 5.9% respectively in the two groups. This indication of a relatively high prevalence of hyperacusis is not congruent with clinical experience and an alternative estimate is derived below.

A coincidence of tinnitus complaint and of experiences of hyperacusis has been widely noted. There is a consensus regarding the prevalence of hyperacusis in patients attending a Tinnitus Clinic with a primary complaint of tinnitus, approximating 40% (Sood and Coles, 1988; Bartnik et al., 1999; Jastreboff and Jastreboff, 2000; Baguley and McFerran, 2011), and in some studies up to 60% (Andersson et al., 2001). In patients with a primary complaint of hyperacusis, the prevalence of tinnitus experienced has been reported as 86% (Anari et al., 1999). However, in the epidemiological study by Andersson et al. (2002b), only 21% of the Internet group and 9% of the postal group with hyperacusis responded affirmatively to the question about tinnitus. Hyperacusis has also been suggested to be a precursor for the development of tinnitus (Hazell and Sheldrake, 1992), and as tinnitus develops it may be the case that hyperacusis becomes worse. However, in a longitudinal follow-up of tinnitus patients, sensitivity to noise became more common with time, increasing from 38% (Andersson et al., 1999) to 85% of the respondents (Andersson et al., 2001) five years later, which suggests that tinnitus can precede hyperacusis.

In a study of self-reported hearing problems in a random study of 850 Finnish adults (based on the city of Oulu) Hannula et al. (2011) reported that 17.2% replied affirmatively to a question about hyperacusis:

> Are you particularly sensitive to loud sounds?

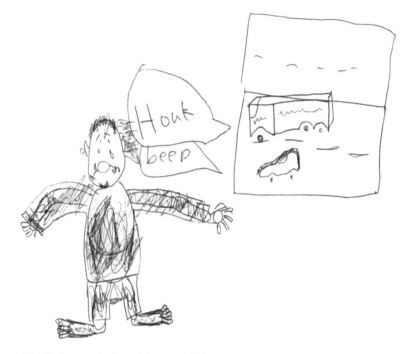

Figure 12.1   Self-portrait of an eight year old boy with hyperacusis.

This might be expected to sample persons perspectives on their reactions to intense sounds rather than to moderate- or low-intensity sound, and as such may illustrate noise sensitivity rather than hyperacusis.

The coincidence with tinnitus allows an alternative estimate to be made of the prevalence of hyperacusis (Baguley and Andersson, 2007). If 5% of the population have troublesome tinnitus and 40% of those have significant hyperacusis, then an estimate of 2% of the population having decreased sound tolerance can be derived. This is still higher than many clinicians would estimate, but in the absence of data, this proposal may be used to estimate demand for clinical services.

Since epidemiological findings suggest that hyperacusis is a common problem in the general population, the issue of psychiatric co-morbidity merits exploration. At the moment there is a paucity of information regarding the extent to which psychiatric conditions overlap with hyperacusis. There are some findings in allied disciplines and, for example, it is known that sleep problems interact with noise sensitivity in a negative way (Job, 1996). It would not be surprising if this was also relevant in hyperacusis.

Even less is known about the prevalence of hyperacusis in childhood. A drawing by a child illustrates the negative impact this may have (Figure 12.1). There is some evidence regarding an association between sound tolerance issues and children identified with Autism Spectrum Disorders (ASD), but there is much work to be done in this area. There are indications that hyperacusis in ASD may be a form of auditory hypervigilance, and as such phenomenologically different from general adult hyperacusis experiences (see Gomot et al., 2008, for example). This is further discussed in Chapter 18.

Measurements of hyperacusis

Although some proposals have been made regarding how to measure the severity or impact of hyperacusis in affected individuals, there is no consensus or empirical data today as to where to draw the line for abnormal levels of loudness discomfort levels for everyday sounds, nor of how to quantify the associated distress.

In an audiological setting, it may seem obvious that following a pure tone audiogram, rather than no measure of loudness discomfort testing should be undertaken. There are two salient areas of concern, however. The first is that it is well recognised that loudness discomfort levels have high within-subject and intersubject variability (Stephens et al., 1977; Valente et al., 1997), and are influenced by how the instructions are given in the test situation (Bornstein and Musiek, 1993), making reliable measurements difficult. It may well be then that information gained in this way is not sufficiently reliable to add clinical value. Loudness scaling techniues may be more reliable (Sherlock and Formby, 2005). However, there is some evidence that self-reported hyperacusis is accompanied by lowered thresholds for discomfort (Anari et al., 1999), and this is an area that needs more work. The second concern is that of the impact upon the patient. Intense sound is the specific thing that they fear, and the source of their complaint, and so subjecting such a person to uncomfortable sound intensities may well be corrosive to building a therapeutic rapport. Discussion continues, and at present each clinician must come to a view of the value of the assessment of loudness discomfort measures in each individual case.

Several measures of noise sensitivity exist in the wider literature (Zimmer and Ellermeier, 1999), including Weinstein's Noise Sensitivity Scale (Weinstein, 1980), but none of these tools particularly target hyperacusis. Recently it has become possible to quantify the handicap associated with hyperacusis, and three instruments have been developed for this purpose (Table 12.2).

Khalfa et al. (2002) reported data from a self-report Hyperacusis Questionnaire with 14 items, which used normative data from 201 individuals who had answered an advertisement placed for subject recruitment. Principal component factor analysis indicated a three-factor solution accounting for 48.4% of the variance, and the three factors were identified as attentional, social and emotional. Nelting et al. (2002) reported on a questionnaire with 27 items, which used normative data from 226 patients with hyperacusis. Principal component factor analysis again indicated a three-factor solution (accounting for 50.6% of the variance) identified as cognitive reactions, actional/somatic behaviour and emotional. This latter questionnaire has been validated by Blasing et al. (2010) who provide an English translation. An alternative approach to quantification of the severity of hyperacusis has been provided by Dauman and Bouscau-Faure (2005) who formulated a multiple activity scale for hyperacusis (MASH), which measures the impact of reduced sound tolerance upon everyday activities. While this undoubtedly captures an aspect of the disability associated with hyperacusis, in that patients may describe a major impact upon family activities such as supermarket shopping or cinema attandance, it should be noted that what is a commonplace activity for an individual in one culture may be exceptional in another context.

None of these instruments has as yet been shown to be sensitive to treatment effects. However, the existence of such instruments is a step forward in the investigation of this

Table 12.2 Self-report instruments for hyperacusis.

Authors (date)	Type	Items	Validation set	Comments
Khalfa et al. (2002)	Questionnaire	14	201 individuals from general population	
Nelting et al. (2002)	Questionnaire	27	226 hyperacusis patients	Validated by Blasing et al. (2010)
Dauman and Bouscau-Faure (2005)	Rating scale for difficulty of activities		249 tinnitus patients	

symptom. Meeus and colleagues (2010a) investigated the correlations between the Hyperacusis Questionnaire and the MASH, and with measures of uncomfortable listening levels. The HQ and the MASH had some correlation ($r^2 = 0.34$), but no such relationship was demonstrated between either the Hyperacusis Questionnaire or the MASH with uncomfortable listening levels.

The type of sounds that produce hyperacusis are also pertinent: using the data from Andersson et al. (2002b) on different kind of sounds, principal components analysis shows a clear two-factor split with noise, music and mechanical, monotonous sounds forming one factor and talk, paper noises and clatter forming a second separate factor.

Without any doubt there is a need to develop better objective measures and behavioural tests of hyperacusis, as well as further validation of self-report measures. In the literature on specific phobia, it is common to conduct behavioural tests when the phobic object is approached (Öst, 1997). This is usually also done in CBT with hyperacusis patients, but the procedures have not been tested or described in any detail in the literature. Moreover, the actual emotional and cognitive effects of exposure to sounds are virtually unexplored in hyperacusis. Another issue meriting further examination is the temporal characteristics of the sounds, as research has found that sudden noises are more likely to be viewed as aversive rather than constant sounds (Job, 1996).

Causes and mechanisms

A review of the medical conditions in which hyperacusis has been reported as a symptom was been undertaken by Katzenell and Segal (2001), and the conditions identified by these and other authors are listed in Table 12.3. It should be noted, however, that of the peripheral conditions identified, several involve facial nerve dysfunction. As the facial nerve innervates the stapedial reflex, which is a mechanism for reducing the perceived intensity of rapid onset sound, these conditions may reduce the efficacy of that reflex and hence increase the perceived intensity of sound. As such this does not meet a strict definition of hyperacusis.

Lyme disease is a systemic bacterial infection that targets specific body organs, and in which both peripheral and central neurological involvement has been observed (Coyle and Schutzer, 2002). The agent responsible is the tick-borne spirochete *Borrelia*

Table 12.3   Medical aetiologies associated with hyperacusis.

Peripheral	Central
Bell's Palsy	Migraine
Ramsey–Hunt Syndrome	Depression
Stapedectomy	Post Traumatic Stress Disorder
Perilymph Fistula	Head injury
	Lyme disease
	Williams Syndrome
	Fibromyalgia
	Addison's disease

burgdorferi and the disease is associated with particular geographical regions where the ticks and their hosts thrive and come into contact with humans. Hyperacusis has been reported as a symptom of Lyme disease, but some caution must be exercised in view of the fact that some patients also experience a facial palsy, and hence stapedial reflex dysfunction as described above. There are reports, however, of hyperacusis in Lyme disease without facial nerve dysfunction (Nields et al., 1999).

Williams Syndrome (WS), which is also sometimes known as Williams–Beuren Syndrome, is a developmental disorder of neurogenetic basis (Levitin et al., 2003) with a prevalence of 1 in 20 000 live births. The deletion of an element of chromosome 7 (which includes the Elastin gene) has been implicated (Baguley and McFerran, 2011). Diagnosis is accomplished by detecting the abnormal gene sequence using *fluorescence in situ hybridization* (FISH test). Affected individuals with the WS phenotype exhibit deficits in conceptual reasoning, problem solving, motor control, arithmetic and spatial cognition (Levitin et al., 2003). Hyperacusis had been associated with WS in up to 90% of individuals (Table 12.4), but a study using the Khalfa hyperacusis questionnaire in a WS population found a much lower prevalence (Blomberg et al., 2006).

Traditionally it was assumed that auditory thresholds in WS were normal. There is now a body of evidence that this is not the case and indications are that WS is often associated with a progressive sensorineural hearing loss (see Marler et al., 2005; Zarchi et al., 2010). Additionally there are reports that in individuals with WS and normal audiometric thresholds there may be subtle cochlear dysfunctions (Marler et al., 2010; Paglialonga et al., 2011) and that these may render the person more vulnerable to noise-induced hearing loss. A proposal is made by Matsumoto and colleagues (2011) that sound tolerance issues arise in WS because of outer hair cell dysfunction, but this presently remains a hypothesis. A central mechanism of hyperacusis in WS has been suggested as 5-HT (serotonin) dysfunction (Marriage and Barnes, 1995), but experimental evidence in support of this proposal has not yet been forthcoming.

Within the literature there are reports of hyperacusis being associated with such rare conditions as middle cerebral artery aneurysm (Khalil et al., 2002) and migrainous infarction (Lee et al., 2003). Although hyperacusis is not commonly associated with multiple sclerosis, a case study series has been published (Weber et al., 2002b). Thus while hyperacusis is rarely a symptom of significant or sinister pathology, it would seem prudent that an informed clinical opinion is sought in such cases.

Table 12.4 Reports of hyperacusis in Williams Syndrome. (Adapted from Baguley and McFerran (2011)).

Authors (date)	N	% with hyperacusis	Comments
Klein et al. (1990)	65	95	
van Borsel et al. (1997)	82	95	Subjects complained of sensitivity to 'noise': example cited of a power saw
Levitin et al. (2005)	118	91	
Blomberg et al. (2006)	38	13	Applied Khalfa Questionnaire
Gothelf et al. (2006)	49	84	Used a Hyperacusis Screening Questionnaire
Bedeschi et al. (2011)	45	11	Young adults with WS, aged 17–39 years

Reports are emerging of hyperacusis associated with fibromyalgia and other pain disorders (see Geisser et al., 2008, and de Klaver et al., 2007, respectively) and this can be observed clinically. At present one is only able to note an association and any thought of causality would be speculative. The idea that sensory sensitivities are problematic in such conditions is worthy of further consideration however.

Another issue that has been raised is that of hyperacusis (and tinnitus) in patients with semantic dementia (Mahoney et al., 2011). These authors state that these symptoms are commonly present in such patients, but do not substantiate this with prevalence data for this population, which would be a useful undertaking.

Mechanisms

There are several potential mechanisms of hyperacusis. These are not mutually exclusive and may be a reflection of heterogeneity of the patient population. There are at least three distinct mechanisms by which auditory gain may be modulated in humans. The first involves the motile function of outer hair cells (OHC) in the organ of Corti within the cochlea, which is involved both in increasing the amount of activity on the basilar membrane associated with low intensity sound and with the fine tuning of that activity (see Fuchs, 2010, for a review). OHC are innervated by efferent fibres from the central auditory system in large part, which analyses the sound environment and influences cochlear function accordingly. Cochlear blood flow may also be important in this process: if the cochlear blood supply is compromised the highly metabolically active OHC are unable to function effectively. The second mechanism is the ability to set auditory gain within the central auditory system (Florentine, 2011), based upon the observations that the range of change in gain is greater than can entirely be accounted for either by OHC activity or the firing rate of auditory nerve fibres (Epstein and Marozeau, 2010; Young, 2010). Thirdly, auditory gain (and specifically auditory startle) is influenced by mood state, particularly anxiety, agitation and fear. Reciprocal links between the auditory system and the reticular formation (which influences agitation and arousal) are present at the brainstem level, specifically in the superior olivary nuclei (FitzGerald and Folan-Curran,

2002). In addition, a functional connection involving the amygdalae, which are involved in fear and anxiety, and higher brainstem auditory nuclei has been described, and is thought to be involved in fear conditioning (Fredrikson and Furmark, 2003; Armony and LeDoux, 2010).

Several additional theories exist as possible explanations of hyperacusis. The high presence of hyperacusis in individuals with Williams Syndrome led Marriage and Barnes (1995) to consider the mechanism in that condition and the extent to which that might be generalised to other individuals. They suggested that a disturbance of 5-hydroxytryptamine (5-HT, serotonin) may be implicated in hyperacusis, based in part upon the clinical observation that hyperacusis is commonly coincident with conditions where 5-HT is involved, specifically migraine, depression and post traumatic stress disorder (Katzenell and Segal, 2001; Westcott, 2002). Serotonin does appear to have a role in the central auditory system (Altschuler and Shore, 2010), including modulating auditory gain and determination of the significance of sound (Thompson et al., 1994; Hurley et al., 2002). It has been suggested, however, that the serotonin disturbance involved in hyperacusis is nonspecific (Phillips and Carr, 1998) and would be difficult to subject to empirical investigation.

Another potential mechanism is that of auditory efferent dysfunction. An auditory efferent system is common to all mammals, and in humans consists of both a lateral and a medial efferent system. The lateral system is characterised by having its cells of origin in or around the lateral superior olives and terminating via the inferior vestibular nerve on the primary afferent dendrites beneath the inner hair cells. The function of the lateral auditory efferent system is as yet unclear. In contrast, the cell bodies giving rise to the medial system are located medially within the superior olivary complexes and terminate on the bases of outer hair cells. The function of the medial efferent system appears to include the modulation of auditory gain (Sahley et al., 1997) and the behavioural response to sound, possibly mediated through anatomical links with the reticular formation. A role for medial auditory efferent system dysfunction in both hyperacusis and tinnitus has been mooted. It has been suggested that such dysfunction might impair the ability to modulate central gain such that the auditory system might remain at high sensitivity even in the presence of noise of moderate to high intensity when the gain would normally be reduced (Jastreboff and Hazell, 1993). The experience of hyperacusis in patients with no apparent dysfunction or involvement of the peripheral auditory apparatus is circumstantial evidence for such central hyperexcitability. Jastreboff and Hazell (1993) further speculated that such central hyperexcitability, manifesting as hyperacusis, might represent a precursive state to troublesome tinnitus, though they did not substantiate this with data. Similar reasoning regarding central hperexcitability has been undertaken in the field of chronic pain (Peters et al., 2000). There is evidence against this hypothesis, however, in that patients who have undergone vestibular nerve section, usually for symptoms of vertigo refractory to other treatments, do not complain of increased tinnitus nor loudness intolerance (Baguley et al., 2002) and indeed psychoacoustic testing of such patients has failed to identify any decrement in auditory performance (Scharf et al., 1997).

Sahley and Nodar (2001) considered the observation that hyperacusis (and tinnitus) appear to increase in extent when one is tired, anxious or stressed. This led to the consideration of changes in the biochemical status of the cochlea, and specifically the role of endogenous dynorphins. Sahley and Nodar proposed that during stress endogenous dynorphins might be released into the synaptic region beneath inner hair cells. This might potentiate the neurotransmitter glutamate, with the results that sound might be perceived as louder than is in fact the case – this applying both to externally generated and internally generated (tinnitus) sound. Empirical evidence in support of this theory has not yet been forthcoming.

Important work by Craig Formby and colleagues (2003) has demonstrated that the perception of loudness can be up- or downrated by a two week use of earplugs and wideband sound generators respectively. There are important clinical implications of these findings: firstly, that the continuous wearing of hearing protection may worsen decreased sound tolerance, but, secondly, that sound tolerance can be increased with the use of sound therapy. These themes will be explored further below, but one should also note in passing that Munro and Blount (2009) have demonstrated that the use of earplugs, and of hearing aids (Hamilton and Munro, 2010), can decrease and increase stapedial reflex thresholds in humans, this being additional evidence that the perception of loudness is plastic.

A psychological model for hyperacusis uses the concept of classical conditioning of emotional responses to sound (Schwartz et al., 2002). Sounds can become associated with aversive responses involving the limbic and autonomous nervous systems although the auditory system is functioning normally (Jastreboff, 2000). This 'fear of sound' is commonly seen among patients with hyperacusis and the aversive reactions may occur in response to certain sounds whereas other sounds of similar level are not feared. However, the idea that hyperacusis may involve fear of injury to the auditory system has not been explored. In the literature on chronic pain, the fear-avoidance model (Lethem et al., 1983; Vlaeyen and Linton, 2000) has become well established. This model predicts that the fear of pain may serve a causal role in leading to disability, in that fear of injury leads to inactivity and that inactivity in itself leads to even more pain and disability. The parallel in hyperacusis is that avoidance of auditory stimulation is likely to sensitise the auditory system, which in turn exacerbates the hyperacusis. Hence, as gradual exposure to feared movements have been endorsed in pain management programmes (Vlaeyen et al., 2001), gradual exposure to sound has been recommended in the treatment of hyperacusis (Sammeth et al. 2000; Jastreboff, 2000; Vernon, 1987b). A comprehensive model for understanding hyperacusis should involve consideration of sensitivity, annoyance and fear of injury. The first two have been extensively researched in the literature on noise sensitivity (Stansfeld, 1992) and fear of injury could be a distinguishing factor in hyperacusis. Following this reasoning, hyperacusis can be seen from three different angles, depicted in Figure 12.2. In this model the experience of hyperacusis can involve annoyance and irritation, without necessarily having a sense of being harmed (e.g. irritation caused by neighbours playing music). It can also involve somatic sensations of pain and otalgia when sounds are experienced as pain in the ear. Finally, hyperacusis may involve a sense of hearing being harmed or, in the case of concurrent tinnitus, that tinnitus might become worse. The fear may concern specific sounds or for sound in general. The links between the central auditory system and areas of the brain implicated with anxiety and fear are currently investigated. Specifically, anatomical and functional links between the central auditory system and the amygdalae have been identified (Bhatnagar, 2002), this being an essential element of fear conditioning.

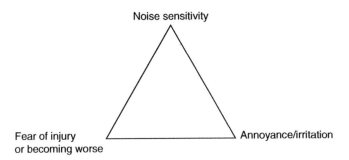

Figure 12.2   A three-component model of hyperacusis.

A further perspective (Dubal and Viaud-Delmon, 2008) has linked hyperacusis with 'magical ideation', which is a conceptual understanding of 'nonrational' beliefs about the world. Magical ideation is used by some psychiatry researchers as a basis for understanding the distorted beliefs held by persons with psychosis. Dubak and Viaud-Delmon found an association between hyperacusis and magical ideation, but this does not imply a causal relationship between the two, and further careful consideration of this issue is required.

Treatment

For many patients the first reaction to hyperacusis is to use earplugs, ear muffs or other hearing protection devices in order to protect them. As most of the theories of hyperacusis suggest that it is a disorder of central gain, the use of such devices, which decrease the intensity of sound entering the auditory system, may actually increase central gain further, and thus exacerbate the problem rather than improve it, as would be indicated by the findings of Formby et al. (2003).

An important self-help resource for persons with hyperacusis is the Hyperacusis Network (www.hyperacusis.net). This site comprises excellent information and a messageboard, which at the time of writing is well moderated.

Clinicians have frequently failed to recognise hyperacusis as a genuine symptom and seem unaware of therapeutic options. This is understandable given the dearth of published research regarding hyperacusis and the complete absence of randomised controlled trials. However, there are some management strategies and preliminary findings are promising. The most commonly used techniques are Tinnitus Retraining Therapy (TRT) and Cognitive Behavioural Therapy (CBT), but pharmacologically based treatments might be helpful in cases associated with specific pathology such as Lyme disease.

TRT has been advocated as a treatment for hyperacusis as well as tinnitus (see Chapter 14). Following audiological and medical evaluation, the treatment protocol (Jastreboff and Jastreboff, 2000; Jastreboff and Hazell, 2004) requires classification of the patients according to their hyperacusis state, and then 'directive counselling' about the auditory system and understandings of mechanisms of hyperacusis and the associated distress. Sound therapy in the form of binaural ear level wideband sound generators is undertaken, even when the symptoms are unilateral. The mechanism by which this sound therapy might be effective is said to be desensitisation, where the sound intensity is increased from a low level very gradually over time. Retraining therapy for hyperacusis has not yet been subject to randomised placebo controlled trials, but Sammeth et al. (2000) found some evidence of its effectiveness in a few cases. In addition, several observational studies (Gold et al., 2002; Hazell et al., 2002) indicate improvements in loudness tolerance, but these have not been published in peer review journals.

The approach taken by TRT practitioners of encouraging the understanding and insight of patients about their situation, and the use of low-level, nonthreatening, wideband noise seems based on common sense. Unfortunately, because the natural history of hyperacusis is poorly understood, placebo effects cannot be excluded. Although most reports of the use of TRT in the management of hyperacusis are positive, there is one report by Axelsson et al. (1995) that is less convincing. In spite of this, the TRT approach is promising.

Hyperacusis has also been treated using CBT, which can be used to treat the emotional, anxiety and stress issues involved in hyperacusis using information, counselling, relaxation therapy and sound therapy. Advice regarding hyperacusis is included as a standard component in the CBT treatment of tinnitus provided at the Universities of Uppsala and Linköping, Sweden, but there is a shortage of studies specifically targeting hyperacusis in isolation. However, Scott (1993) reported beneficial results in a conference case report involving gradual exposure. There is also an unpublished controlled trial on CBT for hyperacusis showing promising results (Jürisa, Andersson, Larsen and Ekselius, unpublished, 2012).

Similarly, evidence regarding the efficacy of sound therapy in hyperacusis is sparse. Gradual exposure to sound has been recommended for hyperacusis, and a few case studies have been reported showing beneficial results (Gabriels, 1993; Vernon, 1987b). A more formal approach using wideband sound generators is possible, either as an element of Tinnitus Retraining Therapy (TRT) or in conjunction with less prescriptive counselling and relaxation therapy. In the TRT context (see Chapter 14), patients with hyperacusis are either category 3 (hyperacusis without prolonged enhancement from sound exposure) or 4 (hyperacusis with prolonged enhancement from sound exposure): in both cases it is advised that wideband noise be introduced at a low level and then increased. The idea is that this gradual increase in intensity is analogous to desensitisation (Jastreboff and Hazell, 2004). An alternative approach (Baguley and Andersson, 2007) is to introduce the wideband noise at a comfortable level, and then leave it there so that the gain of the auditory system can recalibrate using this as a reference. Neither approach has been rigorously tested. Norena and Chery-Croze (2007) used an 'enriched auditory environment' with patients with hyperacusis: this was similar to the sounds in the Norena and Eggermont (2006) study ameliorating the effects of NIHL in kittens. No placebo control was used and the results that improvements in measurements of loudness scaling were seen should be interpreted with caution. Newer sound therapy approaches (such as Neuromonics, see Chapter 13) are anecdotally said to benefit tinnitus, but firm evidence is not yet available.

There has been a certain amount of controversy between the respective advocates of TRT and CBT. However, in the management of hyperacusis the differences between the two techniques are not marked and elements of both approaches may be appropriate.

Summary

While this area has previously been under-researched there has been considerable progress evident in recent years. Terminology is becoming better defined and hypotheses regarding mechanisms of hyperacusis are becoming better constructed and congruent with modern neurophysiological and biochemical insights. Treatment strategies are available and evidence regarding their efficacy is emerging. Although there are very significant gaps in knowledge regarding hyperacusis, this review of current perspectives gives hope for increased understanding and treatment efficacy. However, further progress necessitates that different communities communicate better, and hyperacusis is a typical example of an area in which researchers and clinicians have as yet failed to communicate across their interdisciplinary boundaries.

Chapter 13

Traditional treatments

A large number of therapeutic options have been considered in the management of tinnitus, including surgical treatments, drug treatments, psychological techniques and physical therapies. Many are still practised though often the evidence base is weak or completely lacking. In this chapter some of the more commonly used modalities are considered. Therapies that fall outside the umbrella of conventional medicine are discussed in Chapter 14, which focuses on the use of complementary medicine in tinnitus management.

Surgical treatment

Surgery has a definite role to play in those patients whose tinnitus arises as part of syndromes such as Ménière's disease, otosclerosis and vestibular schwannoma. This is discussed in Chapter 5, as is the surgical management of objective tinnitus. Only surgery for nonsyndromic tinnitus is considered in this chapter. There are two main types of surgery that have been tried for nonsyndromic tinnitus: destructive procedures on the auditory system and operations that decompress the auditory nerves.

Destructive operations

Attempts to cure tinnitus surgically by creating lesions within the auditory system have generally concentrated on the cochlea and the cochlear nerve, though in 1965 Beard investigated the effects of leucotomy on tinnitus. Surgical management of tinnitus by nerve section has been reported, with either division of the whole eighth nerve or selective division of the cochlear nerve, sparing the vestibular nerves (Wazen et al., 1997). By retaining the vestibular nerves the incidence of post-operative nausea, vomiting and vertigo is reduced. Results of cochlear neurectomy are variable and generally improve the

Tinnitus: A Multidisciplinary Approach, Second Edition. David Baguley, Gerhard Andersson, Don McFerran and Laurence McKenna.
© 2013 David Baguley, Gerhard Andersson, Don McFerran and Laurence McKenna.
Published 2013 by Blackwell Publishing Ltd.

tinnitus in about half of the patients. In 1995 Pulec reported a series of 151 patients who had undergone cochlear neurectomy for tinnitus. Total resolution or partial improvement of the tinnitus was reported in 95% of the patients, but unfortunately the results were not based on established outcome measures. There is an international consensus that cochlear neurectomy should only be considered for those patients who have no useful remaining hearing in the affected ear and have exhausted absolutely all nonoperative treatment options. If the patient has bilateral complete hearing loss, cochlear implantation is undoubtedly a better option as it offers the chance of both improved communication and reduced tinnitus.

Decompressive operations

Microvascular decompression surgery has been used in a small number of patients in whom the cause of their tinnitus has been thought to be a neurovascular conflict affecting the vestibulo-cochlear nerve. Moderately encouraging results have been presented but the numbers of patients studied are small, the studies have been uncontrolled and the surgery required carries significant risks. This topic is discussed in greater detail in the section on vascular loops in Chapter 5.

As most patients with nonsyndromic tinnitus have neither a profound sensorineural hearing loss nor vascular compression of the eighth cranial nerve the role of surgery is extremely limited.

Pharmacological

Undoubtedly from a patient's perspective the ideal solution to tinnitus would be to take a tablet or short course of tablets that would eliminate the problem in the same way that penicillin deals with a streptococcal sore throat. It is therefore salutary to note that there is currently no drug recommended by the drug licensing authorities of Western Europe or North America for the treatment of nonsyndromic tinnitus. Over the years considerable effort has been put into trying to find such a pharmacological solution (Murai et al., 1992; Simpson and Davies, 1999) but relatively few potential tinnitus drugs have received the rigorous scrutiny of a randomised controlled trial (Dobie, 1999). Even when drugs have undergone randomised controlled trials much of the research has been of poor quality and those trials of higher quality have generally given negative results. Research into drug treatment of tinnitus should be relatively easy to undertake, as it is much easier to perform randomisation and to select suitable controls for drug therapy than for treatments such as surgery, psychological therapies or tinnitus retraining therapy (TRT). Study design in tinnitus drug trials has often been flawed with poor randomisation techniques, inadequate blinding, lack of power calculation and incomplete data reporting (Hoare et al., 2011). Follow-up has often been far too short for a chronic condition. All extant tinnitus drug trials have used inactive placebos and many of the drugs studied, such as antidepressants or benzodiazepines, have marked side effects, which alerts the patient as to whether they are receiving the active or inactive preparation and effectively unblinds the supposedly blind trial. It is possible to design trials that use active placebos that mimic some of the side effects of the genuine drug; interestingly, when antidepressant drugs have been tested for efficacy in treating depression using such active placebos, the therapeutic effect is vastly reduced (Moncrieff et al., 2004). There has been no standardisation of outcome measures for tinnitus drug trials, which makes it difficult or impossible to perform meta-analysis on trials. Additionally, there are many different pathophysiological processes that can result in tinnitus and individual patients with tinnitus can have very different experiences of the symptom. Tinnitus patients are likely to present very heterogeneous characteristics in a similar way to chronic pain patients (Møller 1997). This heterogeneity bedevils research into drug treatment of tinnitus. Many large studies of both conventional and complimentary drug therapies fail to show statistical benefit to the treatment group. However, it is possible that small subgroups of patients with specific aetiological factors are deriving benefit but the effect is being lost within the larger population. The pharmacotherapy of tinnitus has been the subject of several review articles (Darlington and Smith, 2007; Langguth et al., 2009; Salvi et al., 2009; Langguth and Elgoyhen, 2011) and an up-to-date registry of many of the active tinnitus drug research projects is kept at the US National Institute of Health website (http://clinicaltrials.gov). Although the history of drug research for tinnitus is too often a tale of poor science and negative outcomes, it is important to consider the subject in more detail.

Local anaesthetics

One of the tantalising success stories of tinnitus treatment is the positive, albeit temporary, response of many patients to an intravenous bolus injection of either amide or ester local anaesthetic agents. This effect was first recognised serendipitously by Bárány in 1935 when procaine being used as a local anaesthetic in a nasal operation caused tinnitus relief in the patient. This effect was investigated by Lewy in 1937, with the conclusion that procaine was effective in treating tinnitus associated with normal hearing, sensorineural hearing loss or the deafness of otosclerosis, but was ineffective against pulsatile tinnitus. Fowler (1953) showed that this tinnitus suppressing effect also worked in patients with Ménière's disease. Lidocaine, also known as lignocaine, was developed in the early 1940s and was subsequently shown to have the same tinnitus suppressing properties as procaine (Englesson et al., 1976; Israel et al., 1982; Duckert and Rees, 1983; den Hartigh et al., 1993). Other local anaesthetic agents, with similar modes of action, such as bupivicaine (Weinmeister, 2000) are also able to temporarily suppress tinnitus. Although the tinnitus reducing qualities are seen in several members of this class of local anaesthetic agent the effect has become known as the lidocaine effect. Lidocaine ameliorates tinnitus for a limited period of time in approximately 60% of sufferers (Simpson and Davies, 1999). The chief therapeutic application of lidocaine is as a local anaesthetic agent, in which case it is given topically or regionally. It is also useful, given intravenously, in the treatment of some cardiac dysrhythmias. In these circumstances lidocaine is thought to have its action as a membrane stabilising agent due to antagonism of sodium channels. This mechanism may not apply to its effect in tinnitus and certainly lidocaine also affects some potassium and calcium channels (Josephson, 1988). It has also been suggested that the action on tinnitus could be mediated by altering serotonin (5-hydroxy tryptamine or 5-HT) function (Simpson et al., 1999). When used in the experimental treatment of tinnitus, lidocaine is generally given at a dosage of 1 mg/kg of body weight, as a slow intravenous injection over a period of several minutes. Any tinnitus suppressing effect is usually brief due to the short half-life of the drug within the circulation. There are also potentially serious side effects of administering the drug intravenously, with convulsions, respiratory depression, hypotension, bradycardia and cardiac arrest all possible. Unsurprisingly lidocaine is not licensed for treatment of tinnitus in most countries and is not suitable for general tinnitus management. Baguley et al. (2005) used a randomised double-blind controlled trial to study the effect of intravenous lidocaine on 16 patients who had tinnitus secondary to a vestibular schwannoma. These patients had all retained their tinnitus despite successful surgery to remove their tumour. The surgery had included cutting the auditory nerve, suggesting that any remaining tinnitus was central; 75% of patients had a reduction in loudness, pitch and distress of their tinnitus and it was concluded that lidocaine has a central effect in relieving tinnitus, although additional contralateral cochlear effects could not be excluded. Interestingly lidocaine has also been reported as effective in turning off auditory verbal hallucinations in an elderly patient with hearing loss but no psychiatric symptoms (Plewnia et al., 2007). When given by its normal and safer routes of tissue infiltration or topically to mucosal surfaces, lidocaine does not affect tinnitus. Intratympanic injections of lidocaine were investigated by Coles et al. (1992) with negative results. A study by Podoshin et al. (1992) was more optimistic but only nine of the 52 subjects who started the trial finished it. Side effects, particularly vertigo and vomiting, were common. Lidocaine can be administered topically to the skin for certain types of pain, most notably post-herpetic neuralgia. There is a case report of a patient using lidocaine patches who fell asleep against a heat pad (Shemirani et al., 2010). This caused temporary tinnitus reduction but also resulted in severe dizziness and ataxia.

There are some sodium channel antagonists that can be administered orally and there was initial hope that these would prove efficacious in the management of tinnitus. Tocainide (Blayney et al., 1985) and mexiletine (Kay, 1981) were tried to no avail. A small trial has shown that if a subgroup of patients who respond to lidocaine is selected, these patients are also likely to demonstrate temporary tinnitus reduction when given intravenous mexiletine (Berninger et al., 2006). Mexiletine has significant side effects and this observation has not advanced the treatment of tinnitus.

Psychoactive drugs

The psychoactive drugs include compounds that act on receptors that are common within the central auditory pathways and therefore some of these drugs might be expected to be active against tinnitus. However, both depression and anxiety are commonly seen in tinnitus patients and it is frequently impossible to decide if the mood change has followed the tinnitus or vice versa. It is similarly very difficult when conducting trials on psychoactive drugs to ascertain whether the drug is affecting the tinnitus directly or is affecting the mood disturbance and thereby having a secondary beneficial effect on the tinnitus. Consequently there are conflicting reports of the efficacy of psychoactive drugs in the management of tinnitus.

Tricyclic antidepressants

In the first published trial of the use of tricyclic antidepressants in the treatment of tinnitus Mihail et al. (1988) found no clear effects when using trimipramine. Sullivan et al. (1993) reported positive effects in a study involving 92 tinnitus patients who were given either nortriptyline or placebo. Interestingly some reductions in loudness were observed. Also of interest was the size of the placebo effect in this trial: 40% of the group receiving the placebo reported benefit. If tinnitus patients have associated depression and insomnia, amitriptyline remains useful as it has quite marked sedating effects. A trial by Bayar et al. (2001) showed amitriptyline to be beneficial in the overall management of tinnitus but no attempt was made to separate the depressive symptoms from the tinnitus complaint. Overall it seems likely that tricyclic drugs alleviate the distress of tinnitus rather than having any specific effect on the condition.

Selective serotonin reuptake inhibitors (SSRIs)

Serotonin is a common neurotransmitter in the central auditory system and has a suggested role in the pathogenesis of some forms of tinnitus (Chapter 4). Therefore drugs that modulate serotonin activity might be expected to influence tinnitus. Folmer et al. (2002) found that 33.8% of 957 patients attending a tinnitus clinic reported that they had depression at the time of referral to the clinic. At that time, 11.0% of the total were taking SSRI medication; 30 patients who had started the SSRI after the onset of the tinnitus were examined in more detail and it was discovered that both the depression and tinnitus improved while on the SSRIs. However, the patients also received psychotherapy during this period so it is not possible to ascribe all the benefit to the drugs. Robinson et al. (2005) described a well-constructed randomised double blind trial of 120 patients who were given paroxetine or placebo. Overall this SSRI drug had no effect on the tinnitus. Zöger et al. (2006) looked at another SSRI, sertraline, and concluded that it did have an effect on tinnitus. However, this study had a large dropout rate and some but not all of the participants received a benzodiazepine in addition to the sertraline, making it difficult to draw reliable conclusions. Trazodone is an antidepressant that has features of both tricyclic and SSRI drugs. A trial of this drug by Dib et al. (2007) showed no specific tinnitus effect. A Cochrane review on tinnitus and antidepressants (Baldo et al., 2006) concluded that there was no robust evidence to suggest that antidepressants have an anti-tinnitus action.

Neurokinin antagonists

Vestipitant is the first example of a novel class of drug that acts on neurokinin1 (NK1) receptors – one of the receptors for the neurotransmitter, Substance P. It has been investigated as a possible antiemetic and as an anxiolytic. A randomised placebo controlled double-blind trial was conducted on 24 adult patients with tinnitus (Roberts et al., 2011) but no beneficial effect was seen for multiple tinnitus parameters.

Benzodiazepines

Benzodiazepines such as diazepam, lorazepam and alprazolam are drugs with sedating and hypnotic properties. They bind to a subunit of one of the receptors for the inhibitory neurotransmitter gamma aminobutyric acid (GABA) and have been used extensively in the management of tinnitus. A trial by Johnson et al. (1993) attempted to separate direct tinnitus suppression from the generalised anxiolytic actions of alprazolam and demonstrated tinnitus loudness reduction in 76% of the trial patients, though reanalysing the data on an intention-to-treat basis reduced this figure to 65%. In tinnitus terms the duration of this trial was short at 12 weeks. Jalali et al. (2009) undertook a randomised controlled trial of alprazolam and found that there was no improvement of two outcome measures, namely the Tinnitus Handicap Inventory questionnaire and patient perceived loudness, but there was improvement of a visual analogue scale of tinnitus severity. Clonazepam has been examined for a possible therapeutic effect in tinnitus patients, but the relevant trials have been a retrospective observational study (Ganança et al., 2002) and an inadequately blinded study (Bahmad et al., 2006) so little scientific conclusion can be reached. Meeus et al. (2011) studied patients who were given clonazepam and placebo or clonazepam and a drug that is a mixture of flupentixol and melitracen. Tinnitus was reduced on the flupentixol and melitracen combination. No change was seen with placebo or clonazepam. The mixed flupentixol and melitracen preparation is not licenced for use in many countries. A small trial of diazepam (Kay, 1981) gave negative results. Szczepaniak and Møller (1996) suggested that benzodiazepines might suppress tinnitus by reducing neural overactivity in the inferior colliculus. Unfortunately benzodiazepines have proved to induce both physical and psychological dependence, limiting their usage.

Antipsychotic drugs

The use of sulpiride in the treatment of tinnitus is discussed later in this chapter.

Antispasmodics

Baclofen is a GABA agonist that has antispasmodic properties. Because its mechanism of action has similarities to the action of the benzodiazepines it was hoped that it would be effective in tinnitus control but free of addictive side effects. Unfortunately trials have shown it to be ineffective in tinnitus management (Westerberg et al., 1996).

Neuropathic pain drugs

Gabapentin is another GABA agonist though it remains unclear whether this action on GABA receptors is the mechanism for its therapeutic properties; some work suggests it acts on calcium ion channels. It is used for certain types of seizure and in pain management. Zapp (2001) reported a single patient whose tinnitus improved while receiving gabapentin for an unrelated condition. Since then, several trials have examined its effect on tinnitus (Bakhshaee et al., 2008; Bauer and Brozoski, 2006; Piccirillo et al., 2007; Witsell et al., 2007). All have found no effect on tinnitus with the exception of Bauer and Brozoski (2006), who observed improvement in tinnitus annoyance scores among patients whose tinnitus was secondary to acoustic trauma. This may be an example of subgroup activity and merits further investigation. A recent report suggested that gabapentin might be useful for treating tinnitus caused by neurovascular conflicts, caused by vascular loops abutting the eighth nerve (Russell and Baloh, 2009), but this was based on observation of two patients. A systematic review of gabapentin as a tinnitus treatment (Aazh et al., 2011) concluded that the evidence was insufficient to reach any firm judgement.

Glutamate antagonists

Glutamate is the main excitatory neurotransmitter in the auditory system and it might therefore be expected that blocking its effects would reduce neural activity and could potentially improve tinnitus. However, it is also the main excitatory neurotransmitter for many other pathways in the central nervous system and a blockade of glutamate receptors carries significant risk of inducing side effects. A placebo controlled randomised trial of memantine which blocks the *n*-methyl-D-aspartate (NMDA) subgroup of glutamate receptors showed it to be ineffective against tinnitus (Figueiredo et al., 2008). A small open trial of flupirtine, which is a glutamate antagonist but also active on potassium channels, showed no tinnitus effect (Salembier et al., 2006). Caroverine is a compound that has glutamate antagonist properties against both NMDA and α-amino-3-hydroxy-5-methyl-4-isoxazolepropionic acid (AMPA) receptors. Caroverine is also a calcium channel blocker and antioxidant. A trial by Denk et al. (1997) showed some therapeutic effect but the drug had to be administered by intravenous infusion and, in any case, caroverine is not available in most countries. Neramexane is a molecule that possesses NMDA antagonist properties but can also block nicotinic acetylcholine receptors. A randomised controlled trial showed a tendency towards tinnitus improvement compared to placebo, though this trend did not reach statistical significance (Suckfüll et al., 2011). Work continues to try and find other glutamate antagonists that are specific to the auditory system or to discover whether other routes of administration such as the intratympanic route are efficacious.

Acamprosate

Acamprosate is a drug with a slightly contentious mode of action: it probably stimulates GABA and inhibits NMDA. Its chief clinical use is in alcohol dependency. A pilot trial for tinnitus in Brazil (Azevedo and Figueiredo, 2005) gave optimistic results but present indications are that more rigorous study has shown it to be ineffective as a tinnitus therapy (Martin, personal communication).

Antiepileptics

Because anticonvulsant medications act by reducing hyperexcitability within the central nervous system it was hoped that they would also prove active against hyperexcitability within the auditory system. Carbamazepine is a sodium channel blocker, in many ways similar to the local anaesthetic drugs and active when taken orally. Unfortunately, a study by Donaldson (1981) showed little useful effect in tinnitus. However, Sanchez et al. (1999) have suggested that if patients are selected on the basis of a positive response to a trial dose of intravenous lidocaine they are then likely to respond favourably to carbamazepine. Carbemazepine has been recommended as a treatment for what has been described as 'typewriter tinnitus', a specific form of tinnitus that sounds like a typewriter, popcorn popping or ear clicking (Levine, 2006; Nam et al., 2010a). This type of tinnitus is thought to be associated with vascular compression of the eighth nerve, but this observation and the apparent efficacy of carbamazepine is based on observational studies of a handful of patients. Further work is required to confirm these observations. Other anticonvulsants including amino-oxyacetic acid (Reed et al., 1985) and lamotrigine (Simpson et al., 1999) have been assessed for tinnitus suppressing activity, with negative results.

Drugs acting on dopamine receptors

Dopamine is one of several neurotransmitters to be found in both the peripheral and central auditory systems. Its role within the auditory system is not clear but there have been suggestions that dopamine is an inhibitory neurotransmitter in the cochlea and that dopamine antagonists improve filtering of sensory inputs in the thalamus. Therefore roles for both agonists and antagonists have been suggested. A model of tinnitus based on dopaminergic pathways has been generated (Lopez-Gonzalez and Esteban-Ortega, 2005). Two trials have tested this model using the antipsychotic dopamine antagonist, sulpiride (Lopez-Gonzalez et al., 2003; Shiraishi et al., 1990), and reported optimistic results. However, the methodology of both of these studies was poor and, as yet, no firm conclusions can be drawn. Dopamine antagonists can produce significant side effects and are unlikely to ever enter common usage for tinnitus management. Dopamine agonists have also been assessed: de Azevedo et al. (2009) conducted a randomised placebo controlled trial of piribedil but concluded that it was not superior to placebo and there was a high incidence of side effects reported among those receiving the active drug. Sziklai et al. (2011) undertook a randomised placebo controlled trial and reported that pramipexole was effective against tinnitus associated with presbycusis. However, there was a 34.4% dropout rate among participants and the results were analysed on those who completed the study rather than on an intention-to-treat basis.

Melatonin

Melatonin is a naturally occurring hormone that is produced in the pineal gland and some other tissues and helps to regulate the body's circadian rhythms. It has been used for sleep disturbance and because sleep problems feature highly as contributors towards tinnitus distress melatonin has been tried both as a standalone treatment for tinnitus (Megwalu et al., 2006; Rosenberg et al., 1998; Hurtuk et al., 2011) and in combination with other agents, including dopamine antagonists and anticoagulants (Lopez-Gonzalez et al., 2007; Neri et al., 2009). Mixed results have been obtained though the overall impression is optimistic and there is a repeated suggestion that melatonin is helpful for tinnitus-associated sleep disturbance. It would be extremely useful for the use of melatonin in tinnitus to be subjected to a systematic review and meta-analysis.

Drugs affecting the circulation

Tinnitus is more prevalent with increasing age and with increasing hearing disability. Various mechanisms may underlie these observations but one suggested cause is reduced blood supply to both the central and peripheral auditory systems, allowing deficiency of oxygenation, reduced nutrient supply and a build-up of toxic metabolites. Consequently various drugs that might improve the microcirculation of the auditory system have been evaluated.

Vasodilators

The rationale for using vasodilators in the treatment of tinnitus is that they should increase the blood flow, thereby enhancing the supply of oxygen and nutrients and reducing any dysfunction. The cochlea derives its arterial supply from the inferior cerebellar artery, which is part of the cerebral circulation. The cerebral circulation possesses a robust autoregulation mechanism, which keeps perfusion within quite tight parameters irrespective of the state of the peripheral circulation. Therefore it is unlikely that many vasodilators can have significant effect on cochlear function. Nimodipine is a calcium L channel blocking drug that possesses activity for cerebral blood vessels. One study (Theopold, 1985) suggested that it was effective in tinnitus management but a later study (Davies et al., 1994) failed to replicate these findings. Betahistine is a histamine analogue that has been promoted for the treatment of Ménière's disease and is postulated to improve cochlear blood flow. There is no evidence that it helps the tinnitus of Ménière's disease and similarly no evidence of any beneficial effect among patients of tinnitus due to other pathophysiological processes. Despite this it is frequently dispensed by primary care physicians for subjective idiopathic tinnitus – just under a third of a million prescriptions for betahistine were written in Western Europe in 2001 for the treatment of tinnitus (Langguth et al., 2009). Many clinicians feel that betahistine is essentially a form of placebo treatment but at least it has the benefits of being reasonably cheap and free of serious side effects.

Diuretics

Diuretics such as furosemide, previously known as frusemide (Jayarajan and Coles, 1993), and osmotic diuretics such as mannitol and glcerol (Filipo et al., 1997) have been studied but do not seem to be of major benefit in the treatment of tinnitus.

Anticoagulants

It has been suggested that tinnitus can be caused by small thrombi within the vessels supplying the auditory pathways – both peripheral and central. There have been various trials of heparin and similar agents, the most recent being a trial of sodium enoxaparin (Mora et al., 2003). Although this suggested that there was benefit from using this agent, the trial had sufficient methodological flaws to render the conclusions unreliable.

Prostaglandins

Synthetic prostaglandins are used in the treatment of ulcers and induction of labour. They have vasodilator effects and therefore could have an effect against ischaemia within the auditory system. There are several trials that have investigated whether one of these drugs, misoprostol, is effective against tinnitus (Akkuzu et al., 2004; Yilmaz et al., 2004). To date the trials are small and are best regarded as preliminary studies.

Botox

Botulinum toxin has proved useful in some pain conditions and migraine. Although the primary action of botox is to block acetylcholine receptors it also possesses activity against a variety of other receptors. The exact mechanism by which it is active against pain remains unclear (Dressler et al., 2005). Hypothesising that tinnitus has similarities to some types of chronic pain, Stidham et al. (2005) undertook a randomised, controlled, crossover trial of botulinum toxin A versus placebo ($n=30$). After injecting drug or placebo behind the pinna, a statistically significant improvement of tinnitus disability was seen using the active compound. However, this was a small trial and an inert placebo was used. Further work is required before this drug can be recommended.

Intratympanic drugs

Although modern theories of tinnitus generation have increasingly focused on the central auditory system, most people with tinnitus have a degree of cochlear impairment and, even among those with normal audiograms in the 250–8000 Hz range, cochlear defects are often detected when more sophisticated tests of cochlear function are employed. For this reason there continues to be interest in trying drugs that are directed at the peripheral auditory system and intratympanic delivery is one way of achieving cochlear drug administration. This route has several potential advantages over routes such as oral or intravenous therapy (Herraiz et al., 2010). One advantage is being able to achieve adequate drug levels in the cochlea without having to have large circulating levels of the drug and hence avoid systemic dose-related side effects; some drugs do not easily cross the blood–labyrinth barrier but may be easily absorbed through the round window; drugs that are too toxic for systemic administration may be suitable for administration intratympanically. Intratympanic drugs can be given as a simple injection through the tympanic membrane or a grommet (ventilation tube or tympanostomy tube) can be surgically inserted and the drug can then be applied through the lumen of the grommet. Alternatively, a small wick or a microcatheter can be surgically implanted, allowing a more sustained or even continuous delivery of the drug to the round window. Other largely experimental ways of providing slow-release medication are the use of hydrogels or nanoparticles (McCall et al., 2010). Intratympanic injections already have a proven role in the management of the vertigo associated with Ménière's disease. The main group of drugs that have been investigated with regard to intratympanic therapy in subjective idiopathic tinnitus are steroids. Cesarani et al. (2002) reported favourable results when using dexamethasone, but this was an uncontrolled observational study. Shim et al. (2011) undertook a trial with three arms: one group received alprazolam; one group received alprazolam and four intratympanic injections of dexamethasone; one group received alprazolam, four intratympanic injections of dexamethasone and four intravenous injections of lipoprostaglandin (PG) E1. Patients in the latter two groups reported significantly better tinnitus outcomes. This trial, however, was inadequately controlled as there was no placebo for the intratympanic and intravenous injections. Two trials have used satisfactory experimental techniques: Araújo et al. (2005) investigated dexamethasone using saline injections as a placebo; Topak et al. (2009) tested methyl prednisolone injections against a saline placebo. Both of these trials concluded that there was no advantage to using intratympanic steroids in the treatment of idiopathic tinnitus. Other groups of drugs that have been tested include local anaesthetic agents and drugs that stimulate cholinergic receptors. Pilocarpine and carbachol are cholinergic agonists and a single study showed that intratympanic injection resulted in brief tinnitus improvement, lasting between 12 and 72 hours (DeLucchi, 2000). However, the study was uncontrolled. Trials of intraympanic administration of glutamate receptor antagonists are currently underway. The NMDA antagonist known as AM-101 has successfully undergone safety testing (Muehlmeier et al., 2011) and reports on its efficacy against tinnitus are awaited.

Otoprotective agents

One intriguing answer to tinnitus is to try and prevent the symptom developing in the first place. There are known risk factors for developing tinnitus including noise exposure, receiving cancer chemotherapy, particularly platinum-based chemotherapy, and receiving aminoglycosides. Some noise exposure, such as might be experienced in a factory or recreationally in a nightclub, is predictable and wearing personal protective equipment in these situations is helpful. Some noise, however, is unpredictable – for example the deployment of an air bag in a road traffic accident or the sudden noise of a fire alarm. Military personnel are particularly at risk of developing noise-induced hearing loss and tinnitus (Chapter 19). Chemotherapy and aminoglycoside antibiotics are drugs that are generally only given when there is no alternative course of action. Considerable work has therefore been done trying to find ways of protecting the ear in these situations by administering otoprotective agents prior to exposure or in the immediate aftermath of exposure. Cochlear hair cell death has been shown to be mediated by a process of apoptosis or programmed cell death. This is a complicated chain of events that can be triggered by a build-up of reactive oxygen species within the cell and involves a cascade of biochemical events mediated by several proteins including enzymes called caspases (Cotanche, 2008). Caspase activation is the common final pathway of cell death due to aminoglycosides, noise trauma and platinum-based chemotherapy drugs. Most of the agents that have been assessed for otoprotective potential are antioxidants, administered in the hope that by dealing with excess reactive oxygen species the apoptotic process will be avoided. Campbell et al. (2007) have demonstrated the effectiveness of D-methionine in the prevention of aminoglycoside, chemotherapy and noise-induced hearing losses. Work from the same institution showed that D-methionine can prevent noise-induced hearing loss in an animal model, even when given up to 7 hours post noise exposure (Campbell et al., 2011). D-Methionine was compared against *N*-L-acetylcysteine and ebselen, a selenium containing compound, for its ability to prevent ototoxicity after cisplatin exposure (Lorito et al., 2011). D-methionine was found to be the most efficacious of the three compounds in this animal model. Le Prell et al. (2011) reported on the use of a supplement consisting of beta-carotene, vitamin C, vitamin E and magnesium in preventing noise damage to military personnel during a training exercise. None of the participants demonstrated enough hearing change to say whether or not the supplement was beneficial, but it was well tolerated. This combination is currently being investigated in several other situations where noise-induced hearing loss is expected. Another way of preventing hair cell death is by pharmacologically blocking the caspase proteins and other mediators of apoptosis either by administering inhibitory drugs or by pharmacogenetically modifying the levels of endogenous protective molecules (Knauer et al., 2010). Gene therapy and stem cell administration are also being investigated as ways of repairing damage to the cochlea (Cotanche, 2008). This research into otoprotective agents is still very much in its infancy, but some of the results are exciting and hopefully the research will produce clinically relevant applications in due course.

Sound therapy for tinnitus

The use of sound to relieve tinnitus is not new. Whispered incantations were advised for those with troublesome tinnitus in Ancient Babylon in circa 650 BC, and since that time many clinicians and authors have advised the use of soft sound. Examples of sound sources suggested as long ago as Itard have included watermills, waterfalls and crackling logs in a fire (Stephens, 2000). Modern patients have often come to the same common-sense conclusion, using fans, environmental sound CDs, iPods or one of the range of inexpensive environmental sound generators that is now available.

Vernon was a pioneer of tinnitus research and is credited with the invention of the tinnitus masker in the 1970s, following the observation of a colleague with tinnitus who gained relief sitting near a fountain (Vernon, 1977). Tinnitus masking involves the use of wearable ear-level devices that deliver sound to the patient's ears. The purpose is to produce a sense of relief by making the tinnitus inaudible or by changing its characteristics. Masking has been one of the most commonly applied means of dealing with tinnitus (Vernon and Meikle, 2000) and was suggested as early as 1928 (Jones and Knudsen, 1928). Total masking of tinnitus is at best tedious and sometimes impossible. Sound therapy is used at much lower levels in TRT, in which case it is referred to as sound enrichment, and to help distinguish between masking and the TRT approach, exponents of TRT use the term sound generator instead of masker. Use of sound therapy in TRT is discussed below. In this section classical masking is discussed.

Masking devices and their effects on tinnitus have been studied extensively (Vernon, 1977) and much of the research questions their efficacy, though the quality of that research is not high. In a systematic review, Hobson and colleagues (2010) failed to find compelling evidence of the benefits of masking for tinnitus patients – though these authors do indicate that lack of evidence is not evidence of ineffectiveness. In an ambitious multicentre study (Hazell et al., 1985) few positive effects were found and even fewer in a controlled study embedded within that study (Stephens and Corcoran, 1985). In another controlled study, with placebo maskers, Erlandsson et al. (1987) found no differences between masking and placebo. Finally, masking has not been found to boost the benefits of psychological treatment (Jakes et al., 1992). As another caveat, it has been observed that many patients (up to 50%) do not accept masking as a treatment (Vernon et al., 1990; Henry et al., 2002a). In theory, total masking is said to prevent habituation (Jastreboff and Jastreboff, 2003). There is little if any experimental research on tinnitus patients to support this hypothesis although it remains plausible. Studying masker treatment is hindered by the observation that masking was rarely practised in isolation and patients receiving maskers have often received other treatment modalities such as counselling (Henry et al., 2002a).

Henry and colleagues have introduced a framework for the management of troublesome tinnitus which is in use in the USA Veterans Administration (VA) and which is entitled 'Progressive Tinnitus Management' (Henry et al., 2010). Sound therapy is an essential element of this, and

> … can involve three objectives: (a) producing a sense of relief from tinnitus-associated stress (using soothing sound); (b) passively diverting attention away from tinnitus by reducing contrast between tinnitus and the acoustic environment (using background sound); and (c) actively diverting attention away from tinnitus (using interesting sound). Each of these goals can be accomplished using three different types of sound — broadly categorized as environmental sound, music, and speech — resulting in nine combinations of uses of sound and types of sound to manage tinnitus (Henry et al., 2008).

Essentially, Progressive Tinnitus Management is a stepped care model, with a clear protocol, which facilitates its use within a large organization like the VA.

The Neuromonics technique uses customised sound therapy in a framework of structured counselling and follow-up: the sound stimulus is a spectrally modified piece of chamber music. The technique was developed by Paul Davis during his doctoral studies in Perth, Australia, and then commercialised with backing from venture capital. Neuromonics is presently available in Australasia and the United States, in which latter country it has some influential beacon sites. It is not presently available in the EU, for reasons that are unclear. Customised music (adapted both to fit the audiogram of the patient and in intensity characteristics) is used to promote habituation, while support and structured counselling are also provided. The technique of modification of the music stimulus is mentioned in a patent, though proposals that this may be a beneficial strategy predate the patent

(Baguley et al., 1997). Initial results of Neuromonics (Davis et al., 2007) indicate that this technique should interest the tinnitus clinician, though some important caveats remain. Perhaps the greatest concern lies with the cost efficacy of the technique. If, as reported, Neuromonics produces benefits broadly in line with other sound therapy approaches embedded in counselling, is the extra cost of the device justified over that of an mp3 player or ear-level wideband sound generator (Newman and Sandridge, 2012)?

Hearing aids

The possible benefit of using hearing aids to obtain relief from tinnitus was commented on in 1947 by Saltzman and Ersner. Initial uncontrolled studies suggested that tinnitus patients were helped by hearing aids (Stacey, 1980; Surr et al., 1985), but in a later controlled study no positive effects were found (Melin et al., 1987). In a more recent uncontrolled study by Surr et al. (1999) hearing aid use was found to be associated with reduced tinnitus handicap, but the authors admitted that the effect was small. There are also combination instruments, in which a hearing aid and a masker are housed in the same unit. There is a dearth of good experimental evidence regarding their efficacy and they remain a challenge difficult to fit optimally as there are no clear protocols for this. The published evidence regarding the benefits of hearing aid fitting for people with tinnitus has been reviewed by Noble (2008) who found that the effect might be to 'slightly reduce its prominence'. In clinical practice the effects can exceed this moderate aspiration! This observation is supported by Trotter and Donaldson (2008) who report a 25-year series of tinnitus and hearing aids, with strongly positive results. Moffat and colleagues (2009) investigated the benefits of high bandwith ampification (e.g. extended range hearing aids) upon tinnitus, but did not demonstrate any change in the loudness or spectral characteristics of tinnitus. Andersson et al. (2011) found that tinnitus patients with hearing aids (compared to those without tinnitus) reported slightly less benefit and more problems with their hearing aids, in particular in relation to background sounds and aversiveness of sounds. The question of how to fit a modern hearing aid optimally for tinnitus has begun to be addressed. Searchfield (2005) proposed that one should:

- Disable directionality
- Disable any noise suppression algorithms
- Use low knee point compression.

Such strategies will render speech in noise more difficult to discriminate, so a 'tinnitus-specific' programme would be needed in order to switch between different listening objectives.

Electrical stimulation and cochlear implants

Electrical stimulation of the ear, especially when direct current stimulation is used, can reduce or abolish tinnitus (Dauman, 2000). However, it has proved problematic trying to turn this experimental observation into a clinically useful tool as it is difficult to get sufficient electrical power to the inner ear without causing damage. External electrical stimulation has proved beneficial in the treatment of chronic pain and has given rise to the clinically useful technique of transcutaneous electrical nerve stimulation (TENS). Similar techniques have been assessed in tinnitus patients (Chouard et al., 1981; Lyttkens et al., 1986; Schulman, 1985). In a placebo-controlled trial by Dobie et al. (1986), 20 patients were given either proper stimulation or placebo in a double-blind crossover trial. Severity of tinnitus decreased for two patients following the active treatment, but four patients in the placebo condition also reported improvement, suggesting that any positive response could be explained by the placebo effect. Interestingly, however, one patient derived marked benefit and a prolonged study with this patient seemed to suggest that the effect was not attributable to placebo in this individual. Therefore there may be a limited role for this type of therapy. Following observations on chronic pain patients, there have been other studies in which sites distant from the ear have been stimulated in an attempt to alleviate tinnitus. Kaada et al. (1989) applied low-frequency electrical stimulation to the arms of 29 patients with tinnitus. Nine reported reduced tinnitus and, of these, seven had improved hearing. However, the study was inadequately controlled and it is difficult to extrapolate generally. There have been some anecdotal reports of stimulation of the deep external auditory canal supplying tinnitus relief and this area probably merits further research.

Surgical implants into the middle or inner ear are too invasive to be considered for widespread usage among tinnitus patients who have useful hearing. However, such objections do not apply to patients who have already lost all their hearing: ever since cochlear implantation became possible there has been much interest in its effect on tinnitus among patients with profound sensorineural hearing loss. Initial reports studied the effects of promontory stimulation and then single-channel cochlear implantation. The effects of multichannel implants upon tinnitus have been reviewed several times (Quaranta et al., 2004; Baguley and Atlas, 2007; Punte et al., 2011) with similar observations. Tinnitus is experienced by up to 86% of adult cochlear implant candidates, but is not universal and is only bothersome in a small proportion. Cochlear implant electrode insertion may induce tinnitus in a small (up to 4%) number of patients, but this is rare. Cochlear implant device usage is associated with reduction of tinnitus intensity and awareness in up to 86%, and rarely with exacerbation (up to 9%). There are some indications in the literature that the more complex the simulation strategy the larger the beneficial effect. Despite the reported benefits of CI for tinnitus, there are indications of a substantial residue of adult CI patients with tinnitus handicap – data for children is not available. Di Nardo and colleagues (2007) reported a series of CI users in whom 30% indicated a moderate or greater tinnitus handicap on the THI and in 5% this was severe. This is congruent with data from Sweden, where 25% of an adult CI series had moderate or greater THI scores (Andersson et al., 2009b). It is incumbent upon services providing CI services to proactively identify patients with troublesome tinnitus and to offer therapy and support.

Interestingly, unilateral cochlear implant usage (in the bilaterally deaf) is generally associated with reduction of contralateral tinnitus (in up to 67% of individuals) rather than exacerbation, which undermines the assertion (Jastreboff, 2000) that unilateral sound therapy for tinnitus is contraindicated.

It should be noted that cochlear implant stimulation strategies are designed to optimise speech perception, but they may not be optimal for tinnitus inhibition. Dauman and Tyler (1993) undertook some preliminary experiments with two cochlear implant subjects with tinnitus in an attempt to identify which combination of stimulation rate and location was most effective in suppression of tinnitus. Rubinstein et al. (2003) reported the efficacy of electrical stimulation with 5000 pps pulse trains via cochlear implant (three subjects) and via a transtympanic electrode (11 subjects), reporting that 'between a third and a half of them achieve clinically significant tinnitus suppression without a sustained percept. Vernon and Meikle (2000) reported a case where masking bilateral tinnitus with noise (6–14 kHz) via a Nucleus 22 cochlear implant was helpful, leading to some residual inhibition lasting 2–3 minutes and some reported contralateral suppression. In a further case study Zeng and colleagues (2011) report suppression of tinnitus in a patient with a CI in a unilaterally deaf ear in whom tinnitus was suppressed by a low-rate stimulus (<100 Hz). This remains an interesting area. The use of CI in single sided deafness and tinnitus is considered in Chapter 19.

Biofeedback

In some patients who find traditional relaxation therapy unhelpful, biofeedback has clinical utility. This technique allows the patient to monitor the stress level, usually measured by a galvanic skin response, with either an auditory or visual signal (Young, 2000). The literature in this area is equivocal (Dobie, 1999; Andersson and Lyttkens, 1999). Biofeedback can be useful for tinnitus patients who are profoundly deaf and who find the 'eyes closed, lying on the bed' methods of relaxation therapy troubling. Early studies using a biofeedback method in which warmth of the fingers and muscle tension in the forehead were monitored produced optimistic results (House et al., 1977; House, 1978). However, these trials were not controlled and along with other uncontrolled studies (Carmen and Svihovec, 1984; Walsh and Gerley, 1985; Ogata et al., 1993) the positive findings reported must be interpreted with caution. Among the available controlled trials the findings are less supportive, with a trial by Haralambous et al. (1987) showing nonsignificant effects. A trial by Podoshin et al. (1991) showed that biofeedback techniques were more efficacious in tinnitus control than the use of acupuncture or cinnarizine. White et al. (1986) studied 22 patients who received biofeedback for their tinnitus and concluded that the results in the test group were significantly better than those in the control group. However, the test group also received relaxation therapy, which somewhat dilutes the findings.

In one interesting study by Ince et al. (1987) an auditory matching-to-sample feedback technique was used for training self-control of tinnitus. Patients were trained to decrease the volume of their tinnitus by first matching to an external sound and then decreasing the volume of that sound while simultaneously trying to decrease their own tinnitus sound. It was reported that 84% managed to decrease the loudness of the tinnitus between 10 and 62 decibels. Unfortunately, this study has not been replicated and raises several concerns regarding measurement of loudness and residual inhibition. Still, the approach was innovative and could potentially be helpful.

In a trial that compared a combined CBT/biofeedback-based intervention for tinnitus (12 sessions over 3 months) with waiting list controls, Weise et al. (2008b) reported significant improvements in tinnitus annoyance, diary ratings of loudness and in feelings of controllability in the treatment group. This result replicated a previous controlled trial by the same research group (Rief et al., 2005).

Some emergent findings regarding neurofeedback for tinnitus are of interest (Dohrmann et al., 2007; Hartmann et al., 2011). Information derived from the EEG is fed back to the patient, in real time. Aspects of the EEG that may be used include the delta frequency range (1.5–4 kHz), where increased power has been reported in tinnitus patients, and the alpha frequency range (8–12 kHz), where reduced power has been observed (Crocetti et al., 2011). Haller et al. (2010) used fMRI to train tinnitus patients to reduce activity in primary auditory cortical areas and report that two of six patients benefited. Initial results regarding neurofeedback for tinnitus are positive, but as no randomised placebo controlled trials have yet been reported, great caution is required in interpreting these results.

In summary, biofeedback has been sparsely researched with regard to its effect on tinnitus and is sometimes overly criticised (Howard, 2001; see Baguley and Andersson, 2002).

Relaxation training therapy

Relaxation therapy has long been viewed as an important part of tinnitus management. Therapy may be delivered in groups, or by individual instruction, or administered through use of tape recordings. Modest evidence for the efficacy of relaxation therapy is available (Andersson ad Lyttkens, 1999; Dobie, 1999). However, relaxation can be presented in many different ways, and it is therefore important to look at the evidence of how well relaxation works as the sole intervention. Commonly, relaxation is presented as one out of many treatment ingredients in the psychological management of tinnitus (Chapter 13), and in particular the method of applied relaxation (Öst, 1987), which forms part of the treatment protocol in Uppsala and Linköping, Sweden (Andersson, 2001). There are two controlled studies in which relaxation has been studied as an isolated treatment modality. There were only minor effects of relaxation in a study by Ireland et al. (1985), but this study was of limited statistical power (for meta-analysis of the findings, see Andersson and Lyttkens, 1999). In another small trial, Davies et al. (1995) compared cognitive therapy, passive relaxation and applied relaxation. Results showed a superior outcome of cognitive therapy and applied relaxation compared to the passive relaxation but, at a four-month follow-up, improvements had disappeared. Again, as previously stated, relaxation has often been included as an element of other treatment approaches (Dineen et al., 1997b), but from the literature it appears as if relaxation on its own is of marginal benefit for tinnitus patients. Results regarding applied relaxation fare better, but this is a more comprehensive treatment in which daily practice is encouraged. It is not an easy task to disentangle different approaches to relaxation, and, for example, Yoga (Kröner-Herwig et al., 1995) has been considered under the umbrella of relaxation therapy. Beneficial effects on immune functioning were observed in a study on the effects of progressive relaxation for tinnitus patients (Weber et al., 2002a).

Hypnotherapy

Hypnotherapy was first suggested as a therapeutic option for tinnitus by Pearson and Barnes (1950) and there has been background interest since that time (Dobie, 1999; Cope, 2008). There are striking similarities between hypnosis and some techniques used in cognitive behaviour therapy for tinnitus, but in the present context it is important to underscore the fact that hypnosis is a well-established treatment technique (Kihlstrom, 1985), which is not to be mistaken for the way hypnosis is presented in show business. The aim of hypnosis is to let the mind reach a more focused and relaxed state. In addition, hypnosis can alter somatic experience to the extent that pain is decreased. There are methods in which self-hypnosis is used, which for some patients is easier to grasp than the concept of being hypnotised. The literature regarding the evidence for hypnotherapy in tinnitus has been reviewed by Cope (2008), who concluded that there were indications of benefit for some patients, but that this was difficult to quantify. There are a number of case reports on the use of hypnosis for tinnitus (Marlowe, 1973; MacLeod-Morgan et al., 1982). In a Swedish open study, Brattberg (1983) described the application of hypnosis supplemented by tape-recorded relaxation instructions. She noted that 22 out of 32 patients benefited from the treatment, but no established outcome measures were used. In a crossover study, Marks et al. (1985) studied 14 patients and used three different forms of relaxation. Only five patients reported that the treatment had helped them. Interest in hypnosis has continued and Attias and co-workers in Israel conducted two studies on the effects of self-hypnosis. In the first study, they included 36 patients who were randomised to three groups: self-hypnosis, masking and waiting list control (Attias et al., 1990). The treatment groups received four sessions and then the outcome was evaluated. In addition, a two-month follow-up was included. Results showed that 73% were improved and that the results were maintained at follow-up. In a replication, the same research group included 44 patients and randomised them into three groups (Attias et al., 1993b). The main difference was that they did not include a waiting-list control group, but instead an attention control group who had the opportunity to discuss their tinnitus in a group without any direct intervention. All participants received five weekly sessions. The self-hypnosis group also received a cassette tape and were instructed to listen to the recording of the session and to practise. Again, self-hypnosis resulted in improvements, whereas the masking did not have any effect. Surprisingly, the attention control group improved on some measures. One problem with the studies by Attias et al. is that they did not utilise well-established or validated outcome measures. Other studies suggest that hypnosis can be considered in the treatment of tinnitus (Kaye et al., 1994; Mason and Rogerson, 1995; Mason et al., 1996).

Psychodynamic and supportive therapy

Although cognitive behavioural psychotherapy has dominated the psychotherapy research scene with regard to tinnitus and many other areas, psychodynamic approaches are widely spread worldwide and still represent a commonly practised form of psychotherapy (Fonagy, 2005). Psychodynamic approaches are heterogeneous, influenced to a variable extent by the writings of the founder of psychoanalysis, Sigmund Freud. In the main, therapy is targeted towards underlying conflicts and relationship issues. Concepts such as transference (patient's attitude towards the therapist) and countertransference (how the therapist reacts towards the patient) are central for treatment. Commonly, psychodynamic treatments are less symptom oriented (Weiner and Bornstein, 2009). No psychodynamically informed treatment has been developed for tinnitus, but early case studies have been published (Schneer, 1956; Weinshel, 1955). In spite of the lack of empirical support, it is likely that some aspects of psychodynamic and supportive therapies could be beneficial for tinnitus patients. For example, Granqvist et al. (2001) found a relation between attachment and tinnitus distress. Overall, interpersonal issues have not been targeted in treatment research on tinnitus and the role of nonspecific support is not clearly established.

Individual or group care?

The traditional setting for tinnitus therapy is one to one, with family members in attendance as the patient desires. In some clinics a form of group work has been instigated, wherein, following individual diagnostic assessment, the explanation of tinnitus can be effectively delivered to several persons (and family members) at once, and discussion of impacts and coping strategies involves peer sharing (Newman and Sandridge, 2006). There are benefits for the clinician, in that it can be cost effective, and for the patient, in that the peer support can be invaluable. There are some caveats however. Firstly, not all individuals will benefit from group care, and a tinnitus group session needs setting in a framework of stepped care, so that patients needing more intensive and individual therapy can be identified and graduate into such care. Secondly, the group dynamics need careful management, and the facilitator should be experienced in running groups as well as carrying out tinnitus therapy. Tinnitus patients can be very angry and distressed, and exposure to one another's emotional pain can be destructive if not handled carefully. Finally, in the authors' experience, it is a rare tinnitus patient who does not vouchsafe personal information in an individual session: indeed, it is often through such vulnerability that progress can be made. Such exposure is much less frequent in group work and so potentially something is lost in that context.

Another issue is that of having students or other observers in the clinic. Tinnitus patients are often very keen that trainee Audiologists, Otolaryngologists or Psychologists are learning about tinnitus, but the dynamic of the clinic will be changed. Care should be taken to get the explicit permission of the patient and introduce the student, with an explanation: 'This is my student *name*, they are here to learn about tinnitus, and they are watching me rather than you' may be helpful. There is a benefit to have observers in the clinic, be they students or support staff: many tinnitus clinicians work on their own and would optimally have others in the clinic who can share the emotional burden. This is not, however, a substitute for clinical supervision, meaning having someone with whom the tinnitus clinician can debrief themselves, which is good practice in all aspects of clinical work.

Summary

Numerous treatments have been tried in an attempt to cure or ameliorate tinnitus. Sadly few seem to have any beneficial effect and even those that at first glance seem to help rarely stand up to rigorous scientific scrutiny. Surgical treatments of nonsyndromic tinnitus are rarely justified, with the notable exception of cochlear implantation for profoundly deaf tinnitus sufferers. There have been tantalisingly optimistic results from drug therapy, particularly with lidocaine and some psychoactive medications. More research is needed in this area. Treatment with maskers has failed to demonstrate long-term success but does allow some patients to obtain temporary respite from their symptoms. Biofeedback and relaxation training are related methods that do offer some help, but evidence that they work as standalone treatments is poor and they probably need to be embedded within a more comprehensive management plan. Despite the poor evidence base for genuine effectiveness of conventional treatments, the strong placebo effect in tinnitus management ensures that many people treated with these modalities do appear to derive benefit. The simple fact that a health care professional is trying to help, and doing so in a caring and understanding fashion, cannot be underestimated.

Chapter 14

Tinnitus retraining therapy

The publication of the Jastreboff neurophysiological model (Jastreboff, 1990) represented a synthesis of knowledge about the auditory system, and of related systems of emotion and reaction, and how these are involved in the development and persistence of distressing tinnitus (Chapter 9). Published as it was in a neuroscience journal, it would have been read and cited by that community, but it is unlikely that it would have attracted such widespread interest, particularly from the clinical community, if it had not been for the interaction between Pawel Jastreboff and Jonathan Hazell, an English otolaryngologist who had long specialised in tinnitus. Their early discussions had resulted in three review papers (Hazell and Jastreboff, 1990; Hazell, 1990a, 1990b) that contained information about the medical and surgical management of tinnitus, and also on the practical, clinical implications of the neurophysiological model. Further influence upon the development of a clinical protocol congruent with the Jastreboff model was provided by Jacqui Sheldrake, a UK-based audiologist who had lengthy experience in the treatment of tinnitus patients.

A detailed consideration of the practical implications of the Jastreboff model was undertaken by Jastreboff and Hazell (1993), this paper being more accessible to clinicians than the original publication (Jastreboff, 1990). Fundamental to the neurophysiological model is the concept that tinnitus is perceived because of a failure of filtering mechanisms at a subcortical level and that the symptom becomes distressing because of the involvement of systems of emotion and reaction, the limbic system and autonomic nervous systems, respectively (Chapter 9). The implication, therefore, is that the filtering mechanisms might be modified or retrained so that they once more become effective at filtering the tinnitus. Furthermore, the emotional and reactive components of tinnitus complaint might be reduced by influence upon the meaning of the tinnitus. Both then (Jastreboff and Hazell, 1993) and since (Jastreboff and Jastreboff, 2003; Jastreboff and Hazell, 2004; Jastreboff, 2007), the originators of tinnitus retraining therapy have promoted the theory that the development of tinnitus-related distress involves a traditional conditioned response paradigm.

Tinnitus: A Multidisciplinary Approach, Second Edition. David Baguley, Gerhard Andersson, Don McFerran and Laurence McKenna.
© 2013 David Baguley, Gerhard Andersson, Don McFerran and Laurence McKenna.
Published 2013 by Blackwell Publishing Ltd.

In their 1993 consideration of the clinical implications of the neurophysiological model Jastreboff and Hazell proposed intervention for distressing tinnitus with a protocol that should include:

- 'Cognitive therapy' (Jastreboff and Hazell, 1993, p. 13), which they also entitled 'directive counselling' to facilitate understanding of tinnitus.
- Sound therapy to promote the plasticity of brainstem filtering systems using white noise delivered by ear-level devices.

This approach was first described as 'tinnitus retraining therapy' in the mid-1990s (Hazell, 1996). Criticism was soon evident, initially pointing out that white noise when transformed by the human ear canal and by any significant hearing loss no longer exhibited the flat frequency characteristics defining it as 'white' (Baguley et al., 1997), followed by critiques of the fundamental premises of the counselling technique (Wilson et al., 1998; Kröner-Herwig et al., 2000). The theories and implementation of tinnitus retraining therapy have evolved somewhat since its initial conception. For example, the insistence on white noise was dropped and later protocols recommended broadband sound therapy (Jastreboff and Hazell, 2004). Therefore it would seem prudent to concentrate on the later, and presumably evolutionarily more advanced, works. There is a difference between the neurophysiological model and its clinical implementation as tinnitus retraining therapy and it is important to recognise that many clinicians offer a management strategy that they call tinnitus retraining therapy because it is to a greater or lesser extent based on the neurophysiological model. However, in many cases the therapeutic process does not adhere to the fairly strict principles espoused by Jastreboff and Hazell. Because of these terminological inexactitudes, tinnitus retraining therapy is sometimes criticised unfairly, when the treatment that is being performed is not true tinnitus retraining therapy.

Clinical protocol of tinnitus retraining therapy

While tinnitus retraining therapy proponents often assert that it has not changed since its inception, publications since 1995 have elaborated and expanded the protocol and have clarified the associated terminology. In particular, the early use of 'cognitive therapy' to describe directive counselling ceased entirely (Jastreboff, 1999). The current definition of tinnitus retraining therapy consists of two elements: directive counselling and sound therapy. The only means by which one could become a formal tinnitus retraining therapy practitioner was to attend a training course with one of the originators (Henry et al., 2002a; Jastreboff and Jastreboff, 2003). Since 2005 tinnitus retraining courses have not been run in the UK and there is currently only one available course, in the USA. Although this does little to reassure one about the independence of validation studies, it does at least ensure purity of clinical practice. Initial research on tinnitus retraining therapy was not conducted following a published structured manual and it is often claimed that the papers describing tinnitus retraining therapy are insufficient for its implementation (Jastreboff and Jastreboff, 2000). A full manual became available in 2004 and it was hoped that this would foster more rigorous and replicable research (Jastreboff and Hazell, 2004).

Table 14.1 Patient categories and suggested instrumentation. (Based on Jastreboff and Jastreboff (2003)).

Category		Instrumentation
Category 0	Tinnitus weak or short lasting	No instruments
Category 1	Bothersome tinnitus	Sound generators
Category 2	Tinnitus and hearing loss	Combination instruments or hearing aids
Category 3	Hyperacusis with or without tinnitus:	
	Without hearing loss	Sound generators
	With hearing loss	Combination instruments or sound generators followed by hearing aids
Category 4	Hyperacusis or tinnitus with sound-induced exacerbation	Sound generators or combination instruments

A detailed history is taken of tinnitus and hyperacusis, taking appropriate steps to identify and treat those patients who require specific surgical or medical intervention. Formal tinnitus retraining therapy questionnaires are available for this purpose (Henry et al., 2002b), facilitating a standardised, structured interview and enabling the subsequent allocation into tinnitus categories. Suitable audiological assessments are also conducted, including pure tone audiometry from 125 Hz to 8000 Hz, estimation of loudness discomfort levels over the same frequency range and tympanometry. However, in contrast to masking treatment, assessment of residual inhibition is not recommended (Henry et al., 2002b). The patient is then identified as belonging to one of five categories (Jastreboff and Jastreboff, 2003) (Table 14.1) described in the protocol.

Patients in Category 0 do not have tinnitus with a severe impact, and treatment is titrated to that involving counselling and the use of environmental sound for sound enrichment. Category 1 patients receive retraining counselling (Jastreboff, 1998) and ear-level sound generators set with their output below but close to the perceived tinnitus intensity. This point, at which the external sound source and the tinnitus appear to be at the same level, is referred to as the 'mixing point'. Patients in Category 2 have a hearing loss in addition to tinnitus, though the level at which such an associated hearing loss becomes clinically relevant has not been clearly defined. Category 2 patients are treated with hearing aids or combination instruments, which incorporate a hearing aid and a wideband sound generator, in conjunction with counselling. Categories 3 and 4 include patients with hyperacusis, either without or with marked exacerbation on sound exposure, respectively, and are treated with a desensitising programme of sound (see Table 12.1), with an appropriate protocol for each category.

A somewhat expanded version of this categorisation was presented by Henry et al. (2002a). Unfortunately, neither the categorisation nor the structured interview has been validated scientifically, which is essential if the tinnitus retraining therapy interview is to be utilised by the wider tinnitus community. The difficulties performing categorisation as part of tinnitus retraining therapy was acknowledged by Jastreboff and Jastreboff (2003, p. 331), who wrote: 'The previously mentioned categories provide general approach guidance, and patients might be on the border of two categories.' Despite these criticisms, the approach taken to categorise patients was a welcome innovation in the tinnitus community. Tinnitus retraining therapy also recognises that categorisation can change during the natural history of the patient's condition or during the therapeutic management process. Thus it is important to regularly re-evaluate each patient, as a change of category may require a change of treatment plan. The specific treatment given to each patient is detailed below. Although the treatment varies according to the patient's category one common element is directive counselling (Jastreboff, 1998, p. 92) to teach the patient about:

- The physiology of the auditory system
- The basic principles of brain function with focus on the mechanisms of perception, attention and emotions
- The role of the autonomic nervous system
- The mechanism behind creating and retraining conditioned reflexes.

This introduction to auditory neuroscience can be time consuming and the expertise required is considerable. When it is done well, directive counselling helps to educate the patient, which, in turn, helps to demystify tinnitus and hence to remove negative associations with tinnitus. The use of sound therapy alone without directive counselling is not sufficient (Jastreboff and Jastreboff, 2000), demonstrating that the counselling is a vital component of tinnitus retraining therapy. In tinnitus retraining therapy the use of sound devices is not obligatory, but sound input is deemed necessary to achieve habituation (Jastreboff and Jastreboff, 2000). Unsurprisingly, therefore, sound generators are used in most cases, with 70% being fitted with an instrument from a restricted range of sound generators approved by Jastreboff (Jastreboff, 2000; Henry et al., 2002b). Devices are always fitted bilaterally according to the guidelines produced by Jastreboff (2000) and should have open ear moulds (Henry et al., 2002b) to avoid occluding the ear canal and creating a conductive hearing loss. When using sound generators in the management of tinnitus the volume is adjusted to the mixing point at the beginning of the day and is then not touched for the rest of the day. When using sound generators for categories 3 or 4 patients with significant hyperacusis, different instructions are issued. These patients are advised to set their sound generator to a level that is always just audible. Therefore, as the environmental noise levels fluctuate the patient needs to regularly readjust the output level of their devices. Instructions are given to use the sound generators for at least eight hours per day or hearing aids (including combination units) for all waking hours. All patients undergoing tinnitus retraining therapy are advised to avoid silence and to enrich their sound environment. This can include all means of auditory stimulation, such as bedside sound machines, music, water features, wind chimes and so on (Jastreboff, 2000). It is also recommended that patients should have an enriched sound environment during the night (Jastreboff and Jastreboff, 2003). The tinnitus retraining therapy protocol requires that the patient adheres to the regimen for 12–24 months and specifically points out that habituation is a long-term process (Jastreboff et al., 1996). Regular follow-up appointments are recommended (Jastreboff and Jastreboff, 2003).

Criticism of tinnitus retraining therapy

A number of criticisms of the neurophysiological model, and of tinnitus retraining ther- apy, have been voiced. Wilson et al. (1998) noted that written descriptions of the neuro- physiological model (citing Jastreboff and Hazell, 1993) use terms such as 'attention', 'coping' and 'perception' in an ill-defined and obscure manner. They further asserted that the directive counselling component of tinnitus retraining therapy is a 'weak' form of cognitive therapy (Wilson et al., 1998), given that the explicit objective is to change beliefs. These criticisms called into question the adequacy and novelty of the Jastreboff neurophysiological model, which Wilson et al. (1998, p. 70) rather damned with faint praise: 'We are in broad agreement with the neurophysiological model – to state other- wise would be to refute the very basis of modern psychology'. An opposing viewpoint is that the neurophysiological model may indeed be somewhat simplistic, but this can be viewed as a positive attribute as it facilitates communication of the concepts to patients (Baguley, 2002). A more disturbing possibility is that the model is incorrect and that there are missing links in the description of unconditioned stimuli and conditioned responses, as has been suggested by researchers in the psychological community (McKenna, 2004; Andersson, 2002a). Further, although less cogent, criticism was forthcoming from Kröner-Herwig et al. (2000), who again criticised the neurophysiological model for lack of novelty and inadequacy and advised caution regarding the use of tinnitus retraining therapy, describing public praise for the technique as 'premature' (Kröner-Herwig et al., 2000, p. 77). The directive counselling technique contains elements of persuasion and so could, in the hands of inexperienced clinicians, be misunderstood and even insensitive to the idiosyncrasies of the individual patient. The literature on tinnitus retraining therapy acknowledges the deep distress experienced by some tinnitus patients, but it does not fully or explicitly take this into account in directive counselling. Onward appropriate referral to other clinicians is a critical issue in tinnitus management. According to Henry et al. (2002b, p. 526), 'Audiologists must use their professional judgement to assess whether a tinnitus patient should be referred to a counsellor for a psychological or psychi- atric evaluation.' Clearly, this is not evidence-based advice and more careful assessments could easily be recommended using the readily available validated self-report screening instruments. Given the natural course of depression and the long duration of treatment in tinnitus retraining therapy, it is plausible that at least some of the effects of tinnitus retraining therapy could be attributed to a nonspecific antidepressant effect. This would be relatively straightforward to determine in trials on tinnitus retraining therapy by the incorporation of psychiatric assessments. The usefulness of both the neurophysiological model and tinnitus retraining therapy to clinicians is as difficult to ascertain as their rele- vance to patients. At its outset, the neurophysiological model represented, and still does to this day, a clinically useful synthesis of knowledge about the human auditory system and of reciprocal links with systems of reaction and emotion. It has been widely taught and understood by audiologists and its overall value appears good. Of tinnitus retraining therapy specifically, things are less clear. Henry et al. (2002b) claim that tinnitus retrain- ing therapy is in use in over 100 centres worldwide, which is impressive until one realises that there are approximately 240 audiology centres in the UK alone. Thus, the adoption of tinnitus retraining therapy in pure form is not wide and the insistence that one can practise tinnitus retraining therapy only if trained by one of the originators is not likely to further that adoption.

Evidence of efficacy

There is a dearth of robust experimental evidence regarding the efficacy of tinnitus retraining therapy. Most of the initial evidence comprised case series studies, was published in conference proceedings and had not undergone a proper peer review process. Subsequently there have been several randomised controlled trials purporting to test tinnitus retraining therapy. When many of these are examined, however, they turn out to be treatment protocols based on the Jastreboff neurophysiological model but not adhering to the full definition of tinnitus retraining therapy.

A Cochrane review (Phillips and McFerran, 2010) investigated tinnitus retraining therapy and an initial literature search identified 335 potential articles on the subject. The majority of these were excluded, mainly because they were not randomised controlled trials. Six articles were identified as possible studies to include but four were excluded because the treatment that had been administered did not constitute tinnitus retraining therapy as defined by Jastreboff (1999). The two remaining articles (Henry et al., 2006b, 2006c) turned out to be separate reports on a single study that tested tinnitus retraining therapy against tinnitus masking. This study was subjected to the Cochrane process and was criticised with respect to using a form of quasi-randomisation: the first patient in the study was randomly allocated to a treatment arm and subsequent patients were then allocated in an alternating fashion. The conclusion of the Cochrane review was that tinnitus retraining therapy appeared much more effective than tinnitus masking but the study quality was low.

Since the publication of the Cochrane review on tinnitus retraining therapy there have been two further studies published that adhere to the rules of tinnitus retraining therapy and use adequate scientific rigour. Bauer and Brozoski (2011) compared tinnitus retraining therapy with group counselling and placebo sound therapy. Because of small numbers of participants they used a process of urn randomisation (see Wei and Lachin, 1988, for further details of this type of randomisation process) to ensure balanced groups. Both tinnitus retraining therapy and control groups showed improvement, with the tinnitus retraining therapy group showing a significantly larger treatment effect. Zetterqvist Westin et al. (2011) studied the effects of acceptance and commitment therapy against tinnitus retraining therapy and a waiting list control group. This study is by far the most rigorous study testing tinnitus retraining therapy to date. The main outcome measure was Tinnitus Handicap Inventory scores and participants in both the acceptance and commitments therapy and tinnitus retraining therapy groups showed improvement, with 54.5% of patients in the former group experiencing a statistically reliable improvement compared to 20% in the latter.

The available evidence suggests that tinnitus retraining therapy is effective but perhaps not as beneficial as the latest forms of psychological intervention. Clearly further work in this area is required.

Summary

The contributions of Pawel Jastreboff and Jonathan Hazell to tinnitus research and therapy have been enormous. The concept that one had to look beyond the classical auditory system, or indeed the cochlea, for an understanding of tinnitus was radical for many in the field. This change of viewpoint has had a lasting impact upon both professional and public knowledge about tinnitus. The neurophysiological model has now been utilised in teaching many audiologists and has been widely applied to tinnitus therapy. There is some limited evidence that it is an effective method of managing tinnitus. The longer-term contribution of tinnitus retraining therapy is hard to determine at the present time and may be somewhat constrained by an insistence that trainees should be taught about tinnitus retraining therapy only by its originators. As one of these two originators is no longer teaching the technique very few clinicians outside North America are now learning how to perform tinnitus retraining therapy. However, there remains the potential for clinicians and researchers with a holistic and neuroscientific-based understanding of tinnitus to build upon these foundations to the benefit of patients and clinicians alike.

Chapter 15

A cognitive behavioural treatment programme

Cognitive behaviour therapy (CBT) is a psychological treatment approach directed at identifying and modifying unhelpful thoughts and behaviours (Barlow, 2001). CBT rests on a model of psychological distress that underscores the importance of thinking or cognition and emotion. The importance of behaviour change is also a part of CBT. The therapeutic relation between therapist and patient in cognitive behaviour therapy is collaborative in the sense that an outline of each session and the treatment as a whole are negotiated; the therapeutic process aims to equip patients with the tools for self help rather than regarding them as passive recipients of treatment. Motivation to change habits and to alter behaviour is crucial, and it is made clear to the patient that work is required for the treatment to have any effect. The focus is on applying behavioural and cognitive techniques in real-life settings, and CBT often involves testing out coping strategies when facing difficult situations. The efficacy of cognitive behaviour therapy for psychological conditions such as anxiety and depression has been clearly demonstrated (Persons et al., 2001); the approach has also been found to be effective in the management of patients afflicted with somatic conditions, such as chronic pain (Turk et al., 1983) and insomnia (Morin, 1993). The value of CBT in these other areas provides an inspiration for its application to tinnitus.

The cognitive behavioural treatment model and its rationale

The cognitive behaviour therapy approach to tinnitus management is based on a cognitive behavioural model of tinnitus that has been outlined by several authors (see Chapter 8), but the first steps were taken by British psychologist Richard Hallam. Some early work was also conducted by Scott and colleagues (1985) in Sweden and by Sweetow (1984) in the USA. The Swedish group, however, had a strong behavioural emphasis in their work. The model proposed by Hallam et al. (1984) provides the main source of

Tinnitus: A Multidisciplinary Approach, Second Edition. David Baguley, Gerhard Andersson, Don McFerran and Laurence McKenna.
© 2013 David Baguley, Gerhard Andersson, Don McFerran and Laurence McKenna.
Published 2013 by Blackwell Publishing Ltd.

inspiration for the use of cognitive behaviour therapy in the management of tinnitus patients. Their psychological model of tinnitus (see Chapter 7) suggested that the natural history of tinnitus is characterised by the process of habituation. In seeking to understand tinnitus it is therefore important to investigate factors that impede habituation, for example arousal and novelty. The model suggests that psychological treatment should focus on reducing patients' arousal and on changing the emotional significance of the tinnitus. A stress–diathesis model has been proposed for understanding the severity of tinnitus (Andersson and McKenna, 1998; Schulman, 1995) and is used in clinical practice. This suggests that the strength of the stress interacts with the person's vulnerability to stress. For example, a 'vulnerable' person might develop tinnitus distress following the onset of relatively 'mild' tinnitus, whereas a more stress-tolerant person might bear louder tinnitus before seeking help. Vulnerability does not equal 'psychiatric disturbances', but can result in all sorts of stresses in life, including somatic conditions that may exist before the onset of tinnitus.

The model proposed by Hallam et al. (1984) stresses the central role of beliefs in the distress experienced by tinnitus patients. Thoughts and beliefs about tinnitus are important and can strengthen the association between negative emotions and tinnitus. The meaning attached to tinnitus influences how annoying it is perceived to be. Many tinnitus patients report difficulties with concentration. Hence it can be suspected that tinnitus 'demands attention'. When using cognitive behaviour therapy in the treatment of tinnitus an effort is made to help the patient to accept tinnitus and to adopt the attitude that it is not deserving of all the attention it gets (Andersson and Kaldo, 2006). Patients are helped to distinguish between futile attempts to try to control something that cannot be controlled (as often is the case with loudness of tinnitus) and successful ways of controlling reactions and emotions when faced with difficulties (e.g. the consequences of tinnitus).

A treatment package based on the cognitive behaviour therapy approach is outlined in Table 15.1. It is usually presented in six to 10 sessions on a weekly basis. Although individual treatment often is required, cognitive behaviour therapy can also be successfully used in a small group setting with tinnitus patients (Kröner-Herwig et al., 1995). Homework assignments are necessary for the treatment to make a difference in the patient's life. As the treatment focuses on the ways in which tinnitus affects everyday activities, such as work, family and leisure activities, it is important to obtain information about these areas and to encourage the patient to try out the skills taught in therapy in these relevant situations. Another important aspect of the treatment is the simple notion that 'What is good for life in general, is usually good for your ability to cope with tinnitus.' This includes living a healthy life, with respect to food, exercise, social contacts, etc. One related aspect is that it may be important for the tinnitus patient to establish regular routines in life. Before the onset of tinnitus, it might have been possible to have irregular working hours and sleep patterns, but often adaptation to tinnitus requires regular habits, in particular when it comes to maintaining sleep. As the effects of psychological treatment of tinnitus are most apparent directly after the treatment, it is crucial to schedule follow-up visits, for example at three months after the end of treatment, to assess tinnitus distress at this point. Follow-up sessions are also used to summarise the treatment and to encourage continued use of treatment strategies, in order to prevent a return of tinnitus distress.

Table 15.1 Overview of a cognitive behavioural treatment programme (not all aspects will apply to every clinical situation).

- Structured clinical interview
- Treatment rationale and information
- Treatment
  - Applied relaxation (progressive relaxation, short progressive relaxation, cue-controlled relaxation and rapid relaxation)
  - Positive imagery, sound enrichment by means of external sounds, hearing tactics and advice about noise sensitivity
  - Modification of negative thoughts and beliefs
  - Behavioural sleep management
  - Advice about concentration difficulties, exercises of concentration (mindfulness) and physical activity
- Relapse prevention
- Questionnaire assessment
- Follow-up (personal interview)

Psychological assessment

At least one medical consultation including audiological tests should precede the first meeting with the patient who is referred for cognitive behaviour therapy. This is to provide 'a solid medical context' within which to provide the psychological therapy. Then the cognitive behaviour therapist interviews the patient using a structured interview including questions on tinnitus history and characteristics, psychological and physical consequences (e.g. sleep disturbance), exacerbating and relieving factors, related symptoms and previous treatments (see Chapter 8). Typically, 1.5 hours is needed to interview the patient. The aim of the interview is to establish good therapeutic contact and to collect enough information in order to be able to decide if the patient is suitable, or not, for psychological treatment. This is typically done in the format of a functional analysis (Sturmey, 1996), which for tinnitus involves collecting information about factors that influence the tinnitus annoyance and investigating causal links between the things that the patient does and experiences and how tinnitus is perceived. In this first session a rationale is presented that incorporates the idiosyncrasies of the patient and also gives some preliminary goals of the treatment (McKenna, 1987). The end result of the interview can be expressed in terms of a case formulation where the major problems, goals and obstacles are presented (Persons and Davidson, 2001). The case formulation can later be revisited with new information, from self-report questionnaires, for example, supplementing the information obtained in the interview (see Chapter 11).

Applied relaxation

Applied relaxation is a set of methods by which the patient is gradually taught to relax quickly and to use self-control over bodily and mental sensations (Öst, 1987). The purpose of relaxation is to deal with the consequences of tinnitus and not to reduce tinnitus loudness (for a detailed description see Andersson and Kaldo, 2006). It is important to point this out at an early stage, as the patient who expects a reduction in tinnitus loudness is likely to be disappointed. There are some patients for whom applied relaxation does decrease tinnitus loudness, and such experiences should of course not be dismissed as irrelevant. It should be noted, however, that the opposite can happen initially, with temporary increases in loudness when learning relaxation. Experience suggests that it is best to prepare the patient that the most likely outcome is no change in loudness. Interestingly, there are cases in which a clear association with loudness and tension is observed, supporting the somatic modulation hypothesis of tinnitus (Cacace, 2003; Møller and Shore, 2011).

Applied relaxation can be compared to any other skill, such as learning to swim, ride a bike or drive a car, in that it takes time and practice to learn, but once it has been mastered it can be used everywhere. The goal is to obtain a relaxed physical state. This can help promote a relaxed state of mind and so break the vicious circle of tension leading to more focus on tinnitus. Learning applied relaxation training is usually the first task that the patient is assigned in the treatment protocol described by the authors of this book and in use in Linköping and in London. Although other CBT clinicians (Henry and Wilson, 2001) do not use relaxation techniques to the same extent as UK and Swedish psychologists, proponents argue that it has considerable face validity in tinnitus management and represents an easily learnt sense of control for patients. The technique is taught in stages over four to six sessions, and the last stage is practised for the rest of the treatment once it is mastered. Usually, four components are included:

- Progressive relaxation (tense and release body parts)
- Release-only relaxation without tension
- Cue-controlled relaxation (controlled breathing)
- Rapid relaxation in everyday situations.

Imagery techniques are taught in association with the relaxation training.

Although there are few studies on the differential effects of different forms of relaxation for tinnitus (see Chapter 13), there are indications that the combination of elements of applied relaxation is slightly superior to other alternatives such as progressive relaxation (Davies et al., 1995). It should be mentioned that there have been more recent studies on biofeedback as well that indicate good outcomes (Rief et al., 2005; Weise et al., 2008a).

Distraction and focusing

The use of attention-diversion techniques, imagery by using 'inner pictures' and exercises directly aimed at reinterpreting tinnitus as something less painful (Henry and Wilson, 2001) form part of the treatment protocol. The goal is for the patient to learn these techniques in the clinic and then to apply the skills in real-life settings. Exposure techniques, inspired by the principles used in the treatment of phobias (Zlomke and Davis III, 2008), are also often included. These techniques have been used with chronic pain patients (Linton et al., 2002) and it appears that they may be applicable for a proportion of tinnitus patients. Strong emotional reactions, particularly involving fear and avoidance, are sometimes associated with tinnitus. They can lead to a negative view of tinnitus and can occasionally develop into panic-like attacks when the patient seeks to escape from tinnitus. Apart from advice about sound enrichment, the programme deals with adverse reactions to silence (when this is a problem) and this is an instance where exposure techniques can be helpful. A list of distraction techniques was recommended by Henry and Wilson (2001). For example, one such technique is 'thought stopping', which involves deliberate attempts to suppress thoughts about tinnitus. As stated by Henry and Wilson (2001), the idea is not so much to stop thinking about the tinnitus as it is to learn to direct attention both to and from the tinnitus. It is questionable if this works in the long term and, theoretically, it could even be counterproductive (Wegner, 1994). In the short term, however, there is evidence to suggest that it can be a helpful strategy. Problems with concentration are often a source of great distress for the tinnitus sufferer and are targeted in the treatment. Methods for improving concentration and memory training have been developed by neuropsychologists (Wilson, 2008). The techniques involve structuring material to ensure encoding (e.g. to focus on one element at a time), elaboration (thinking things over, maybe using notes) and retrieval of information (e.g. using hints to aid memory). As yet these techniques have not been evaluated systematically with tinnitus patients.

Sound enrichment

The therapeutic implications of sound and the patient's attitude towards masking, partial masking, silence and fluctuations in environmental sounds are important considerations within the treatment. This element was introduced following the development of tinnitus retraining therapy (Jastreboff and Hazell, 2004), but in cognitive behaviour therapy specific tinnitus instruments, such as sound generators, are rarely used. Sound enrichment can include analysis of sound environments in the patient's daily life, tapes or CDs, but, more importantly, advice and analysis of fluctuations in tinnitus loudness and explanation of the risks associated with trying to mask (i.e. cover) the tinnitus. Thoughts and beliefs in relation to sounds are an integral part of the cognitive therapy component of the treatment. For example, selective attention is described and exemplified by illustrating that tinnitus can either be masked or be made very noticeable in the same environment, depending on whether attention is directed towards or away from it (Andersson, 2002a). In some cases the use of sound enrichment can represent a form of avoidance that maintains anxiety about tinnitus and efforts are made to help the patient reduce this avoidance and become more tolerant of their tinnitus.

Sleep management

Sleep hygiene, bedtime and worry-time restriction, relaxation and cognitive restructuring can be helpful for patients with sleep problems (McKenna, 2000; McKenna and Daniel, 2006). These methods are tailored according to the special needs of the tinnitus patient. Obviously, sleep management in the case of tinnitus must include the role of sounds and how to handle wake-ups. In general, psychological treatment of insomnia often consists of stimulus-control techniques (such as going to bed only when tired and/or getting up at

Table 15.2 Components of a sleep management programme.

- Week 1: Information about insomnia and sleep. Introduction to sleep restriction and stimulus control strategy I
- Week 2: Sleep restriction and stimulus control strategies II–VI. Information about sleep medication
- Week 3: Sleep restriction and stimulus control strategies continued. Information on negative automatic thoughts and introduction to cognitive restructuring
- Week 4: Sleep restriction and stimulus control strategies continued. Further elaboration on cognitive techniques.
- Week 5: Sleep restriction and stimulus control strategy repetition. Continued use of cognitive restructuring techniques. Information about sleep hygiene
- Relapse prevention

---

the same time every day), sleep restriction (e.g. staying in bed only for an expected sleep period rather than lying in), relaxation techniques, sleep hygiene and cognitive behaviour therapy programmes. The latter often combines approaches such as stimulus control and cognitive restructuring (Morin et al., 1999). An example of a comprehensive sleep management programme is outlined in Table 15.2. Briefer consultations, however, may also be beneficial for some patients (Hauri, 1993) and sleep management is a field for which self-help methods have been successfully applied (Mimeault and Morin, 1999). Two meta-analyses have documented the effects of stimulus control therapy, sleep restriction, relaxation and a number of different educational and cognitive strategies (Morin et al., 1994; Murtagh and Greenwood, 1995). Compared with pharmacological treatment protocols, studies have shown that nonpharmacological interventions are perceived as not only more acceptable but they also produce more lasting improvements (Morin et al., 1999; Smith et al., 2002). The efficacy of multicomponent approaches has been found to give slightly better results than single-component treatments (Morin et al., 1999). To date, there is no controlled outcome study of insomnia management specifically targeted towards tinnitus patients with insomnia.

Hearing tactics

The field of hearing tactics deals with different ways of facilitating communication, such as optimizing signals and using conversational strategies (Brooks, 1989). A cognitive behavioural adaptation of hearing tactics has been developed (Andersson, 2000c) and has been found to have positive results in controlled trials (Andersson et al., 1995b). It is important to note that hearing tactics do not represent an alternative to hearing aid fitting but, rather, should be viewed as one of many ways to assist the hearing-impaired person. A condensed form of hearing tactics is commonly used in tinnitus treatments. A key feature is communication skills training, in which the participant is encouraged to focus on one person and concentrate on communication with that individual. This includes proper positioning in relation to the other person, moderately expressive body language and being active in the conversation. When hearing fails, repair strategies are practised (Tye-Murray, 1991), including ways of handling missing information and asking for confirmation if the participant has understood things correctly. This necessitates active listening and focusing on meaning instead of the details of the message. Assertive responses are practised, such as informing others about the hearing loss and anticipating their reactions. Moreover, waiting for your turn, reinforcing the behaviour of the communication partner and the advantages of talking on a topic about which you have knowledge are highlighted. Distribution of a leaflet with advice on communication with hearing-impaired people that is to be presented to relatives is set as a homework assignment. The role of relatives and the ways they can help is discussed further (e.g. identification of the social skills needed in good communication).

Cognitive therapy

Cognitive restructuring of thoughts and beliefs associated with tinnitus is a central and necessary feature of cognitive behaviour therapy with tinnitus patients. Patients are helped to identify the content of their thoughts and are taught ways to challenge or control those thoughts that are unhelpful or even inaccurate. It is important to note that this is not equal to 'positive thinking'. Some patients find the cognitive model difficult to understand at first, and it is therefore crucial that time is taken to educate them and to check that the model is understood properly. As with many other physical symptoms, tinnitus can be accompanied by negative beliefs that are not necessarily irrational. On the surface, beliefs such as 'I have tinnitus', 'It will never go away' or 'I shall never hear silence again' are reasonably accurate. Although the beliefs first expressed can be correct, it is sometimes the case that more catastrophic beliefs exist in the background. This can be in the form of 'I shall never be able to enjoy life again' or 'Tinnitus affects me very badly; I must be a very weak person'. Such unrealistic beliefs are targeted by cognitive therapy (Persons et al., 2001). It is common practice to combine the challenging of unrealistic beliefs with education about the natural course of tinnitus and a comprehensive assessment of quality of life in general. The truth is that most patients have at least a part of their life that is not affected by tinnitus. However, the clinician needs to identify and distinguish irrational beliefs from accurate ones, and in particular to be careful not to go too fast when evoking thoughts (e.g. core beliefs) that might be very distressing for the patient to discover. For many patients, it is relatively straightforward to discover the content of their beliefs about tinnitus.

Relapse prevention

Relapse prevention includes a discussion of risk factors for developing more severe tinnitus and hearing loss, and devising a plan for what to do should the tinnitus become worse (Henry and Wilson, 2001). High-risk situations may also involve psychosocial aspects, such as work-related problems and marital difficulties. As part of the secondary prevention, the importance of regular practice of therapeutic techniques is covered. During treatment, or immediately afterwards, tinnitus can become temporarily louder and more noticeable. This effect, however, is often temporary and the beneficial effects of treatment outweigh the small fluctuation in loudness the patient may perceive. One crucial aspect of cognitive behaviour therapy is to foster generalisation from the treatment setting to the daily life of the patient. One way to secure continued treatment gains is to refer to matters of everyday life during treatment and to discuss how the patient can use the skills taught in treatment in different settings in life (e.g. on holiday). Lastly, one way to prevent relapse is to make sure that the patient is not abandoned once treatment has ended. Therefore the plan should include identifying whom to contact if the annoyance increases again.

Self-help and use of the Internet

It is interesting and important to reflect on the idea that CBT ultimately seeks to equip the patient with the tools to solve his or her own problems. In this sense CBT directs the patient towards self-help. The idea of self-help in further pushed by the fact that there is a relatively small supply of CB therapists compared with the demand for their services. This is particularly true in the field of tinnitus. There has therefore been some interest in the idea of minimal therapist contact and self-help treatments for tinnitus. For example, Kröner-Herwig et al. (2003) found that two minimal contact interventions led to positive results with reductions in disability.

There is a huge market in self-help books for a vast range of medical and psychological problems. A substantial proportion of these books are based on CBT. These books have the advantage of being easily accessible and there is evidence that they can be helpful (Watkins and Clum, 2008) and, overall, self-help is well validated in outcome trials (Cuijpers et al., 2010). In parts of the UK where there is little provision of formal psychological therapy such books are available on prescription, from local libraries, for common mental health problems such as anxiety and depression. There are only a few CBT-based self-help books for tinnitus (e.g. Henry and Wilson, 2002; Kaldo and Andersson, 2004; McKenna et al., 2010). The effectiveness of using one of these books (Kaldo and Andersson, 2004) compared with a waiting list control was assessed by Kaldo et al. (2007). The use of the self-help book was supported by seven brief (weekly) phone calls during which the therapist evaluated treatment progress and provided advice on how to continue the programme. Although there was a 20% attrition rate from the treatment group the study revealed both statistically significant and clinically significant improvements associated with the self-help programme. The outcome was measured using tinnitus complaint questionnaires (i.e. TRQ and THI), a questionnaire of emotional state (HADS), a measure of insomnia (ISI) and a number of visual analogue scales (see Chapter 11 for more information on these instruments). The subjects in the waiting list control later went on to receive the self-help book but with less therapist support. They then also showed significant reductions in tinnitus distress, although again there was a high attrition rate. The improvements observed in this study were maintained at one year follow-up. The effectiveness of Henry and Wilson's (2002) self-help book was investigated by Malouff et al. (2010). These researchers compared the use of the book, unsupported by contact with a therapist, with a waiting list control. Their aim was to assess the effect of using the self-help book in the way that a person might do if buying the book from a book shop. They did not exclude any participants who volunteered for the study. Participants were asked to complete the book within two months. All subjects were assessed at the beginning and end of this two-month period and then the waiting list control group was provided with the book and two months after this all participants were assessed again. The outcome was assessed using tinnitus complaint questionnaires (i.e. TRQ and TSS) and a measure of general psychological distress (GHQ-12; Goldberg, 1978). As with the Kaldo et al. (2007) study, there was a considerable attrition rate among the intervention group. Statistically significant changes in the outcome measures were observed, however, among those subjects in the treatment group who did complete the study. A nonsignificant trend towards improvement was observed in the control group after they had completed the book. There was not a significant difference in the number of subjects in the treatment group and the control group who reported clinically significant improvements. A statistically significant reduction in tinnitus distress was observed at 12 to 18 months follow-up among subjects who remained within the study and who had received the book.

The interventions in the Kaldo et al. (2007) study revealed a moderate effect size (Cohen's $d=0.42$). In the Malouff et al. (2010) study a small effect size ($d=0.28$) was observed. These findings suggest that although the outcomes were positive they were less so than those associated with regular CBT for tinnitus (Martinez-Devesa et al., 2010; Hesser et al., 2011a).

The Internet offers a way of delivering treatments involving self-help or minimal therapist contact. Such Internet-based therapy have been shown to be helpful in the treatment of a range of disorders including: panic disorder, social anxiety disorder, post-traumatic stress disorder, depression, headache, chronic pain and eating disorders, just to name a few examples (Andersson, 2009). Internet-based CBT has also been developed and used in the treatment of people with tinnitus. The studies have mostly been carried out by a group of Swedish researchers; one study has been carried out in Australia using a translation of the Swedish protocol and there is also an unpublished study conducted in Germany. The Swedish protocol clearly demands that all patients need to have access to a computer, an Internet connection and should be able to print out the training instructions. Although it is possible to go through all the steps without any personal contact, in clinical practice the patient is seen for a first assessment session, and later on for a follow-up; there are ethical and medicolegal problems associated with treating patients who have not been assessed in a clinic. All registration forms and rating scales are converted into web pages and are filled out via the Internet. Web pages are not 'open' and are only accessible with a password, given by e-mail to the patient. In cases when the Internet fails to work or when patients have problems with their connection, the therapist can be contacted by telephone. The programme is set up in six separate modules (or weeks) that basically mirror the face-to-face treatment offered in the clinic. All modules involve homework assignments and reports on a web page, to be submitted weekly. Patients are encouraged to ask questions about the treatment and all queries are answered as promptly as possible by the therapist or the physician. An example of a web page is given in Figure 15.1. When submitting a week's report the patient is sent an encouraging e-mail, with the instruction to go to the next module (and is given the code to that module). Some automatic processing of reports is possible, but it is generally recommended that the clinician should read all the submitted material from the patient. In the latest version of the treatment patients are encouraged to plan their treatment. Some ingredients, such as applied relaxation, are

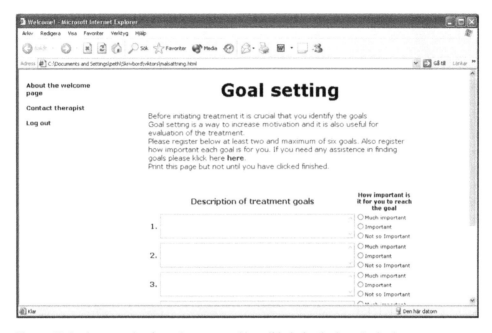

Figure 15.1 An example of a web page used in self-help for tinnitus via the Internet.

obligatory, whereas others, including hearing tactics and sleep management, are selected depending on the unique needs of each patient. In order for the programme to have any effect, it is crucial that patients go through all the appropriate exercises and that they contact the therapist if there are any questions or technical problems.

In the first study of Internet-based CBT for tinnitus distress (Andersson et al., 2002c), participants were recruited through web pages and newspaper articles, and they were then randomly allocated to a cognitive behaviour therapy self-help manual in six modules, or to a waiting list control group. All treatment and contact with participants was conducted via the Internet with web pages and e-mail correspondence. The participants were 117 people with tinnitus of at least six months' duration. In the first phase of the study 26 subjects completed all stages of treatment (49%) and 64 subjects from the waiting list control group provided measures. At one-year follow-up all participants had been offered the programme and 96 provided outcome measures, yielding an 18% dropout rate from baseline to follow-up. Tinnitus-related problems were assessed before and after treatment, and at the one-year follow-up. Daily diary ratings were included for one week before and one week after the treatment period. Results showed that tinnitus-related distress, depression and diary ratings of annoyance caused by tinnitus decreased significantly. Immediately following the first study phase (with a waiting list control group), significantly more participants in the treatment group showed an improvement of 50% on the Tinnitus Reaction Questionnaire. At follow-up, 27 (31%) had achieved a clinically significant improvement.

In a subsequent study, Kaldo-Sandström et al. (2004) demonstrated the effectiveness of an Internet-based CBT approach in a naturalistic setting. Kaldo et al. (2008) again found that Internet-based CBT was effective in relieving tinnitus distress; the Internet-based approach was found to be as effective as face-to-face group CBT. Hesser et al. (2012)

provided further evidence that Internet- based CBT is effective in relieving tinnitus distress and that Acceptance and Commitment Therapy (one of the latest developments of CBT) can also be successfully delivered through the Internet. Abbott et al. (2009), however, reported that Internet-based CBT was not more effective in the treatment of tinnitus in a industrial setting than an information only control condition; they had a high attrition rate, which almost certainly affected the outcome. A detailed description of an individual case using Internet-based CBT is set out by Andersson and Kaldo-Sandström (2004).

Evidence base for cognitive behaviour therapy

Cognitive behaviour therapy is among the most, if not *the* most, thoroughly validated treatment approach to tinnitus (Hesser et al., 2011a). However, there is still a lack of large-scale studies, with the exception of trials conducted in Australia by Henry and Wilson (2001). Meta-analysis is a technique of combining results from different trials in order to obtain estimates of effects across studies (Hedges and Olkin, 1985). The effect size, Cohen's d, is a standardized difference between groups or within groups (Cohen, 1988). A positive effect size indicates that the treatment group achieved better outcomes than the control group (or post-treatment improved over pre-treatment). An effect size of 0.20 is considered small, 0.50 is considered medium and 0.80 is considered large for clinical research (Cohen, 1988).

A number of meta-analyses have now been published on the effects of cognitive behaviour therapy for tinnitus.

The outcomes of 18 studies of psychological treatments were summarised by Andersson and Lyttkens (1999). Their meta-analysis included a total of 24 samples and up to 700 subjects. Studies on cognitive behaviour therapy, relaxation, hypnosis, biofeedback, educational sessions and problem solving were all included. Effect sizes for perceived tinnitus loudness, annoyance, negative affect (such as depression) and sleep problems were calculated for randomised controlled studies, pre–post design studies and follow-up results. The results showed strong to moderate effects on tinnitus annoyance for controlled studies (Cohen's $d=0.86$), pre–post designs (Cohen's $d=0.50$) and at follow-up (Cohen's $d=0.48$). The results on tinnitus loudness were weaker and disappeared at follow-up. Lower effect sizes were also obtained for measures of negative affect such as depression and for sleep problems. Exploratory analyses revealed that cognitive behaviour therapy (Cohen's $d=1.1$) was more effective than other psychological treatments (Cohen's $d=0.30$) on ratings of annoyance in the controlled studies.

A Cochrane library review of studies using CBT for tinnitus patients was carried out (Martinez-Devesa et al., 2007). This review was restricted to only six randomised controlled trials. The review identified 21 possible trials but excluded 15 primarily because of concerns about the allocation of subjects to one condition or another and high dropout rates among subjects. All the treatment trials involved group therapy studies. The primary outcome under consideration was subjective tinnitus loudness with tinnitus severity (a more global measure of distress referred to as 'quality of life') and depression acting as secondary outcomes. Analysis covered data from 285 participants. The review found that CBT had no statistically significant effect on the subjective loudness of tinnitus. It can be argued that the loudness of tinnitus is a curious thing to have as a primary outcome, as the purpose of CBT is usually to help the patient manage their tinnitus rather than to make it go away; a measure of loudness may not necessarily be taken within a CBT setting (e.g. Henry and Wilson, 1998). The analysis did reveal a statistically significant effect on the measure of tinnitus-related distress. When CBT was compared to a waiting list control then an effect size of 0.7 was observed and when it was compared with another intervention such as yoga or standard education strategies an effect size of 0.64 was observed. The analysis revealed that CBT did not have a significant effect on depression. The findings therefore are similar to those of Andersson and Lyttkens (1999). The Cochrane review concluded that CBT has a positive effect on the way in which people cope with tinnitus.

The Cochrane review was updated in 2010 (Martinez-Devesa et al., 2010). This review considered eight studies out of a possible 27 studies. Again, the remaining 19 studies were excluded from the review because the allocation of subjects to one or other condition was not considered sufficiently rigorous or because of a high dropout rate among subjects. Again, the primary outcome under consideration was subjective tinnitus loudness and tinnitus-related distress (referred to as the quality of life) and depression acted as a secondary outcome. As with the previous Cochrane review CBT was not found to have a significant impact on subjective loudness of tinnitus. The analysis did suggest that CBT has a significant effect on tinnitus-related distress (effect size of 0.91 when compared with a waiting list control and of 0.64 when compared with other interventions). In this review CBT was found to have a mild but significant impact on depression when compared with a waiting list control (effect size = 0.37).

Another meta-analysis has been conducted by Hesser et al. (2011a). These researchers examined 15 randomised controlled trials including a total of 1091 subjects; the number of subjects involved makes it the largest meta-analysis to date. They used a broader definition of CBT than that used by the Corchrane reviews. Arguably, the Corchrane reviews were overly restrictive in excluding some well-conducted studies. Hesser et al.'s (2011a) review included a small number of studies that were specifically excluded by the Cochrane review, but it also includes an equal number of studies not identified by the Cochrane search strategy. Hesser et al. (2011a) compared CBT treatments with active (e.g. treatment as usual or education) and passive control conditions (e.g. waiting list or no treatment) on measures of tinnitus distress. CBT was found to have a significant positive impact on tinnitus-related distress. This was more evident when CBT was compared to passive control conditions when a large effect size was observed (Hedge's $g = 0.70$), but was still the case when CBT was compared with active treatments (Hedges $g = 0.44$). Interestingly, these researchers also reported that CBT led to significant positive effects on measures of mood. When compared with both active and passive control conditions a mild to moderate effect size was observed (Hedge's $g = 0.42$ and 0.35, respectively). Their analysis also suggested that although the benefits of CBT declined slightly over time they remained significant at follow-up. This is a more positive finding than that of the Cochrane review. It is interesting that both this and the 2010 Cochrane review reveal more positive findings for CBT than the earlier reviews. Importantly, the meta-analysis by Hesser et al. (2011a) includes two studies involving Acceptance and Commitment Therapy (ACT), a recent development within the broad cognitive therapy school of thought.

In recent years it has become increasingly popular within clinical psychology research to assess effectiveness in outcome studies in terms of clinical significance (Ogles et al., 2001). This followed criticisms that statistical significance does not indicate whether treatments make a palpable, worthwhile difference in people's everyday lives and, secondly, does not indicate the proportion of individuals that improve. The use of the effect size statistic does address the issue of magnitude of change; however, the size of an effect is relatively independent of its clinical significance (Jacobson and Truax, 1991). Within the tinnitus literature there have been only a few references to clinical significance (e.g. Hesser et al., 2012; Londero et al., 2006). Clinical significance might be defined in terms of crossing a defined cutoff point, usually one that distinguishes one degree of severity from another on a given measure. Using the Tinnitus Handicap Questionnaire, Londero et al. (2006) defined clinical success in terms of a final score of less than 500. They reported that 75% of their patients could be regarded as clinically improved using this criterion. A problem with this approach, however, is that simply crossing a cutoff point does not take account of the size of the change.

The effect of cognitive behaviour therapy on insomnia in relation to tinnitus has not been investigated in any depth. Clinical experience attests to the usefulness of sleep management (McKenna, 2000; McKenna and Daniel, 2006), but in the meta-analysis only two controlled studies were identified in which sleep problems had been measured before and after treatment (Jakes et al., 1992; Kröner-Herwig et al., 1995). Andersson et al. (2002c) collected diary recordings in an Internet-based study but found no effects on insomnia. More recently, Kaldo et al. (2008) found significant reductions on the Insomnia Severity Index (Bastien et al., 2001), suggesting that sleep can improve after cognitive behaviour therapy for tinnitus.

The third wave of behaviour therapy

Recent trends within CBT have focused on methods of increasing acceptance of distressing thoughts, emotions and bodily sensations (Hayes et al., 1999). These approaches have been referred to as the 'Third Wave' of cognitive therapy. Acceptance-based therapies highlight the idea that suffering is a normal part of life and that people's attempts to resist or change it often lead to the perpetuation of suffering or even to greater degrees of suffering (see Chapter 6 for more information). There are two broad and heavily overlapping strands to this approach: Acceptance and Commitment Therapy (ACT) and Mindfulness therapies such as Mindfulness Based Cognitive Therapy. Acceptance and Commitment Therapy (ACT) aims to teach people to accept private experiences and to 'defuse' or distance themselves from private events by focusing carefully on and observing the processes of thinking and emotional feelings. There is now a body of evidence to suggest that acceptance is associated with less distress in a range of medical conditions such as chronic pain, epilepsy and Type II diabetes (to name a few examples) (Hayes et al., 2011). A small number of studies have investigated the use of acceptance-based treatment in the management of tinnitus. A cross-sectional study by Andersson et al. (2004b), a cross-sectional study by Schutte et al. (2009) and a longitudinal study by Westin et al. (2008a) indicate that this approach has beneficial effects on the impact of tinnitus. The study by Hesser et al. (2012) indicated that ACT is as effective as conventional CBT in alleviating tinnitus distress and a study by Zetterqvist et al. (2011) indicates that it is superior to a Tinnitus Retraining Therapy based approach in this respect. Acceptance and Commitment therapy has also been provided via the internet to tinnitus patients and has been found to have therapeutic benefits on tinnitus related distress (Hesser et al., 2012). Studies by Hesser et al. (2009, 2012) have identified acceptance as an active ingredient in the process of change in tinnitus therapy and indicate that the level of acceptance behaviour within treatment sessions predicted improvements in the level of tinnitus distress.

In addition to the emerging evidence base for ACT, evidence is also building for the parallel approach of 'mindfulness'-based treatments. As with ACT, mindfulness-based treatments invite people to become aware of and notice thoughts, emotional experiences and physical feelings and to 'turn towards' these experiences rather than trying to fight or control them. Mindfulness-based treatments rely primarily on meditation techniques to foster this acceptance. The meditation helps people 'pay attention in a particular way: in the present moment, on purpose and non-judgementally' (Kabat-Zinn, 1990). There is an overlap between ACT and a mindfulness approach to treatment and the latter forms a substantial element with ACT. As with ACT there is a body of evidence to suggest that mindfulness is helpful in reducing distress associated with a variety of problems including cancer, generalised anxiety disorder, depression and other psychiatric and physical medical conditions. A meta-analysis by Hofmann et al. (2010) looked at 39 studies involving a total of 1140 participants and found strong effect sizes (between 0.59 and 0.97) on a number of distress-related measures. Another meta-analysis by Bohlmeijer et al. (2010) looked at eight randomised controlled trials for depression, anxiety and psychological distress across chronic medical diseases. These authors found weaker effect sizes (between 0.26 and 0.47). It may be that the stronger effects are associated with a greater cognitive therapy component within the mindfulness training, but this remains to be seen.

The evidence concerning the value of a mindfulness approach in managing tinnitus is emerging. Sadlier et al. (2008) used a combination of CBT and mindfulness meditation in the treatment of patients with intrusive tinnitus. Using a waiting list control study design they reported a significant reduction in patient's Tinnitus Questionnaire scores following treatment and noted that 80% of patients reported that they were 'better' or 'much better' when seen at a four- to six-month follow-up. These authors conclude that mindfulness meditation is a technique that can be used successfully with Cognitive therapy and facilitates the habituation process. Mindfulness meditation, however, was only one element in the treatment offered and it cannot be concluded that it was an active ingredient of treatment. A randomised controlled study using mindfulness-based cognitive therapy has been carried out by Philippot et al. (2011). These researchers offered all subjects a single session of psychoeducation about tinnitus followed by either six weekly sessions of relaxation training or of MBCT. The results indicated that the psychoeducation had benefits in terms of reduced negative emotions, rumination and psychological difficulties in living with tinnitus. These benefits were maintained or enhanced in the MBCT group even though subjects' ratings about the presence of tinnitus increased. The benefits seen following psychoeducation were eroded in the relaxation group at follow-up.

There have been reports of the use of mindfulness-based treatments in conference proceedings. Mazzolli et al. (2010) reported on the effects of mindfulness meditation in the management of tinnitus across three centres in northern Italy. They reported significant improvements in some of the factors within the Tinnitus Questionnaire and noted that 70% of patients reported being better able to relax and control tinnitus during periods of increased annoyance due to tinnitus. They also reported significant changes in patients' EEG recording with an increase in alpha waves post-treatment. McKenna and Love (2011) also reported that mindfulness-based cognitive therapy had a beneficial effect for tinnitus patients. At the start of therapy 78% of their patient group had scores within the clinically significant range on a widely used measure of emotional distress (the Clinical Outcomes in Routine Evaluation – Outcome measure). Of these 67% showed clinically significant improvement on this measure at the end of therapy. Both Mazzolli et al.'s (2010) and McKenna and Love's (2011) reports need to be regarded with caution as neither is a controlled trial but rather clinical audits that do not involve a control group. Nonetheless, these reports reflect the growing interest and optimism in this area.

Who should provide cognitive behaviour therapy?

There is a strong evidence base indicating that CBT is effective in tinnitus management. The idea that it should be an integral part of tinnitus management is supported by the UK Department of Health Good Practice Guidelines (DH Publications, 2009). An important issue, however, is that there are relatively few therapists trained in the provision of CBT and fewer still who work in the field of tinnitus (Coles, 1992; McFerran and Baguley, 2009). Further, few tinnitus patients are referred out of audiology services to psychiatrists or psychologists. Referring to data from a survey of tinnitus management, Coles (1992) noted that only nine of 458 consultants referred patients to psychiatrists or clinical psychologists more than 15 times per year. This is probably still the case today – two decades later. Gander et al. (2011) found that in only one in five audiology services in the UK dealing with tinnitus was there an onward pathway to psychological services. Experiences from the field of chronic pain, however, suggests that multidisciplinary treatments can work very well (Jensen et al., 1995) and that cognitive behaviour therapy principles can be incorporated as long as the staff are trained in the provision of the methods. Training in CBT for audiologists is still in scarce supply; one training course aimed at training audiologists to use CBT with tinnitus patients is available in the UK. This will be an easier task when training manuals that provide step-by-step guidance are available. Supervision by a trained cognitive behaviour therapist should, however, always be part of the arrangement. The need for training is just as important, if not more so, when considering approaches such as mindfulness; these approaches can seem deceptively straightforward but are sophisticated and require careful training. Clearly, each person dealing with tinnitus patients, either directly or via supervision, should have a fundamental knowledge about tinnitus and the auditory aspects involved. Although most patients will not need a psychologist, there are, of course, occasions when a referral is needed. Therefore, it is crucial to know when to refer to a cognitive behaviour therapist. Self-report measures such as the Hospital Anxiety and Depression Scale (see Chapter 11) can be used for initial screening, but sometimes it is necessary to refer for an assessment by a psychologist, or a psychiatrist in the case of suspected psychopathology. For less complicated cases, self-help is an alternative, in particular when support can be given by the staff in the clinic. This can be done via e-mail or telephone calls. It is likely that there will be an increased role for Internet technology in tinnitus management in the future. There are often several different elements within any given tinnitus treatment; this is as true of cognitive behaviour therapy as of other treatment approaches. This makes it difficult to know what treatment ingredients are the most effective, which are necessary and which ones could be omitted. All forms of cognitive behaviour therapy must involve an understanding and caring therapist (even when he or she is on the other side of an Internet connection) and the importance of this in tinnitus management should not be dismissed (Tyler et al., 2001).

Summary

Cognitive behaviour therapy for tinnitus involves identifying and modifying maladaptive behaviours, thoughts and feelings by means of practical hands on work and homework assignments. Cognitive behaviour therapy has been practised for many years, but its use in tinnitus management is still not widespread. This is unfortunate as research suggests that this approach benefits many patients, in particular when tinnitus is a significant source of distress in the patient's life. While there is little evidence that cognitive behaviour therapy has any long-term effects on the perceived loudness of tinnitus, the benefits regarding the distress associated with tinnitus are clearer and have been replicated in many studies. Developments within the field of cognitive behaviour therapy such as acceptance and mindfulness-based approaches are now being applied within the tinnitus field with encouraging results. There is, however, a continuing need to develop and implement cognitive behaviour therapy treatments in which the criteria of clinically significant improvements are met. Other challenges involve the dissemination of cognitive behaviour therapy to a broader multidisciplinary community. Potentially, recently developed self-help approaches might facilitate such progress. Finally, cognitive behaviour therapy can be incorporated with other existing approaches to tinnitus management, such as the teaching component of Tinnitus Retraining Therapy (Hiller and Haerkötter, 2005).

Chapter 16

Emerging treatment approaches

The resurgence in both scientific and clinical interest in tinnitus in recent years has led to the emergence of a number of new approaches to treatment, and in this chapter we take the opportunity to review the main examples. While none have yet become mainstream treatment options, each brings a new perspective to bear on treating tinnitus and deserves careful attention as novel information may be gleaned regarding both treatment options and underpinning mechanisms of tinnitus.

Transcranial magnetic stimulation

The possibility that magnetic stimulation might modulate tinnitus has been of interest for some years, but magnetic stimulation of the ear had been demonstrated not to be beneficial (Coles at al., 1991). Transcranial magnetic stimulation (TMS) is a noninvasive technique whereby rapidly changing strong magnetic fields can be used to induce electrical activity in the human brain. When applied to the cerebral cortex, these changes in activity can transiently activate or inhibit focal cortical areas, which may influence movement, perception or behaviour. The most common clinical application of the technique utilises high-intensity (1.5–2 tesla), brief (100–300 ms) and repeated stimuli through an insulated stimulating coil placed on the scalp, which is described as repetitive transcranial magnetic stimulation (rTMS). While the magnetic field declines rapidly with distance from the coil, so that the direct stimulation effect is limited to superficial cortical areas, the induced stimulation may influence other areas of the brain that are functionally connected to the stimulated areas (Kleinjung et al., 2011).

The frequency of stimulation used influences the way in which cortical activity is modulated. Stimulation at high-frequency rates (5–20 Hz) has been demonstrated to increase the excitability of cortical areas, whereas low-frequency stimulation (<1 Hz) has been shown to decrease excitability. Therefore, it is possible to instigate a focal functional lesion in the cortex using rTMS, and this has been used in studies seeking to associate

Tinnitus: A Multidisciplinary Approach, Second Edition. David Baguley, Gerhard Andersson,
Don McFerran and Laurence McKenna.
© 2013 David Baguley, Gerhard Andersson, Don McFerran and Laurence McKenna.
Published 2013 by Blackwell Publishing Ltd.

structure and function in the human brain. Guidelines exist for the safe application of rTMS (Rossi et al., 2009), and there is a consensus that when these are applied rTMS does not do long-term harm and is reasonably well tolerated, though unpleasant due to perceiving a loud abrupt sound and to facial discomfort. Contraindications for rTMS include electronic implants, previous seizures and the presence of intracranial metal (Kleinjung et al., 2011). The risk of post rTMS seizure is 0.5% (George, 2010) – all reports have indicated that seizure may be induced during or immediately after exposure (George, 2010) but not subsequently. The incidence of post rTMS headache has been estimated at 10% for tinnitus studies (Kleinjung et al., 2011).

One clinical application of rTMS has been in the treatment of clinical depression. Studies have indicated an effect whereby the impact upon symptoms of chronic depression are greater than those of sham treatment (see George, 2010, for a review) (though see below for a caveat regarding the reliability of blinding when sham rTMS is used) and in the United States, FDA approval for the use of rTMS in patients with depression was granted in 2009. The improvements in depression have generally subsided by 12 weeks from the final stimulation (Allan et al., 2011). Major questions remain about how the effect can be optimised, however, and these include the consideration of eligibility criteria and stimulation parameters such as intensity, duration, site and frequency of application (George, 2010).

The extent to which a 'sham' or placebo version of rTMS can be relied upon in a clinical trial is open to question (Allan et al., 2011). When TMS is performed anywhere on the head, the subject perceives a transient sound and facial and scalp discomfort or pain. While there are techniques mimicking the sound sensation, and more recently the discomfort, challenges continue in maintaining the blinding for both subjects and researchers. In the majority of studies considering the effect of rTMS upon tinnitus, the coil is angled away from the head, which induces sound sensation (but not discomfort) and is presumed not to modulate cortical electrical activity to the same extent as a 'real' rTMS. This is problematic, as it is not blinded as far as the researcher is concerned and the size of the angle from the head may be variable. There are indications that the experiment may not be adequately blinded to the subject – in a recent experiment using rTMS for tinnitus subjects were asked to judge whether they had just had 'real' or 'sham' rTMS and the majority of them judged correctly (Kleinjung, personal communication). This issue means that the rTMS/tinnitus literature must be interpreted with caution.

Regarding tinnitus, the investigation of the potential clinical utility of rTMS rests upon the assumption that the perception of tinnitus is associated with anomalous or abberant activity in the auditory cortex, though the ignition site may be upstream (e.g. more peripherally sited). The application of rTMS may potentially be associated with an inhibition or modulation of such tinnitus-related activity, and so reduce the perceived intensity of the tinnitus. If such an effect were demonstrated, then further work would be needed to optimise that affect and to make it as long lasting as possible.

The possibility that one can transiently reduce the perceived intensity of tinnitus using a single exposure to rTMS has been investigated by several studies, which have been summarised by Kleinjung et al. (2011). The literature is hard to interpret as there is marked heterogeneity of method, including different stimulation rates, intensities, sites and characteristics of subjects. Considering the findings, a theme emerges that single-exposure rTMS is able to transiently reduce the intensity of tinnitus in a proportion of individuals (circa 50%), but unfortunately it is not possible to be more specific. These subjective observations have been supported by indications that rTMS influences auditory activity in the auditory cortex, as evidenced by data from PET studies (Meenemeier at al., 2011) and auditory steady state responses (ASSR) (Lorenz et al., 2010). A consensus emerged that the effects of rTMS upon tinnitus warranted further investigation.

Further work consists of studies that investigate whether repeated rTMS can induce some longer lasting inhibition of tinnitus intensity. Once again the heterogeneity of methods of stimulation, subject variables and outcome measures bedevil interpretation. The most commonly used stimulation paradigm is low-frequency stimulation in trains of 1200–2000 pulses repeatedly over 5–10 days (Kleinjung et al., 2011). Regarding the effect, a theme emerges of a modest reduction in over 50% of subjects, though these are highly (self) selected individuals, willing to try such an experimental technique. While there are some reports of rTMS instigating reduced perceived tinnitus intensity for several months (see Kleinjung et al., 2005; Khedr et al., 2009), in the majority of subjects the effect subsided after 2–4 weeks following the final stimulation (Plewnia, 2011). The possibility has been raised that left and bilaterally lateralised tinnitus may be more likely to respond to rTMS delivered on the left (Frank et al., 2010) and that persons with normal hearing and/or short-duration tinnitus may be more likely to have a positive response (Kleinjung et al., 2011).

Following a Cochrane systematic review of low-frequency rTMS in tinnitus, Meng and colleagues (2011) summarised the situation thus:

> There is very limited support for the use of low-frequency TMS for the treatment of patients with tinnitus.

Therefore, TMS for tinnitus should be viewed at the present time as a research technique, worthy of clinical interest but not yet ready for wide application.

A number of strategies have been employed to investigate how the benefits of rTMS can be enhanced. These have included neuronavigation to optimise coil positioning (Langguth et al., 2009, 2010) and the use of the drug levodopa in an attempt to enhace neuronal plasticity (Kleinjung et al., 2009). High-frequency TMS has been utilised to prime the auditory cortex for a low-frequency rTMS (Langguth et al., 2008). None of these enhancement strategies have been effective.

There are a small number of reports of worsening tinnitus following rTMS, but this may in part be an effect of the attention devoted to monitoring tinnitus during a clinical trial and the unpleasant effects of rTMS (albeit transient). One caveat that has been raised regarding rTMS for tinnitus, however, is that the reported effects are modest, and if the understanding is that perceived intensity of tinnitus has at best an indirect relationship with domains such as annoyance, handicap or burden then the benefits for the person (rather than the percept) may be modest indeed. Plewnia (2011) notes that rTMS tinnitus studies that have used a measure of handicap have a weak influence on that domain at the end of treatment.

Direct brain stimulation

Using rTMS to influence cortical activity is at best an indirect endeavour and some researchers have investigated the possibility of direct stimulation of the brain. The literature regarding the largely beneficial effects of stimulation of the cochlear nerve with cochlear implants is an indication that the perceived intensity of tinnitus can be reduced by such electrical stimulation, so the prospect of directly stimulating the auditory brain is of some interest.

A rationale for such stimulation has been proposed by De Ridder and Vanneste (2011). The argument is based upon the hypothesis that troublesome tinnitus is associated with increased synchrony in gamma band activity in the auditory cortex. Considering that rTMS may be effective (to the extent that it is) by disrupting this hypersynchrony, De Ridder and Vanneste proposed that direct electrical stimulation of the auditory cortex may allow this to happen on a long-term chronic basis. They acknowledge that the determination of the exact site of the tinnitus-related activity – and hence the site for stimulation – would be a key factor in success, but argue that MEG and fMRi techniques allow that to happen. Three electrode configurations are in use:

- Extradural, overlying secondary auditory cortex
- Intradural, in an existing groove or sulcus of the primary auditory cortex
- Intradural, inserted into the primary auditory cortex.

A series of 43 patients in whom such procedures were undertaken has been reported (De Ridder and Vanneste, 2011), all having very severe intractable tinnitus and all having a positive response to rTMS. Of the series, 13 (30%) had no benefit from direct brain stimulation. In the 70% who did respond, burst stimulation gleaned better results than tonic stimulation. In this report, which is not in a peer review paper but at the time of writing is the only published report of this study, data regarding handicap is not reported, but an indication that tinnitus reduction was more evident in patients with shorter tinnitus duration was mentioned.

Other groups around the world are investigating this interesting but challenging area. Friedland and colleagues (2007) report a pilot study of eight patients in whom epidural direct electrical stimulation was performed. Intriguingly, while the single blind cross-over trial of electrical stimulation versus placebo stimulation did not indicate benefit, there was a reduction in tinnitus with continuous stimulation following the 4-week crossover period. In a conference report, Dauman et al. (2011) report on a series of nine patients who underwent extradural auditory cortex stimulation; in only four patients was there a reduction in tinnitus handicap, and placebo was felt to have an influence in those cases. While little weight can be given to such a report, this is an indication that direct electrical stimulation of the auditory brain is being undertaken by several groups around the world.

Other brain stimulation

There are two other approaches to brain stimulation that are worthy of note. The first is transcranial direct current stimulation (tDCS), whereby a low-level constant current (0.5–2 mA) flows through the cerebral cortex via scalp electrodes. These small amounts of current are hypothesised to have a neuromodulation effect similar to that of TMS, with brain areas under the anode to have an excitatory effect, whereas those under the cathode an inhibitory effect (Vanneste et al., 2011). The technique is felt to be safe

Table 16.1 Description of studies on transcranial direct current stimulation (tDCS).

Author (date)	N	Design	Method	Results
Fregni et al. (2006)	7	No blinding	Cathodal and anodal stimulation of left temperoparietal cortex; 1 mA, three minutes, single application	Significant reduction in tinnitus intensity after anodal tDCS
Vanneste et al. (2010)	543	Waiting list control (n=65), no blinding	Cathode over left DLPFC, anode right DLPFC (n=448); cathode over right DLPFC, anode left DLPFC (n=30); waiting list control (n=65); single administration, 1.5 mA, 20 min	Group data: significant decrease in tinnitus intensity pre/post for anode right, cathode left; 134 (29.9%) 'tDCS responders'
Frank et al. (2012)	32	Open-label pilot	Cathode over left DLPFC, anode right DLPFC; 1.5 mA, 30 min, 2 days a week for 3 weeks	Significant changes in unpleasantness and discomfort of tinnitus
Garin et al. (2011)	20	Double-blind placebo controlled	1. Anode left temperoparietal cortex, cathode right, 1 mA, 20 min 2. Anode left temperoparietal cortex, cathode right 3. Sham: burst stimulation, three sessions in two weeks	Significant reduction in tinnitus intensity group data following tDCS over sham, tendency for greater effect with anodal tDCS; 7/20 (35%) 'tDCS responders'

(Poreisz et al., 2007): side effects are temporary and include headache and infrequent nausea. Brain areas of interest for treating tinnitus include not only the temperoparietal cortex (e.g. primary auditory cortex), but also the dorsolateral prefrontal cortex (DLPFC), which has been suggested to have a role in top-down auditory processing and auditory memory. Work regarding tDCS for treating tinnitus is preliminary and is summarised in Table 16.1. Caveats about nonblinded designs and unsatisfactory placebo conditions apply here as with other experimental interventions: despite this it does appear that tDCS may have a neuromodulating effect upon tinnitus intensity. Vanneste and colleagues (2011) report data indicating that there is a higher likelihood of a reduction in tinnitus intensity following tDCS in a patient in whom a higher 'functional connectivity' (meaning coherence and phase synchronisation) between right DLPFC and right parahippocampus was identified using gamma band EEG. No placebo tDCS is evident in this paper, and so interpretation of the results await replication with a placebo blinded trial.

An alternative approach to brain stimulation is to consider the effects of caloric vestibular stimulation (CVS). CVS has been demonstrated transiently to modulate a variety of cognitive functions, including binocular rivalry, visual imagery, neglect and other post-lesional conditions, and some pain disorders (see Been et al., 2007, for a review). These effects are associated with the brain activation induced by CVS, involving the temporal–parietal cortex, anterior cingulate cortex and insular cortex, which are thought to form a multimodal vestibular cortical network. Baguley et al. (2011) investigated the effect of CVS upon tinnitus, hypothesising that if CVS were to significantly modulate tinnitus, then the percept was within the multimodel vestibular cortical network – and if it did not, then the percept was extrinsic to that network. It was reported that CVS does not modulate tinnitus and the authors propose that this is an indication that tinnitus is a low brain and perhaps brainstem phenomenon. They note the difficulty many tinnitus patients have in describing their tinnitus as a further pointer towards this suggestion – and if this were the case the ability of tDCS and rTMS to treat tinnitus might be limited.

Phase shift

It is possible to cancel sound in the external environment using another sound of identical intensity and frequency characteristics, but with phase manipulated to be 180 degrees to the original. This technique, known as antinoise or antiphase, was first suggested in the 1930s and was applied to noise inside aircraft in the 1970s (Barratt and Pool, 2008). More recently the ability to perform the calculations required has been possible within noise cancelling headphones, which make lengthy air travel more pleasurable. Many patients, knowing of this technology, ask if this is possible for tinnitus, and a technique entitled Tinnitus Phase-Out aims to do that (Choy et al., 2010). The pitch of the tinnitus is assessed (though see Chapter 10 for the challenges of doing that reliably) and the patient is issued with a device that plays a sound said to be shifted in phase by 180 degrees to that. Some early reports from the clinicians who developed the technique indicated benefits in treatment, and an open independent trial was similarly optimistic (Vermeire et al., 2007), though it was noted that these studies did not include a placebo control arm and did not determine whether phase-shift had a particular advantage over some general wideband sound therapy. In a study with an innovative design, Meeus and colleagues (2010b) compared the benefits of phase-shift for persons with tonal tinnitus (in whom it might conceiveably be effective) to those with a noise-like tinnitus (which would not have a phase to be cancelled). Measures of tinnitus loudness and annoyance did not improve for the noise-like tinnitus patients, and in fact worsened in those with tonal tinnitus. The lack of evidence for efficacy of phase-out for tinnitus is congruent with indications that tonal tinnitus does not beat with an external sound of close but nonidentical frequency, as is experienced when two such external sounds are perceived together (Oster, 1973). This infers that the tinnitus percept does not have phase characteristics, which, if correct, would render the prospects of phase-shift treatment for tinnitus to be modest.

Laser therapy

A number of investigators have considered the proposal that low-level laser stimulation might have a role in treating tinnitus. In such therapy a light source (red to infrared – 630–904 nm) is shone upon the area of interest and there have been reports of benefits in wound healing and chronic pain, though these are preliminary and not consistently replicated. Studies that have considered low-level laser therapy for tinnitus have mainly utilised the laser shone down the ear canal and report varied results, from apparently beneficial to no benefit (Kleinjung, 2011). Few studies published to date have involved any form of placebo control, and those that have generally report little or no benefit (von Wedel et al., 1995; Teggi et al., 2009, for example). An uncontrolled study reported benefit from a combination of rTMS and transmeatal laser stimulation in patients with hyperacusis, but the design of this study is poor. There is one report of acute hearing deterioration following laser therapy for tinnitus (Nakashima et al., 2002) so the possibility of harm should be borne in mind. It is difficult to see how laser therapy might be helpful for tinnitus, given the small amount of energy that might permeate into the cochlea through the tympanic membrane and given the involvement of the central auditory system in tinnitus. A paper by Siedentopf and colleagues (2007) used fMRI to indicate changes in auditory cortex activity following laser stimulation of the ear canal, but this has not been replicated. Generally speaking, the scientific and clinical tinnitus community are sceptical about the possibility that laser therapy may confer substantial benefits for troublesome tinnitus.

Coordinated reset stimulation

For some years there have been research perspectives on Parkinson's disease which view the associated functional defects as involving a loss of segregation of signal processing pathways, setting up abnormal synchronisation (Hauptmann and Tass, 2010). It is further suggested that some forms of deep brain stimulation (DBS) may 'reset' the signalling networks such that the functional segregation is restored. These views are supported by computer modelling data (Lysyansky et al., 2011) and by emergent data from DBS studies in Parkinson's disease patients.

These insights have begun to be applied to tinnitus, taking as a starting point the hypothesis that tinnitus is associated with, and potentially instigated by, anomalous synchronisation of activity in the auditory system (Chapter 5). Rather than using DBS as a reset stimulus, which would be overinvasive for all but a tiny fraction of people with tinnitus, a series of tones distributed around the frequency of tonal tinnitus is proposed as a treatment intervention. At the time of writing initial results from a single-blind trial conducted by the inventor are available (Tass et al., 2012) and more robust trials have begun, while a small number of clinics have also started to offer treatment to patients. As the ANM treatment is limited to patients with tonal tinnitus, there may also be a limit to the numbers that may be eligible for such an approach.

Other sound-based emergent approaches

While the idea that a sound therapy stimulus for tinnitus should be modified to match the audiogram of the individual is not new (Baguley et al., 1997, for example), recent work has considered the extent to which amplitude modulation of the stimulus might increase the acceptability and efficacy of the sound for a patient. In order to understand this one might consider white noise (which can sound rather strident and harsh) and the sound of the rain (pleasant and soothing). These two stimuli are very similar in the frequency domain, but in the amplitude domain there are marked differences, with the rain having much greater variability. There are several groups worldwide investigating the ways in which a tinnitus therapy sound can be modulated and hence customised for an individual; an example is the research by Reavis et al. (2010) that uses various depths of amplitude modulation in sound so that a tinnitus patient can identify which is most acceptable (the researchers then investigating whether this is the most effective in treating tinnitus). An alternative approach is that proposed by Pineda et al. (2008), who produce a 'replica' of an individual's tinnitus and aim by repeated exposure to this to suppress 'overactive circuits', said to be responsible for the tinnitus. As with much tinnitus research, speculation is at least as common as evidence. However, clinical trial data are not yet available for either approach, but this is an area to watch with interest.

Rather than spectrally shaping music such that tinnitus frequencies are enhanced, as is the case in the Neuromonics device (see Chapter 13), Okamoto and colleagues (2010) removed a frequency band from music that surrounded the tinnitus frequency. The subject's choice of music was utilised, and this approach was only tried on persons with a matchable tonal tinnitus. A placebo was implemented in the form of music notched at frequencies distant from the tinnitus. This study is essentially a pilot, and the finding that tinnitus loudness reduced with repeated use of the active condition but not in placebo is of interest but needs replication and further development. A follow-on study indicated that the treatment was only effective when the matched tinnitus frequency was below 8 kHz, and not above (Teismann et al., 2011).

Acceptance-based treatments

Recent advances within the world of cognitive behaviour therapy have involved the development of 'acceptance'-based treatments. The two main therapy approaches are Acceptance and Commitment Therapy (ACT) (Hayes et al., 1999) and Mindfulness Based Cognitive Therapy (MBCT) (Segal et al., 2002); these therapies have been found to be successful in helping people manage a number of other chronic medical conditions (Hofmann et al., 2010; Hayes et al., 2011). Acceptance-based therapies highlight the idea that suffering is a normal part of life and that people's attempts to resist or change it often lead to the perpetuation of suffering or even to greater degrees of suffering. They suggest that rather than trying to continually escape or avoid difficult experiences, allowing such experiences to be present without resistance and, if possible, without judgement, results in them being richer and less destructive. Patients are invited to deliberately and carefully observe their experiences and through this observation to 'defuse' or 'stand back' from their private events rather than being swept along by them. In this context 'acceptance' is distinctly different from concepts such as resignation or defeat. Acceptance is an acknowledgement of the patient's situation, including the ways in which their reaction to their problems helps to maintain those problems and using that perspective as a position from which to pursue their more fundamental goals in life. Much has been made of the fact that the MBCT approach represents a point at which Western psychology overlaps with some ideas from Buddhist philosophy; it should be noted, however, that similar contemplative approaches are utilised in the other mainstream religions and in some Western philosophies.

ACT and MBCT have now been applied to tinnitus management. There are differences between these two schools but in general they will invite a patient to carefully observe their tinnitus without attributing any significance or meaning to it, rather than using continual distraction from these processes. The patient may also be invited to observe a variety of other experiences in life, so allowing a broader perspective rather than maintaining solely a tinnitus focus. To date there have been only a small handful of studies examining the benefits of acceptance approaches in tinnitus treatment. These studies have, however, revealed encouraging results and it is possible that this approach will become more established in tinnitus management. A further account of acceptance-based treatments is provided in Chapter 15.

Summary

It is heartening to see new and emergent treatment approaches for tinnitus. While one might be sceptical about some, and acknowledge that all need to be subject to clinical trials, the breadth of novel interventions and the innovative spirit evident in their instigation is encouraging. Given that (to date) mainstream clinical medicine has not delivered an effective means of inhibiting tinnitus, nor of comprehensively ameliorating tinnitus-associated distress, then the ability of some to look beyond the 'can't get there from here' view is commendable. Time will tell if any of these approaches outlive an initial promise.

Chapter 17

Complementary medicine approaches to tinnitus

Some years ago the UK Royal College of Pathologists won a Silver Medal at the Chelsea Flower Show with an exhibition of plants, both healing and injurious to health, entitled 'Pathologists and Plants Working in Partnership'. A spokesman was quoted as saying 'Plants were the basis of all medicine at one time … .' It is salutary to remember that present medical practice, however evidence-based, derives from folk medicine and custom. Treatments outside the medical domain should be considered with respect, as there may be effects at work that are not yet understood. As individuals, the authors of this book have each personally undertaken or had a close family member undertake a complementary therapy in good faith; as tinnitus specialists it is, however, important to consider critically available evidence of efficacy of treatments for tinnitus, and indeed their potential for harm.

The acronym CAM is in common use for complementary and alternative medicine (Cassileth and Deng, 2004). The use of such approaches is widespread: Barnes et al. (2004) reported that 36% of a large sample of adults in the United States had used a CAM therapy within the last 12 months. Such use is not restricted to the credulous public, as a Danish study found that 68% of medical students surveyed had used a CAM at some point (Damgaard-Morch et al., 2008).

Given the poor record of conventional Western medicine in treating tinnitus, it should not be surprising that many patients have sought recourse to CAM. In an investigation of the treatments patients had sought before being seen by a psychologist in a tinnitus clinic in Sweden, Andersson (1997) found that of 69 consecutive patients seeking help for troublesome tinnitus, only 24 (35%) had not undertaken treatment before seeking clinical help; these treatments included acupuncture, nonspecific relaxation therapy and various other CAM approaches. Analysis indicated that the nontreatment patients showed a statistically significant difference from the treatment group, in that they showed greater acceptability for change. Thus, seeking treatment outside the clinical domain may have an

Tinnitus: A Multidisciplinary Approach, Second Edition. David Baguley, Gerhard Andersson, Don McFerran and Laurence McKenna.
© 2013 David Baguley, Gerhard Andersson, Don McFerran and Laurence McKenna.
Published 2013 by Blackwell Publishing Ltd.

effect in hardening attitudes and beliefs about tinnitus, though it should be noted that the group investigated, by definition, had not benefited from their prior treatment.

When considering CAM one should be mindful of the placebo effect. *Placebo* is Latin for 'I shall please'. In the Renaissance, a placebo was a fake potion or manipulation (Basmajian, 1999; Tyler et al., 2001) and the term became pejorative. The term 'placebo effect' became common with the use of controlled trials that utilise an inert substance or procedure, against which to compare the effect of potentially active treatment. However, according to many sources the placebo effect is fundamental to medical treatment, and the placebo effect is not the same as lack of an effect (Evans, 2003). The use of the term 'placebo effect' in tinnitus treatment does not do justice to the good faith in which attempts are made to improve a patient's situation (Tyler et al., 2001). Indeed, the observation made by Duckert and Rees (1984), that 40% of tinnitus patients reported an effect on their tinnitus following placebo injection, is often quoted as 'evidence' of huge placebo effects in the management of tinnitus. In reality, fluctuations of loudness may be of minimal relief for the tinnitus patient and might even be irrelevant for the annoyance experienced.

Homeopathic remedies

The use of homeopathy is widespread in both Europe and the USA (Eisenberg et al., 1998), despite the fundamental principle of homeopathic therapy being contrary to those of modern pharmacology (Vandenbroucke, 1997). Homeopathy is based upon the principle of similars, in that 'a patient with a specific pattern of symptoms is best treated by a remedy which causes the same or very similar pattern in healthy subjects' (Linde et al., 2001, p. 4), although the remedies are given in high dilution so that they may be 'unlikely to contain any molecules of the originally diluted agents' (Linde et al., 2001, p. 4). Simpson et al. (1998) undertook a well-designed and rigorous study of a homeopathic remedy entitled 'Tinnitus' and the results indicated no benefit of this homeopathic remedy for tinnitus compared with placebo. There are many homeopathic remedies for tinnitus available for sale on the Internet, none of which has been subject to controlled trial evaluation.

Acupuncture

Acupuncture involves the stimulation of defined points on the body by the insertion of needles or manual pressure (acupressure). The principle is based upon traditional Chinese medical concepts wherein the flow of energy around the body (Chi) is the basis of the patient's disorder and can be influenced by stimulation of a relevant point on the body (Linde et al., 2001). Wang and colleagues (2010) made the point that one fundamental principle of acupuncture treatment (for tinnitus in their example) is individualised placement of the needles depending upon the characteristics of the patient and that this does not fit easily into randomised controlled trial methodology.

There have been a number of studies considering the effects of acupuncture upon tinnitus, using variable amounts of scientific rigour. The results are summarised in Table 17.1. A cautionary note should be struck about acupuncture. Not only has it been

Table 17.1   Investigations of the effect of acupuncture upon tinnitus.

Authors (year)	Design	n	Findings
Hansen et al. (1982)	Sham control	17	No advantage over placebo
Marks et al. (1984)	Sham control	14	No advantage over placebo
Axelsson et al. (1994)	Sham control	20	No advantage over placebo
Gu and Axelsson (1996)	Observational	625	'More than 50% were helped'
Furugard et al. (1998)	Control (physiotherapy)	22	Significant improvement, which fell to pre-treatment level after 12 months
Vilholm et al. (1998)	Randomised, double-blind placebo-controlled	52	No advantage over placebo
Nebeska et al. (1999)	Crossover study: placebo (laser), acupuncture	16	Statistically significant reduction of tinnitus loudness following acupuncture but not placebo
Okada et al. (2006)	Single-blind placebo control	76	Temporary improvements in perceived intensity in both study and placebo groups; temporary improvement in treatment group significantly higher
Jackson et al. (2006)	Six $n=1$ trials	6	Very variable responses; authors report a 'trend' for improvement in tinnitus intensity
Wang et al. (2010)	Randomised, single-blind placebo control group ('placebo needles')	50	Some improvements in quality of life measures were reported for subjects undergoing electrical and manual acupuncture compared to placebo

shown not to benefit tinnitus patients in previous reviews (Dobie, 1999; Park et al., 2000), but it has been demonstrated occasionally to have been a factor in the exacerbation of tinnitus (Andersson and Lyttkens, 1996), albeit of a temporary nature.

Starting from a view that acupuncture may have an inhibitory effect upon tinnitus, de Azevedo and colleagues (2007) sought to determine if that intervention influenced cochlear function in persons with tinnitus by analysing transient otoacoustic emission amplitudes before and after acupuncture. A placebo (single blind) was also used, this being a needle placed in a position that was not a recognised acupuncture point. The authors reported a significant increase in TOAE amplitudes following acupuncture in the treatment group, but not in the placebo, but concede that a larger and more rigorous study would be needed before any robust conclusions could be drawn.

Ginkgo biloba

Ginkgo biloba (GB) is an extract from the Chinese ginkgo tree, and has been used in Chinese medicine for thousands of years. Studies suggest that ginkgo has antihypoxic, free radical scavenging, antioxidant, metabolic, antiplatelet and microcirculatory actions (Ernst, 2002). Holgers et al. (1994) investigated the effects of Ginkgo biloba in a trial with an unusual

Table 17.2 Potential drug interactions with Gingo biloba. (Based upon Graham et al. (2008)).

Interacting drug	Interaction severity	Description of interaction
SSRI	Major	Increased risk of serotonin syndrome
Antiplatelet agents (such as aspirin)	Major	Increased risk of bleeding
Nonsteroidal anti-inflammatory agents	Major	Increased risk of bleeding
Nifedipine	Moderate	Increased risk of nifedipine side effects
Trazodone	Major	Excessive sedation
Anticonvulsants	Moderate	Decreased anticonvulsant effectiveness
Buspirone	Moderate	Changes in mental state

design. Firstly, an open study design was used in which 80 patients tried Ginkgo biloba. Then responders ($n=21$) were recruited to a double-blind study. Interestingly, there were six patients who experienced the opposite effect and got worse. However, in the controlled phase no support for the use of Ginkgo biloba was found. The study was later criticised by Ernst and Stevinson (1999), who claimed that the Ginkgo biloba was underdosed. Instead, in their review, they described five randomised controlled trials, which they interpreted as showing that Ginkgo biloba extracts are effective in treating tinnitus. Subsequently, Drew and Davies (2001) conducted the largest trial to date on Ginkgo biloba and tinnitus, with 978 participants. The intervention lasted for 12 weeks and consisted of either 50 mg Ginkgo biloba extract or placebo administered three times daily. Results showed no significant differences between the groups, though critics of this trial have suggested that the dosage of Ginkgo biloba (GB) was below the therapeutic level. In some studies GB has been combined with laser treatment, showing some promise in one uncontrolled trial (Plath and Oliver, 1995) and no effects in a placebo-controlled trial (von Wedel et al., 1995).

Morgenstern and Biermann (2002) published a double-blind pacebo-controlled study of GB in patients with a primary complaint of tinnitus. The primary outcome measure was matched for tinnitus loudness and no significant improvement was demonstrated. Rejali et al. (2004) performed a placebo-controlled randomised trial of GB on patients in a general otolaryngology clinic whose primary complaint was tinnitus. The primary outcome measure was the Tinnitus Handicap Inventory, and no significant improvement was demonstrated over placebo following 12 weeks of use of GB.

A Cochrane systematic review of the published evidence regarding the efficacy of Gingko biloba for tinnitus was undertaken by Hilton and Stuart (2004). They considered the studies of Drew and Davies (2001), Morgenstern and Biermann (2002) and Rejali et al. (2004), concluding that:

> The limited evidence did not demonstrate that Gingko Biloba was effective for tinnitus which was a primary complaint.

A clinician should avoid the view that patients could try Ginko biloba with impunity, 'just in case'. Graham et al. (2008) note possible drug interactions between GB and prescribed medications (Table 17.2).

Table 17.3 Potential drug interactions with St John's Wort. (Based upon Graham et al. (2008)).

Interacting drug	Interaction severity	Description of interaction
SSRI	Major	Increased risk of serotonin syndrome
Oral contraceptives	Major	Decreased contraceptive effectiveness
Bezodiazepines	Minor	Reduced benzodiazepine effectiveness
Statins	Moderate	Reduced atorvasatin and simvastatin effectiveness

Other CAM approaches to tinnitus

To our knowledge, no study has been published on the use of St John's Wort (*Hypericum perforatum* – SJW) in the treatment of tinnitus. SJW is widely available without prescription in Europe and the USA, and is marketed as helpful for depression. Studies of efficacy in this regard have varied in the benefits described: SJW has been held to be beneficial for mild to moderate but not severe depression (Ernst, 2002), but evidence has also cast doubt about whether it is in fact superior to selective serotonin reuptake inhibitors or indeed placebo (Rapaport et al., 2011). The evidence base suffers from a heterogeneity of definitions of depression and its severity, and variations in preparation and dose of SJW.

A recent study of the CAM use of 657 patients who renewed prescriptions with their USA General Practitioner found that 6.9% were also taking SJW (Graham et al., 2008). Given the common use of SJW in the treatment of depression (Nahas and Sheikh, 2011), it could potentially be helpful for at least some tinnitus patients – specifically, those with low mood. Care should be taken though to point out that concern exists about SJW interaction with several conventional drugs, with potentially significant adverse effects (Graham et al., 2008; see Table 17.3).

Melatonin is a hormone secreted at night by the pineal gland and acts as a natural hypnotic in the regulation of the sleep–wake cycle. It is available without prescription in some countries (though not in the UK). Observing the role of sleep loss in tinnitus, Rosenberg et al. (1998) undertook a controlled crossover study on its effects on tinnitus. Included were 30 patients who showed similar improvements following placebo and active treatment. However, a slight difference was found in favour of melatonin for the patients who reported insomnia related to their tinnitus. Similar findings were reported by Megwalu and colleagues (2006) who found an associated improvement in quality of sleep and tinnitus handicap during 8 weeks of use of melatonin. This study did not have a placebo control, however, and the sustainability of the benefits was not determined. Neri et al. (2009) reported improvements in both tinnitus handicap and matched tinnitus intensity associated with the use of melatonin and sulodexide (which has vasodilatory properties, and the authors hypothesised that this might improve the efficacy of melatonin upon tinnitus). The statistical analysis of the results in this study were not sufficiently robust for it to make a major contribution and the effects upon sleep were not considered as a contributory variable, but it is a further signpost to potential benefits of melatonin for persons with troublesome tinnitus in whom sleep is disrupted (and who have not benefited from more conventional sleep management techniques).

Dietary supplements

A variety of dietary supplements have been suggested to have a beneficial effect upon tinnitus. One should bear in mind, however, that it is relatively easy to engender toxic levels of several vitamins and minerals using supplements purchased from supermarkets, health food stores or via the Internet, and caution should be urged by clinicians and exercised by patients. While the absence of evidence of efficacy of specific dietary supplements is detailed below, this can be summarised by saying that no remotely convincing evidence for efficacy of such agents yet exists.

The possibility that vitamin B complex supplements may be beneficial for tinnitus has been raised, and Siedman and Babu (2003) consider that vitamins B1 (thiamine), B3 (niacin), B6 (pyridoxine) and B12 (cobalamin) may have a specific role. The evidence quoted is anecdotal at best, despite the potential for conducting placebo-controlled trials in this area.

Several minerals have been suggested as treatments for tinnitus. Shambaugh (1986) and DeBartolo (1989) proposed zinc deficiency as a mechanism of tinnitus generation and advocated the use of supplements. Hypozincaemia was not supported as a mechanism for tinnitus, however, by Gersdorff et al. (1987), and a placebo-controlled trial of zinc supplements for tinnitus did not demonstrate benefit above placebo control (Paaske et al., 1991). Ochi et al. (1997) reported an improvement in troublesome tinnitus in a group treated with zinc supplements in an uncontrolled study and repeated this study with a control group (Ochi et al., 2003), again eliciting data supporting the use of zinc in tinnitus treatment. Another uncontrolled study was reported to indicate benefit from zinc supplements by Yetiser et al. (2002) and a placebo-controlled trial by Arda et al. (2003) again indicated benefit. In no study, however, has benefit been shown to persist, and neither has the possibility that benefit is specific to patients with demonstrable zinc deficiency been rigorously investigated. Thus, despite several studies in this area, the observation of Ochi et al. (2003, p. 25) that 'the clinical correlation between zinc and tinnitus remains obscure' seems pertinent.

Reports have appeared in the UK popular press indicating that magnesium supplements may benefit individuals with troublesome tinnitus. The only evidence cited in support of this is not relevant and consists of a study by Attias et al. (1994) that tentatively suggested that magnesium supplements may reduce the risk of noise-induced hearing loss in battle combatants. Siedman and Babu (2003) supplemented this evidence with anecdote, but the evidence for efficacy of magnesium supplements in tinnitus is paltry at best.

Antioxidant therapy is not strictly a CAM, but may be considered here in the context of dietary interventions. Savastano et al. (2007) reported the effect upon tinnitus loudness and associated distress in 31 patients undergoing oral reactive oxidant therapy (glycerophosphorylchorine, glycophosphorylethanolamine, B-carotene, vitamins C and E). This observational trial (with no placebo control) indicated reductions in tinnitus loudness and distress after 18 weeks of treatment, but no indication was given as to whether these improvements persisted, and randomised controlled trial evidence would be required before firm conclusions could be drawn.

Stimulation of the ear

Direct electrical stimulation of the ear and magnetic stimulation of the brain are discussed in Chapter 16. Ultrasonic stimulation has been tried for tinnitus, with an initial suggestion of benefit (Carrick et al., 1986), but this was not repeatable (Rendell et al., 1987). Interestingly, in the initial study participants were described as 'an enthusiastic group of 40 patients' (Carrick et al., 1986, p. 153), but despite this observation only 28 of them completed the study.

Ear candles

Ear candling is a practice wherein the recipient lies on the side while a hollow cone that has been soaked in paraffin and has been allowed to harden is placed inside the ear and lit. Claims that the practice originated with the Hopi tribe have been discounted. Anecdotal reports of benefits for cerumen and tinnitus are available, the mechanism being said to be the creation of a vacuum in the ear canal. More formal investigation has determined, however, that not only do ear candles not produce a negative pressure within the ear canal but also that serious harm may befall the participant (Seely et al., 1996). Specifically, burns, occlusion of the external auditory meatus with wax and of perforation of the tympanic membrane have been documented (Seeley et al., 1996), and this has caused the Food and Drug Administration (FDA) to issue a stern cautionary alert about their use (IA 77-01, 1998). Ernst (2004) summarises the situation thus:

> There are no data to suggest that it is effective for any condition. Furthermore, ear candles have been associated with ear injuries. The inescapable conclusion is that ear candles do more harm than good. Their use should be discouraged.

Summary

The question remains as to whether the tinnitus therapist should encourage or discourage patients about undertaking complementary therapy. There is a common misconception that herbal medicinal products are devoid of adverse effects, which is not true (Ernst, 2002), and this is also the case for overuse of vitamin and mineral supplements. Furthermore, the effect of repeatedly trying therapy in the complementary domain may prove not only expensive but repeatedly disappointing, with resultant demotivation. This effect was demonstrated empirically in attenders at a tinnitus clinic who had tried other treatments and who demonstrated significantly less acceptance of change and novel concepts (Andersson, 1997). Caution in the use of complementary therapy should be advised by a tinnitus therapist.

The placebo effect has been invoked repeatedly above. Tyler et al. (2001) advocate harnessing the placebo effect in tinnitus treatment, proposing the following strategy:

- Be perceived as a knowledgeable professional.
- Be sympathetic towards the patient.

- Demonstrate that you understand the problem.
- Provide a clear therapy plan.
- Show that you care.
- Provide feelings of mastery.
- Provide hope.
- Instil confidence in the tinnitus clinician.

While such suggestions are neither new (Fowler, 1948) nor applicable only to tinnitus, they are of such eminently good and common sense that they are commended to tinnitus clinicians, mainstream or complementary alike.

Chapter 18

Tinnitus and hyperacusis in childhood and adolescence

Although tinnitus and hyperacusis are well recognised in adulthood it is widely assumed, even by many health care professionals, that these symptoms either do not exist in childhood or are exceedingly rare. There are certainly more obstacles to obtaining reliable information regarding tinnitus and hyperacusis among children, but the available information suggests that these symptoms are far from rare and that this represents a somewhat neglected clinical area.

Prevalence and incidence of childhood tinnitus

The prevalence of tinnitus in children has been investigated and the findings are worthy of careful consideration. There are, however, methodological problems estimating the prevalence of tinnitus in a paediatric population: it is difficult to ask children about such symptoms and some studies have relied on parental report rather than obtaining information from the children themselves. Moreover, younger children may easily misconstrue what the question entails or may respond in the affirmative to please the adult questioner. Research in this area is further confused by differences in worldwide opinion as to what constitutes the different stages of development and in particular what ages constitute the boundaries between childhood, adolescence, youth and adulthood. The following studies cover a wide gamut of different age ranges covering subjects at very different stages of development. As a generalisation, some experience of tinnitus seems to be common in childhood (Baguley and McFerran, 1999, 2002; Davis and El Rafaie, 2000; Shetye and Kennedy, 2010) but tinnitus impact seems lower than among adults. Far fewer children than adults are seen in tinnitus clinics and it is relatively unusual to see an adult tinnitus patient who reports that their problem has been present since childhood.

Tinnitus: A Multidisciplinary Approach, Second Edition. David Baguley, Gerhard Andersson, Don McFerran and Laurence McKenna.
© 2013 David Baguley, Gerhard Andersson, Don McFerran and Laurence McKenna.
Published 2013 by Blackwell Publishing Ltd.

Tinnitus in the general paediatric population and among children with normal hearing

There are several estimates of the prevalence of tinnitus in childhood in the general population but most can be criticised to some extent for methodological shortcomings. Nodar (1972) surveyed 2000 normally hearing children aged 11–18 years and found a tinnitus prevalence of 15%, with no further specification of annoyance. In a study by Mills et al. (1986), 93 normal-hearing children were screened for tinnitus, 29% reported tinnitus and one-third were said to be bothered by their tinnitus. Stouffer et al. (1992) used a more rigorous interview method and found that in a group of 161 children aged 7–10 years, 6% reported tinnitus, a figure that rose to 13% if less rigorous criteria were used. Holgers (2003) studied 964 school children aged 7 years. The prevalence of tinnitus in this sample was 13% among the normal hearing children, but the possibility of priming cannot be excluded as the children were first given a lecture on hearing loss and tinnitus. The study was later replicated involving 756 7-year-old children (Juul et al., 2012). Results showed that 41% out of 756 children reported either noise-induced tinnitus or spontaneous tinnitus on several occasions (Juul et al., 2012). In a study of primary and junior high school children, Aksoy et al. (2007a, 2007b) found a prevalence of 15.1% in a sample size of 1039 children; 54.4% of the tinnitus group were boys, compared to 45.5% girls, though this gender difference did not reach statistical significance. Tinnitus was central in approximately half and split evenly between left and right ears in the other half. The age group with most tinnitus were aged 14 years. This figure tallies well with a mean age of 15.86 years in a group of 95 children who sought help for tinnitus (Holgers and Juul, 2006). Coelho et al. (2007a) looked at 506 children aged between 5 and 12 years, finding 19.6% with tinnitus that was bothersome or annoying; 8.1% of those who reported bothersome tinnitus also had hyperacusis. A large Polish study (Raj-Koziak et al., 2011) looked at 60 212 children aged 7 years, of whom 8164 (13.6%) reported some tinnitus experience and children with hearing loss were twice as likely to report tinnitus as their peers with normal hearing. Three-quarters of those with tinnitus had not mentioned the symptom to their parents.

Tinnitus in children with hearing impairment

There are several attempts at quantifying the level of tinnitus among hearing-impaired children but, as might be expected, the study populations are even more heterogeneous that when looking at normal-hearing children. Mills and Cherry (1984) found a prevalence of 29.5% in children with sensorineural hearing loss ($n=66$) and 43.9% of children with otitis media ($n=44$). In another study Mills et al. (1986) found a prevalence of 38.5% among children who were seen by otologists and said to have evidence of ear disease ($n=267$). In one interesting study, Nodar and Lezak (1984) found that 100% of children with moderate or severe hearing loss reported tinnitus, whereas in children with profound hearing loss 35% did so. Rather similar findings were made by Graham (1987) who found that in children with moderate or severe hearing loss 66% reported tinnitus, whereas in children with profound hearing loss the figure was 29%. Drukier (1989) studied 331 children with profound hearing loss, of whom 33% reported tinnitus. Viani (1989) found a similar percentage of 23% in a sample of 102 children with severe hearing loss (aged 6–17 years). In association with a study on social competence, parents of children with hearing impairment were asked about tinnitus in their child. Only 13% were aware of any tinnitus in their child (Andersson et al., 2000c). A study by Aust (2002) looked at 1420 children who had current or previously reported hearing loss and found a tinnitus prevalence of 7.2%; 73.5% of these children had hearing loss in one or both ears at the time of tinnitus complaint while 26.5% had normal hearing.

Data concerning the incidence of tinnitus in paediatric populations is starting to emerge. Baguley et al. (in press) reviewed the tinnitus activity of four major European tinnitus centres (Cambridge, Padua, Regensberg and Warsaw), finding that, in 2009, 88 cases of a primary complaint of tinnitus were seen, representing 3.8% of the entire paediatric workload and 0.3% of the total all-age clinical workload in these centres. In 93% of cases the patient was aged 10 years or older. While this is not a true incidence study, it indicates that even in well-established tinnitus centres, complaint of childhood tinnitus is not common.

Prevalence of childhood hyperacusis

Most studies that have examined the prevalence of hyperacusis in childhood have looked at defined populations where there is a condition known to be associated with altered loudness tolerance, such as autism (Rosenhall et al., 1999; Khalfa et al., 2004) or Williams syndrome (Klein et al., 1990). Within a general paediatric population, Coelho et al. (2007b) estimated the prevalence of tinnitus and phonophobia in a study of 506 children aged between 5 and 12 years. They used a combination of interview and loudness discomfort level (LDL) testing to estimate the prevalence, but acknowledged that there is no single agreed definition of what constitutes hyperacusis. They found hyperacusis in 3.2% of the study group and within this subgroup phonophobia was reported in 31%. Among those with hyperacusis, 50% also reported tinnitus.

There are no reliable studies into the incidence of hyperacusis in general paediatric populations but Baguley et al. (in press) determined the proportion of paediatric tinnitus cases in whom hyperacusis was also observed, utilising data from four European tinnitus centres. Of the 88 tinnitus cases, tinnitus was accompanied by hyperacusis in 34 patients (39%).

Impact of tinnitus

Some researchers have argued that tinnitus in children is not annoying and that it will pass (Graham, 1981), and certainly fewer children than adults present at tinnitus clinics despite the apparently similar prevalence of tinnitus percepts in the two populations. It has also been suggested that children notice tinnitus but habituate so rapidly that it does not become a clinical problem. There are, however, some children who become seriously distressed because of tinnitus and in a follow-up study by Martin and Snashall (1994), looking at 42 children with tinnitus, as many as 83% still had their tinnitus when reviewed. Sleep problems are also very prevalent among children complaining of tinnitus (Gabriels, 1996; Aksoy et al., 2007a). Kentish et al. (2000) showed that children with tinnitus can suffer a great deal as a consequence of their symptom and reported that 80% of a group of 24 children referred to a child psychology service for help with tinnitus complained of sleep problems. This extremely high figure may be specific to that particular child psychology service and may not be relevant to all children who experience tinnitus, but does show the importance of asking about sleep when confronted with a child complaining of tinnitus. Headache is also commonly reported among children with tinnitus (Martin and Snashall, 1994; Aksoy et al. 2007a), as is dizziness and vertigo (Aust, 2002; Aksoy et al., 2007a). Holgers and Juul (2006) investigated 95 patients between the ages of 8 and 20 complaining of tinnitus. They used several tools, including the Hospital Anxiety and Depression Scale (HADS); 32% scored above the cutoff level for anxiety disorders while 14.5% scored positively for depressive disorders. This is interesting to observe though it should be noted that HADS has been validated for use in adolescents from the age of 12 but not for younger children. Holgers and Juul (2006) also noted that 54% had developed their tinnitus after noise exposure, most commonly music, and that there was a correlation between the severity of the symptom and the degree of associated hearing loss.

Associated conditions

Martin and Snashall (1994) sent questionnaires regarding 67 children who had previously presented with a complaint of tinnitus. Of the 42 questionnaires returned, among these were diagnoses of migraine (13 cases), juvenile Ménière's (5 cases), other forms of endolymphatic hydrops (3 cases), noise-induced hearing loss (3 cases), chronic suppurative otitis media (3 cases) and brainstem tumour (1 case). Juvenile Meniere's disease has also been reported with tinnitus as one of the symptoms by Hausler et al. (1987) and Telischi et al. (1994). Perilymph fistulae have also been described in childhood (Parnes and McCabe, 1987). Tinnitus in childhood has been reported as a manifestation of vestibular schwannoma, particularly in association with neurofibromatosis type 2 (Evans, 2009). Motion sickness has been reported to be more common in children with tinnitus (Coelho et al., 2007b).

Hyperacusis in childhood has been described in association with autistic spectrum disorders, and this has been raised in Chapter 12. A study by Khalfa et al. (2004) assessed the subjective perception of loudness in 11 subjects with autism compared to 11 age- and gender-matched healthy controls, using two psychoacoustic tests. These tests found smaller auditory dynamic ranges in the autistic group compared to the control group, together with an increased perception of loudness, supporting a diagnosis of hyperacusis in children with autism. Tecchio et al. (2003) hypothesised that autistic patients present abnormalities at the preconscious stages of sensory system cortical processing. They used magnetoencephalography to investigate this theory in a group of 14 autistic patients, which included children, with 10 age- and gender-matched control subjects. Significant differences in cerebral responses between patients and control subjects were detected, supporting the view that autistic subjects exhibit dysfunction of the processing of auditory sensory afferent information. Limbic system structures including the amygdalae and hippocampus were implicated. Another study used tests including auditory brainstem response audiometry, distortion product otoacoustic emissions and acoustic reflexes, and demonstrated no difference in peripheral auditory function between autistic children and matched controls (Tharpe et al., 2006). When these subjects were tested using age appropriate behavioural tests including visual reinforcement audiometry, tangible reinforcement operant conditioning audiometry and conditioned play audiometry, the autistic children performed less well. An alternative view is contained in work by Gomot and colleagues (2008), who demonstrated auditory hypervigilance in young adults with high functioning autistic spectrum disorder (ASD) using fMRI. Essentially wider and more rapid brain activation associated with novel auditory stimulation was observed in individuals with ASD compared with a control group. This fits with the clinical observation that persons with ASD who can report their auditory experiences do not discuss being overwhelmed with the intensity of sound, but continually distracted by new and unexpected sound events. Such observations are glimpses into the complexity of sound tolerance issues. Further robust research is keenly awaited in this area.

Williams syndrome, also known as Williams–Beuren syndrome or WBS (Pober, 2010), is a genetic neurodevelopmental disorder caused by deletion of genes on chromosome 7. It is characterised by hypercalcaemia, growth delay, cardiovascular anomalies and elfin facial features. There are reports that most people with this condition have associated hyperacusis (see Chapter 12 for a detailed discussion of this issue). The exact cause of the hyperacusis in Williams syndrome remains unknown, but efferent system hyperactivity and absent stapedial reflexes have been suggested (Attias et al., 2008), as has deficiency of the enzyme LIM kinase with subsequent outer hair cell dysfunction (Matsumoto, 2011).

Management

There is a dearth of information relating to how to investigate and treat tinnitus in childhood. Commonsense dictates that history taking should be conducted in child friendly surroundings, involving the child as well as the parents. The areas to be covered are the same as for adults, but age-appropriate terminology should be used and it is sometimes useful to ask the child to make a drawing of their tinnitus (see Figure 18.1).

Particular attention should be directed at tactfully finding potential sources of stress both at home and at school: factors such as family illness, bereavement, parental divorce and bullying may be relevant. Because of the high reported prevalence of sleep disturbance among children with tinnitus this should be specifically enquired about. Examination as with adults is often normal but it is important to not only examine the auditory system but also to check for dysmorphic features.

Children who have the communication skills to report tinnitus are generally able to perform adult audiometric tests. Pure tone audiometry together with tympanometry would seem sensible baseline tests, particularly given the prevalence of Eustachian tube dysfunction in childhood. Stapedial reflex testing has been suggested as a routine test, as a measure not only of auditory function but also of brainstem function (Shetye and Kennedy, 2010), but this test should probably be avoided in those children where hyperacusis is suspected. Clearly, if the clinical history suggests another concomitant hearing problem such as an auditory processing disorder, then the appropriate test battery should be applied. If the child has hyperacusis as part of autistic spectrum disorder or

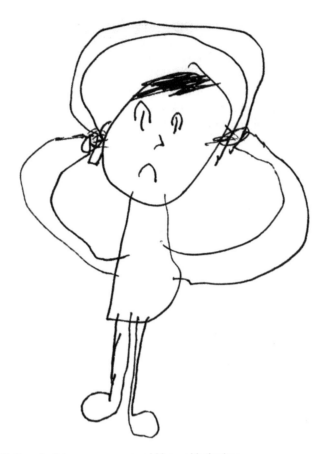

Figure 18.1   Self-portrait by a seven year old boy with tinnitus.

Williams syndrome then other types of hearing tests may be required. The limited available epidemiological evidence suggests that children with clinically significant tinnitus are more likely than adults to have specific underlying otoneurological pathology. Therefore clinicians should not withhold further tests such as MRI scans. The same criteria as in adulthood should apply, namely asymmetry of the symptom, asymmetrical hearing loss or associated neurological symptoms or signs.

If investigation has revealed a specific cause for the tinnitus, this should be addressed. The majority of children with tinnitus will, however, not have specific pathology. Explanation and reassurance is important both to the child and the parents. Viani (1989) studied 24 children with tinnitus and reported that most were both surprised and relieved to know that they were not alone in suffering from this symptom. It would seem sensible to recommend correcting any hearing loss, though surprisingly there is very little evidence base to support the use of hearing aids in the management of tinnitus in all age ranges. Indeed, there is some evidence that hearing aids may be counterproductive in certain cases of paediatric tinnitus (Gabriels, 1996) due to ear canal occlusion by the hearing aid mould, though using open fittings may minimise this. Environmental sound enrichment can be helpful and this can often be managed by use of a quiet radio or story CDs rather than having to resort to environmental sound generators, though when these are offered they are usually readily accepted. Ear-level sound generators have been used in the paediatric tinnitus population but there is no reliable evidence regarding the efficacy of their usage. Where possible, allowances should be made at school and appropriate liaison can be undertaken via the Teachers of the Deaf service. An uncontrolled retrospective study in Poland (Bartnik et al., 2012) looked at 143 children who had been seen in a tinnitus clinic in 2009. This constituted 0.5% of the total number of patients seen with tinnitus; 41.3% of the study group had troublesome tinnitus and, of these, just under half had normal hearing. All the children with troublesome tinnitus were treated with Tinnitus Retraining Therapy and 6 months after the start of therapy 81.4% were reported as having shown statistically significant improvement. Some children require input from child psychologists or psychiatrists.

There is very little evidence regarding drug treatments for tinnitus in childhood. One small uncontrolled study (Gryczyńska, 2007) looked at 55 children who were treated with betahistine for their tinnitus. The conclusion was that betahistine was helpful but in the absence of a more rigorous study it is difficult to recommend this strategy. As sleep problems seem to be common in childhood tinnitus, use of sleep hygiene measures can be helpful, escalating, if necessary, to more formal psychological management (Kentish et al., 2000).

An alternative perspective on the management of childhood tinnitus has been entitled *Narrative Therapy* (Kentish and Crocker, 2006; Edwards and Crocker, 2008). Coming from a psychological perspective, Susan Crocker and colleagues are interested in the stories and meanings associated with tinnitus, and use narrative therapy to consider why tinnitus has become problematic. Within a context of discussion and play, externalising techniques are used wherein the tinnitus becomes viewed as a problem separate from the person. Opportunities exist to address other associated issues in the child's life. Clinical trial data for this approach is not available and it could only sensibly and safely be delivered within psychological services, but it represents an intriguing approach to childhood tinnitus.

Summary

Tinnitus experience is widespread among children with prevalence figures very similar to those seen in adults. Tinnitus distress, however, seems much less common among children: young people make up a tiny fraction of those seeking help for tinnitus. There is some evidence that childhood tinnitus is more likely to be associated with specific otological or neurological pathology, so careful attention should be paid to children who do seek help. Disrupted sleep appears to be a common complaint among children with troublesome tinnitus. Hyperacusis is commonly seen in certain conditions including Autistic Spectrum Disorder and Williams Syndrome. Relatively little work has been done on hyperacusis within the general paediatric population but the limited evidence suggests that this symptom is also quite common in childhood. Although there is little robust evidence regarding the management of tinnitus and hyperacusis in this age group, techniques that are employed for adults can be adapted for use in children.

Chapter 19

Special populations

In this chapter we consider some specific situations in which tinnitus and/or hyperacusis can become problematic. It is hoped that there may be two potential benefits: the first is that clinicians seeing patients in the situation described may be able to rest upon previous knowledge in the area and the second is that in by describing the specific there may be some insight into the wider patient experience of tinnitus and hyperacusis.

Acoustic shock

Since the 1990s it has been recognised that a particular symptom complex can arise among call centre operatives who are exposed to sudden unexpected sounds through their headsets or telephone handsets. The condition has become known as Acoustic Shock Injury, Acoustic Shock Syndrome, Acoustic Shock Disorder or simply Acoustic Shock (McFerran and Baguley, 2007; Milhinch, 2002). The sounds that trigger the condition are known as Acoustic Shrieks or Acoustic Incidents. There is very little written about the topic in the medical literature, with more interest being shown by the legal profession and telecommunications engineers.

Some of the sounds that have triggered acoustic shock have been analysed. A Danish study (Hinke and Brask, 1999) found sounds in the frequency range 100 Hz to 3.8 kHz, with intensities varying from 56 to 100 dB. An Australian study (Milhinch, 2002) found sounds of 2.3 to 3.4 kHz with intensities between 82 and 120 dB. One feature that seemed common was that the rise time of the acoustic incident sound was generally short, usually between 0 and 20 ms. Sound sources that have been reported in association with acoustic shock include sounds generated by faulty headsets, transmission faults, positive feedback from cordless telephones, accidental connection with facsimile machines or modems and sounds deliberately produced by customers such as shouting or blowing a whistle. Work undertaken in 1979 (Alexander et al., 1979) showed that spurious sounds were common in the call centre environment, with 36 signals detected in 2000 hours of recording, though none of the

Tinnitus: A Multidisciplinary Approach, Second Edition. David Baguley, Gerhard Andersson, Don McFerran and Laurence McKenna.
© 2013 David Baguley, Gerhard Andersson, Don McFerran and Laurence McKenna.
Published 2013 by Blackwell Publishing Ltd.

sounds found in this study went on to cause auditory symptoms. There are no reliable figures regarding the prevalence or incidence of acoustic shock but anecdotal reports suggest that only about one in ten of people exposed to an acoustic incident go on to develop any acoustic shock symptoms and of these only about one in six have persistent symptoms. Women seem to be affected more often than men, even after correcting for the skewed gender distribution of call centre employees. Acoustic shock is seen more commonly in those who report stress and pre-existing neck and shoulder pain. There does not, however, appear to be an excess representation of people with previous psychological morbidity (McFerran and Baguley, 2007).

Symptoms generated in acoustic shock can be divided into those that occur immediately or soon after the incident and those that have delayed onset. Among the immediate symptoms, pain is the most common single symptom: 81% have otalgia, 11% pain in the neck or jaw and 7% report pain in the face. Tinnitus and balance symptoms are also common, affecting about half of affected individuals. By contrast hearing loss is less common, being reported in 18%. Where there is hearing loss it is usually temporary and is often not of the typical noise-induced hearing loss pattern. In a few instances, acoustic shock has resulted in sudden collapse. The delayed onset symptoms include anxiety, depression, sleep disturbance, hypervigilance, a sensation of aural blockage or fullness and reduced sound tolerance (hyperacusis or phonophobia).

Examination is often unremarkable. Audiological testing commonly shows normal hearing or age-appropriate symmetrical sensorineural hearing loss. In the minority where hearing loss exists it is often of an atypical pattern and may affect the low or mid-range frequencies rather than the typical 4–6 kHz of noise-induced hearing loss. Patients with acoustic shock are often extremely anxious about further noise exposure and unless there is an extremely compelling clinical reason, loudness discomfort levels should be avoided. To date there does not appear to be any benefit in undertaking more involved audiometric testing such as ABR or OAE. Asymmetric symptoms or test results should be investigated in the normal fashion with appropriate imaging, most typically MRI; it should not be automatically assumed that an asymmetric audiogram is due to the acoustic shock.

The pathophysiology of acoustic shock remains an enigma. Some workers have suggested that tonic tensor tympani syndrome (TTTS) is responsible for many cases (Westcott, 2006), and certainly the predominance of pain as a symptom argues for middle ear involvement. Furthermore, there is evidence that middle ear muscle function is linked to the serotoninergic system (Thompson et al., 1998), with potential links to the startle reflex and emotional pathways. On the other hand, the presence of balance symptoms in almost half of affected patients together with sensorineural hearing loss, albeit in the minority, suggests that the inner ear may be implicated. Changes in the central auditory system have also been suggested and the hypervigilance, sleep disturbance, anxiety and depression point to psychological mechanisms. Clearly further research is required to elucidate these varied hypotheses. The management of acoustic shock patients is equally unclear. Many patients with acoustic shock feel that they are disbelieved because there is nothing to detect on examination and in many cases testing is within normal limits for the patient's age. Anecdotally many patients with acoustic shock are relieved when they have received a diagnosis. Thereafter, using the same techniques as used in patients with hyperacusis and other forms of reduced sound tolerance seems appropriate. Thus, explanation, counselling and desensitisation using low-level sound may be useful.

Psychological techniques may also have a role, particularly for those in whom hypervigilance, anxiety and depression are foremost symptoms.

Ultimately it would be preferable to prevent acoustic shock happening in the call centre working environment rather than having to treat it. Headphones and handsets in UK call centres already have output limiters that restrict maximum output to 118 dB. Many of the sounds that have produced acoustic shock, however, are considerably quieter than this level and would therefore still reach the operatives. Also there is a limit to how much sound can be filtered without excessively reducing intelligibility. Various electronic in-line devices have been produced that remove sounds with rapid rise times in the 1–4 kHz band. Because there are no reliable prevalence and incidence figures it is not clear whether such devices are beneficial. Care with the acoustic environment of call centres, utilisation of techniques to reduce stress in the workplace and staff education programmes may also be helpful in reducing the number of people who develop acoustic shock.

It is not clear whether acoustic shock can only be caused by sounds delivered through headphones or telephone handsets. The authors of this book have certainly encountered patients who have been exposed to some unexpected noise in other situations and have gone on to develop the symptom complex seen in patients with acoustic shock. Causative sounds have included demolition work, impact noise in engineering workshops and the use of air horns at sporting events. Sound sources that are close to the ear seem more likely to result in acoustic shock symptoms than distant sounds.

Single-sided deafness

The term single-sided deafness (SSD) has entered widespread use, and usually refers to unilateral profound sensorineural hearing loss. By reviewing the incidence data for the most common causes of SSD, including viral infection, ischemia, trauma, surgery, Meniere's disease and autoimmune hearing loss, Baguley et al. (2006a) estimated that there may be 8000 new adult cases of SSD arising in the UK each year. In the majority of cases the contralateral ear is unaffected and of normal hearing acuity. Despite this, patients with SSD experience a range of auditory challenges, including poor/absent auditory localisation skills, poor speech discrimination in noise, and may have reduced confidence and quality of life as a result. Presently the best instrument for measuring the auditory impact of SSD is the Spatial, Speech and Qualities of Hearing Questionnaire (SSQ) (Gatehouse and Noble, 2004; Noble, 2010).

The first careful consideration of tinnitus in SSD was undertaken by Chiossoine-Kerdel et al. (2000), who found that of the 21 respondents in a cohort of 38 patients who had undergone a sudden SNHL in preceding years leading to SSD, 14 experienced tinnitus (67%) and in 29% the tinnitus was severe (as determined by the THI).

Interventions for SSD have included CROS hearing aids and bone-anchored hearing aids. The results are not compelling for either of these interventions (Baguley et al., 2006b, 2009), and for bone-anchored hearing aids in SDD in particular it seems that care must be taken to ensure that the patient is both motivated and realistic about the outcome. To the authors' and manufacturer's knowledge, no study has been made of the effect upon tinnitus of CROS or bone-anchored hearing aids upon tinnitus in patients with SSD.

An alternative approach to intervention is to use a cochlear implant (CI) for the treatment of tinnitus in SSD (Baguley, 2010). While this might seem dramatic, for some patients it potentially offers both an inhibition of their tinnitus and the ability to access hearing in the SSD ear. To date there have been two published series describing the use of a cochlear implant in SSD patients with tinnitus. Paul van der Heyning and colleagues have provided information in a series of patients with SSD and severe tinnitus (van der Heyning et al., 2008), the latest update including 26 such individuals (Punte et al., 2011). Self-report group measures of tinnitus intensity and of handicap all indicate significant improvement, and all patients reported that they had benefited. Vermiere and van der Heyning (2009) reported on the effect upon hearing of the CI in 20 subjects from this series. Group data indicated benefits in SSQ scores and in experimental conditions where noise was present from the front and speech from the CI side. The group was spilt into two subgroups, one with normal hearing contralaterally ($n=11$) and the other those who wore a hearing aid contralaterally ($n=9$): the auditory benefit of the CI for the hearing aid wearers was marginally greater than for the normal hearing subjects.

The second series to consider is that from Arndt et al. (2011), who report a series of 11 patients with SSD and severe tinnitus who underwent CI, notably after trialling a CROS hearing aid and declining a bone-anchored hearing aid. Group metrics of tinnitus distress and of quality of life improved, and in some patients an improved auditory localisation ability was demonstrated. SSQ scores improved with CI use. The researchers proposed that not only did CI in SSD not degrade hearing by competing with the normal contralateral hearing but that the CI contributed to improved auditory abilities and that normal and electrical hearing were integrated.

Thus early indications are that CI is a promising treatment for tinnitus in SSD. Future work should focus upon candidacy and demonstrating the cost effectiveness of this intervention.

Low-frequency noise complaint

There are reports that in developed countries there are a small number of people who report being distressed by low-frequency noise (LFN) in their environment (Leventhall, 2003). The disturbance can be so severe that complainants frequently resort to extreme measures, like sleeping in a car or garden shed, to try to avoid the noise. In the majority of such cases, no LFN can be identified by environmental health or acoustic survey professionals. Little is known about the incidence of LFN complaint. Typically two-thirds of LFN complainants are women and the average age is around 55 years (Pedersen et al., 2008; Leventhall, 2003), although this profile may not be significantly different to the profile of complainants about noise in general (e.g. not LFN).

A postal survey of LFN complainants was conducted in Denmark in 2002 (Møller and Lydolf, 2002); 198 respondents reported sounds as deep humming or rumbling. Most reported hearing the sounds but others mentioned a perception of vibration either in their body or in external objects. Secondary effects such as insomnia, headaches and palpitations were often associated with the sounds. In a proportion of cases, surveys were conducted that generally showed LFN levels to be at or below hearing thresholds.

The complaint pattern in LFN appears to be very similar to that of severe tinnitus. The mechanism may be some identification of LFN as anomalous, and then an orientation to that and fixation upon it, with associated distress, involving the limbic and sympathetic autonomic nervous systems, as is the case in tinnitus. Present interventions include CBT (Leventhall et al., 2008), with modest success, and a trial of audiologically based management is presently underway in the UK.

Musical hallucination

Musical hallucination (MH) is defined as the subjective experience of hearing music, or aspects of music, when none is being played (Cope and Baguley, 2009; Sanchez et al., 2011), and persons who complain of this may be referred to a tinnitus service. MH is rare, though robust prevalence and incidence data are not available. Those studies that have been undertaken have tended to consider people with psychiatric treatment services rather than wider populations. Risk factors associated with MH include female gender, old age, significant cochlear hearing loss and social isolation – though these factors are far from independent of each other. The experience of MH can be very distressing, and may involve extreme irritability and insomnia. A number of MH patients are firmly of the belief that the sound arises from a neighbour rather than themselves, and may have attempted retaliation for this imagined assault. MH is often characterised by hearing short fragments of music, which may be familiar tunes such as nursery rhymes, old pop songs or hymns. In some patients the natural history is of a gradual improvement, with shorter fragments of music, but in some patients, the situation continues unabated.

There are likely to be multiple mechanisms of MH, but the association with significant hearing loss has led to the understanding that one perspective is to view MH as a deafferentiation phenomenon (Griffiths, 2000). Reduction in auditory input may trigger a disinhibition of fragments of auditory (musical) memory, which then acquire emotional salience.

The investigation of a patient with MH should exclude neurological disease, and as a number of medications have been associated with MH, a prescription review is indicated. Care should be taken to ensure that the experience is entirely musical, and if there are verbal aspects (other than the expected lyrics) then psychiatric evaluation is indicated, as is also the case in the distorted belief that a malevolent neighbour is responsible (once that has been excluded!). Audiologically based treatment is based upon counselling and hearing aids: evidence is sparse about the efficacy of such an approach but it has face validity.

Armed forces and combat veterans

Military personnel may be exposed to large amounts of noise, both as sudden blasts and chronic exposure, and unsurprisingly there is a high incidence of noise-induced hearing loss. Helfer (2011) reports that around 36 000 US service personnel undergo a permanent and significant NIHL each year while on active service and that this number has risen in recent years. Some personnel may be exposed to chemicals that have ototoxic qualities, and this may further increase the impact upon hearing for this population (Kirk et al., 2011). While hearing protection is issued routinely in many armed forces, the use of such devices is very variable and may actually decrease on the battlefield with the urgent need for environmental awareness (Killion et al., 2011). Research in this area is not of high quality, however (Verbeek et al., 2009), as indicated in a Cochrane review.

Until relatively recently little attention was given to the incidence of tinnitus in the military and veteran populations. It has become apparent that there is a major issue with tinnitus in military personnel, and in the US tinnitus is the most prevalent disability in cases added to the Veterans Affairs Programme (Baldwin, 2009). Of 1.3 million US troops deployed in Afghanistan, 70 000 are receiving benefit for tinnitus related disability, and the numbers of combat veterans who experience troublesome tinnitus is said to be rising (Folmer et al., 2011; Helfer, 2011).

In the military population there is also a considerable incidence of post-traumatic stress disorder (Helfer et al., 2011) and Fagelson (2007) has considered this issue in detail. In a series of 300 referrals for tinnitus to a veterans facility, Fagelson found that 34% also carried a diagnosis of PTSD. The association may be biochemical in that PTSD is thought to involve serotonin dysfunction (as are tinnitus and hyperacusis), but also complicates treatment.

Blast injury may affect not only the cochlea but also the brain. This situation is entitled traumatic brain injury (TBI) and can in itself carry associated hearing loss and tinnitus (Lew et al., 2007; Fausti et al., 2009), and should be borne in mind when assessing blast injury patients.

While some of the increase may be due to more diligent reporting, there do seem to be increases in the incidence of NIHL, tinnitus, PTSD and TBI in the military population, with the most accessible data coming from the US services. With the large population of military veterans with tinnitus in the US, it is not surprising that specific protocols for tinnitus therapy have been developed (Henry et al., 2005a, 2005b, for example).

Functional tinnitus

Functional hearing loss, by which is meant behaving as if one has a hearing loss when auditory function is normal, is surprisingly common. The behaviour can be limited to test situations, or observed also in social interactions, and can be intentional or unintentional (Austen and Lynch, 2004; Peck, 2011). Very little is known about functional tinnitus, but it would be surprising if there were not claims to have tinnitus, or claims about tinnitus intensity, that were not faithful representations of the situation. As with hearing loss, that might be intentional, and there might be some gain for the patient, either in sympathy or adopting an 'illness identity', or financial in the case where there is litigation or disability benefit. It may be unintentional and potentially involves the somatisation of emotional pain associated with events such as bereavement or bullying. Given the lack of an objective measure of tinnitus this area is fraught with difficulty and robust multidisciplinary work is keenly awaited.

Summary

In this chapter we have considered some very specific populations and how their auditory experiences correlate with general tinnitus and hyperacusis. Such detailed attention is worthwhile, not least for benefit to particular patients, but also for insights that may be gleaned into these interesting conditions.

Chapter 20

A multidisciplinary synthesis

In recent years there has been a major resurgence of scientific and clinical interest in tinnitus. This increased interest is of great potential benefit for the millions of individuals who are distressed by this common symptom. Activity in tinnitus research is slowly answering questions regarding the best way to undertake tinnitus management. Within the large number of studies that have been published, however, there are many with unique and sometimes idiosyncratic design, so that comparison between test results or treatments is often nigh on impossible. In brief, the major problem has been and continues to be a lack of large-scale well-conducted randomised controlled trials (Dobie, 1999, 2004; Hesser, 2010; Møller, 2007). On a more promising note, important findings are emerging on the basic mechanisms behind the generation of tinnitus and its consequences (Baguley, 2002; Roberts et al., 2010), and hopefully this bulk of new knowledge will inform treatments and lead clinicians to consider how to develop their protocols further. There are also indications that systematic integrative meta-analyses and other systematic reviews can be conducted on the tinnitus literature (e.g. Hesser et al., 2011a, 2011b; Phillips and McFerran, 2010), which will hopefully bring order into the field of tinnitus research.

Once the acute distress of patients seen in the tinnitus clinic has passed there is often time for reflection and wider ranging discussion. At this point, usually in follow-up appointments, patients may remark 'Why is there no research into tinnitus?' or 'Why does no one really understand this?' The reader will by now have realised that there is much research (for instance 8000 papers currently appear in a Medline search on 'tinnitus' and nearly 500 on 'hyperacusis') and there are many models, so that the challenge facing the tinnitus clinician and researcher is the integration of these insights into a whole that is congruent with personal clinical experience and understanding.

Another common question is 'Why has there been so little progress with tinnitus?" There are of course issues of financial resources and staffing levels, but one major factor has been the lack of interdisciplinary communication and collaboration. The inadequacy of any one discipline or perspective to perceive the tinnitus as a whole can be illustrated by an ancient Sufi story, retold by Senge (1990):

Tinnitus: A Multidisciplinary Approach, Second Edition. David Baguley, Gerhard Andersson, Don McFerran and Laurence McKenna.
© 2013 David Baguley, Gerhard Andersson, Don McFerran and Laurence McKenna.
Published 2013 by Blackwell Publishing Ltd.

> As three blind men encountered an elephant, each exclaimed aloud. 'It is a large rough thing, wide and broad, like a rug,' said the first, grasping an ear. The second, holding the trunk, said 'I have the real facts. It is a straight and hollow pipe.' And the third, holding a front leg, said 'It is mighty and firm, like a pillar.' Given these men's way of knowing, they will never know an elephant.

Thus a cellular physiologist considering tinnitus may see patterns of activity in the cochlear nerve; a psychologist may see emotional distress, behaviour change and cognitive distortions; an audiologist may see hearing loss; and an otologist, possible aural pathology. Working effectively with tinnitus patients, both now and in the future, requires one to find new ways of knowing. In a clinical context the perspectives of otology, audiology and psychology can work together, and in research the additional perspectives of pharmacology and neuroscience are of profound importance. It is only by working together that one can see the whole elephant and then begin to design truly effective therapeutic interventions (Møller, 2007).

There are several practical implications for this call for synthesis on a conceptual level. Firstly, tinnitus patients will be best served clinically by being treated by a multi-disciplinary team (Langguth, 2011). Indeed, the notion of a multidimensional management approach to tinnitus patients is not new (Stephens et al., 1986; Coles and Hallam, 1987), but perhaps seldom put into practice apart from in a few specialist centres. It is not possible to be prescriptive about the exact composition of a tinnitus team because of variations in staffing, skills and experience, both locally and globally. However, underlying this book is the principle that tinnitus patients deserve effective diagnosis by an informed and interested clinician, and that therapy should be undertaken by an experienced professional with a deep understanding of all the different perspectives of tinnitus. Furthermore, there should be clear and explicit referral paths for patients whose issues fall outside the scope of practice of the core team members.

The second implication concerns the knowledge base of the team members. It would not be appropriate to expect an otologist or audiologist to be fully aware of all the details and practical aspects of cognitive behavioural therapy, and neither would one expect a psychologist to be fully conversant with the details of otological or audiological practice. One should expect, however, these professionals to be *literate* in these other disciplines, such that they are aware of the broad scope of practice and are able to integrate insights and concepts from those other disciplines into their own understanding and practice. An example of this has been the writing of this book, in that it should not be assumed that the psychological chapters were written by psychologists and the otology-related elements by an otologist or audiologist. To the contrary, all chapters have had a team approach with much discussion about evidence and conceptual robustness from all disciplines.

Thirdly, it almost goes without saying that this team approach can only be achieved by hard work and dedication, and in an atmosphere of mutual respect and positive regard (Tyler et al., 2001). Finally, it should also be noted that the above is not asking for the moon, in that such multidisciplinary treatment teams and protocols are evident in other fields, chronic pain management being an example. Brooks and Chalmers (1991), in a paper on training in audiology, presented a promising model of the core knowledge needed in audiology and linked professional knowledge that can be attached to this basic

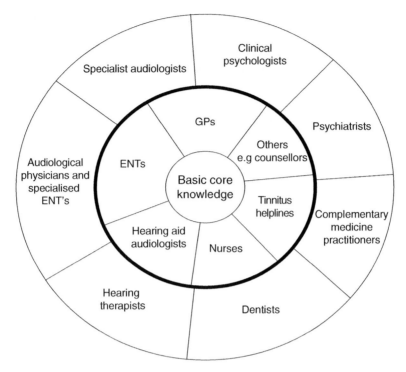

Figure 20.1 Core professional knowledge needed for tinnitus management.

knowledge. Clearly, this is relevant for tinnitus management too. A tentative model is presented in Figure 20.1, outlining what we believe should be the first line of practitioners seeing tinnitus patients and the second tier of specialists to whom difficult clinical problems can be referred. What should this basic core knowledge about tinnitus contain? We hope we have covered not only this basic knowledge but also a portion of information that, although not clinically essential for each professional who sees tinnitus patients, will expand their understanding of tinnitus and its consequences.

Some readers having reached this point may have become concerned that they have not been instructed in what exactly to do or say to a tinnitus patient sitting in front of them. While in Appendices 1 and 2 we indicate some starting positions for clinicians, we believe that a prescriptive, or 'cook book', approach is neither helpful nor respectful to the individual situation of the patient, nor indeed the experience and skills of the clinician or therapist. In any case, such material is readily available elsewhere. It has been of more importance, we believe, to have laid out current understandings of tinnitus incorporating theoretical and practical perspectives, so that the reader may have a wide understanding of the topic that will inform their practice.

What then of the future for tinnitus research and therapy? Baguley et al. (2003) delineated a vision for tinnitus research, wherein novel techniques and insights from neuroscience might be utilised to determine the mechanisms of tinnitus, giving targets for therapy and the means of robust determination of the efficacy of such therapy. The present indications of a collaborative approach to tinnitus research provides evidence that this process is underway.

As has been described above (Chapter 13), the hope for pharmacological therapy is very much alive and the prospect of integration of pharmacological treatment with counselling therapy is intriguing. The future of present therapies is also interesting to consider. Both psychological therapies and TRT are based upon conceptual models of tinnitus that are not fully satisfactory. Furthermore, the therapeutic approaches derived from these models are both limited in their application, in the case of formal psychological therapy by the number of interested psychologists available and in TRT by the insistence on attending a formal TRT training course. What is needed are therapeutic approaches that are widely available and based upon insights from both the psychological and neurophysiological models, which in our view are neither mutually exclusive nor immiscible. It is our hope that this second edition of this book may in some small way promote such approaches and syntheses.

Appendix 1

A treatment protocol for use in primary care, audiology and otolaryngology

The following protocol provides an introduction to the practicalities of tinnitus treatment: for further reading seek out the 'Good Practice Guide for treating adults with tinnitus' (2009) produced by the Department of Health, UK, a publication to which three of the four authors of this book contributed. The intention of this protocol is to supply guidelines rather than rules, not to be overly prescriptive and to identify themes that can be explored and adapted according to local needs and resources. These guidelines propose a stepped approach to tinnitus care, indicating what may be appropriate at primary, secondary and tertiary care levels, and the clinical red flags triggering onward referral. The protocol is designed around the UK healthcare delivery system and details will vary in different countries. For example, in many countries it is possible for patients to refer themselves directly to ENT or audiology services without having to seek referral from their General Practitioner.

Primary care

Although there is a limit to how much otological investigation can be undertaken in a primary care setting, the General Practitioner or Primary Care Nurse is pivotal in identifying which patients need to be referred onwards for further investigation and treatment. The following guidelines list the main reasons for referral to secondary care:

- Unilateral tinnitus or hearing loss
- Pulsatile tinnitus
- Examination showing abnormalities of the ears
- Associated vertigo
- Associated neurological symptoms or signs
- Significant associated symptoms of anxiety or depression
- Significant associated sleep or concentration problems
- Patient anxiety regarding possible underlying pathology such as an intracranial neoplasm
- Distressing tinnitus that is failing to settle despite initial measures
- Patient request for ENT/audiology assessment.

Tinnitus: A Multidisciplinary Approach, Second Edition. David Baguley, Gerhard Andersson,
Don McFerran and Laurence McKenna.
© 2013 David Baguley, Gerhard Andersson, Don McFerran and Laurence McKenna.
Published 2013 by Blackwell Publishing Ltd.

If the patient has none of these factors, has bilateral tinnitus and is not excessively distressed, then it is appropriate to offer initial management within primary care. It is possible to offer considerable help and support to tinnitus patients without having great knowledge of the topic. It is equally possible to do harm: many tinnitus patients report that their tinnitus got dramatically worse when they were given information such as 'You've got tinnitus; there is nothing that can be done for it; you'll just have to get used to it.' This negative counselling is common and to be deprecated. Better to say nothing than to say this. Some positive statements regarding tinnitus are listed below:

- Tinnitus is common. About 1 in 10 of the UK population have tinnitus at any given time. Most of these people, however, are not severely distressed by the symptom. The figure for people who have tinnitus so badly that it is preventing them doing their normal daily activities is much lower, at approximately 1 in 200. More tinnitus is at the mild end of the spectrum than the severe end.
- In many cases tinnitus lessens – or even disappears – with time. Habituation is common.
- Tinnitus is very rarely associated with sinister pathology.

In addition to general reassurance, practitioners in primary care can help by removing any wax that may be blocking the ears and causing conductive hearing loss. Cerumen removal should be undertaken as gently as possible and if removal is proving difficult, patients should be referred to secondary care where more sophisticated equipment is available. When present, simple underlying pathology can be treated. Herein, however, lies another potential pitfall. Many people with tinnitus report that their ears feel blocked and are then treated as if they have Eustachian tube dysfunction, secretory otitis media or even acute otitis media. There is anecdotal evidence that trying treatments that do not help has a negative overall impact on this symptom. Decongestant or antibiotic treatment should only be administered if the diagnosis of middle ear disease is incontrovertible – and these conditions are rare causes of tinnitus. If in doubt, seek advice from ENT. The administration of drugs aimed at specifically reducing tinnitus can also be counterproductive: there are no currently approved drugs for the treatment of idiopathic tinnitus and it is better not to try drugs such as betahistine, diuretics or antispasmodics as failed treatment appears to have a long-term deleterious effect on the course of tinnitus. It is, of course, entirely reasonable to administer drugs for associated symptoms: antidepressants are appropriate for depression, anxiolytics for anxiety and short courses of hypnotics for severe sleep disturbance. It should be made clear to the patient that these preparations are intended to improve the co-morbidities and have no specific anti-tinnitus properties, so that the patient's expectations are not unfairly raised. Everyone presenting with tinnitus should have an assessment of their hearing. In primary care some practitioners have access to pure tone audiometry either within their own practice or via community audiology services. If any degree of hearing loss is detected, consider referral for formal audiological assessment and hearing aid fitting: optimising hearing is generally beneficial for tinnitus patients, even if the hearing is not at a point where hearing aids would normally be considered from a communication perspective. If the hearing cannot be assessed in primary care, the patients should be referred onwards: every tinnitus patient merits a hearing test as the bare minimum investigation. In addition to offering reassurance, those in primary care can offer patient information leaflets and contact details for organisations such as the British Tinnitus Association or Action on Hearing Loss, both of which offer advice on tinnitus via their websites, telephone helplines and written material. If a local tinnitus group is available, the patient can be directed towards that body.

Secondary care

Health care professionals in secondary care encounter patients with tinnitus in various ways and with varying degrees of severity and clinical need. Not every patient requires full tinnitus therapy for what may be a minor irritation in their life. It is up to the health care professional(s) to decide how much input is required.

In the UK, most patients referred to secondary care will be referred to an ENT Surgeon or an Audiovestibular Physician. In some centres direct access from GP to audiology for tinnitus is underway. Such arrangements should be subject to local clinical governance and the principle that sinister pathology should be excluded in a patient with tinnitus should be upheld.

Patients presenting with tinnitus as an incidental symptom

People who have been referred to ENT or audiology with other problems as disparate as hearing loss, dizziness or mid-facial pain may answer in the affirmative when asked about tinnitus as part of the medical history taking process. The clinician should then try and ascertain a ranking of the patient's various symptoms. As clinic time is often very limited it is important to have a few pertinent questions that can ascertain the clinical importance of the tinnitus report. Some of the questions that can be used are listed below:

- What is the nature of the tinnitus? If the tinnitus is pulsatile the patient should be investigated further.
- Where is the tinnitus? If the tinnitus is unilateral the patient should be investigated further.
- Is sleep significantly disturbed?
- Is concentration at work disturbed?
- Would the patient like further input regarding the tinnitus?
- If only one symptom could be cured would that be the tinnitus or another symptom?

Administration of a tinnitus questionnaire could be utilised at this point but there are downsides to using such devices: questionnaires take time to complete and score and questionnaires can result in someone with mild tinnitus feeling worse about their symptom after filling in the questionnaires. The authors of this book do not routinely use tinnitus or mental health questionnaires at this stage of the patient pathway but reserve them for those patients in whom the clinical history suggests that tinnitus is a serious problem. If the tinnitus is judged to be a minor problem then management can be carried out in a very similar way to primary care management. An audiogram should be obtained and if there is more than minimal hearing impairment, ways of improving the hearing should be discussed. Explanation of tinnitus and reassurance can be given – ENT personnel and audiologists have much more in-depth knowledge of the topic that most primary care doctors and nurses, so this discussion can go into much greater detail. This process of information giving can be very powerful: as the Nobel laureate Oliver Smithies said in his Nobel Prize Banquet Speech, 'It is possible to overcome fear with knowledge.' In addition to an explanation of the process by which the tinnitus has developed, simple measures to counteract the symptom can also be discussed. Environmental sound enrichment and basic distraction and relaxation techniques can be suggested. The patient can be given details of tinnitus organisations and self-help groups, as discussed above. The authors of this book do not routinely arrange follow-up appointments for patients in this category but do offer them a way of getting back in touch if they feel they want more input regarding their tinnitus. The method of achieving this will vary according to local protocols and patient preferences but giving an 'open' appointment, offering a telephone number, postal address, email address or giving the patient a business card are all appropriate methods. A letter outlining the details of the consultation should be sent to the patient's primary care team.

Patients presenting with tinnitus as the main problem

Patients may be referred straight from primary care with a history of tinnitus or they may have been filtered out of the group that presented with tinnitus as an incidental symptom because their tinnitus has been found to be a more significant problem than originally thought. This is the group of patients that provides the bulk of the work for a tinnitus clinic.

Some thought should be given to the setting and timing of tinnitus services. It is important to be comfortable and uninterrupted. Time is also important: many clinicians allow 45–60 minutes for an initial tinnitus appointment. If someone with troublesome tinnitus is encountered in a busy ENT outpatient context the patient may require a longer clinic slot on another occasion. Patients with hyperacusis should be given appointments when the clinic environment is quiet – such patients are unlikely to be happy in the clinic waiting area during a busy paediatric clinic. A discussion of tinnitus can unearth some emotionally raw topics, so the clinician should be prepared for this eventuality. Allowing a friend or relative to accompany the patient to the appointment can be very helpful in supplying support and also helping to retain any information that is given to the patient. On the other hand, having the friend or relative present can inhibit the free flow of the patient/clinician dialogue. Occasionally the third party can also rather take over the session and dominate the patient in a counterproductive fashion, supplying answers that the clinician would rather hear from the patient. It is perhaps best to let the patient decide whether or not they want someone else with them. If they do bring someone else with them it can be useful to engineer some time without the third party so that the patient can be asked if there is anything else they wish to discuss. The initial clinical history should be detailed and serves several purposes: to allow diagnosis of underlying pathophysiology, to determine the impact of the tinnitus upon the individual and their family, to identify associated anxiety/depression and to determine the aims of the patient in attending the clinic. The structure of the interview should cover the following areas:

- Nature and site of tinnitus. One noise or several? Constant or rhythmical? If rhythmical, is it pulse synchronous? Musical or voices? Left, right or both ears? Or in the middle of the head? Or appears to be external?
- The onset of the tinnitus and relation to illness and/or life events.

- Does the patient feel there was a specific cause?
- Variability of the tinnitus. Relation to environment and stress. Can the tinnitus be altered by facial movements, jaw movements or other actions? How much of the time is the tinnitus intrusive?
- What is the impact of the tinnitus on normal daily life?
- Is there reduced sound tolerance? All sounds or specific sounds? How does this limit normal daily activities? Protection measures, and do these constitute overprotection?
- Associated symptoms: hearing loss, dizziness, neck problems, temporomandibular joint problems, mental health issues.
- General medical questions.
- Social history including occupational history. Noise levels at work and whether the job required the use of hearing protection equipment. Recreational noise exposure including music, firearms, motorcycles, do-it-yourself tools.
- Details of current medication and allergies.

If desired, this interview can be conducted using a structured interview form such as the Tinnitus Retraining Therapy Initial Interview form. Once the interview is complete, the patient should be examined. This follows standard ENT/audiology practice, particularly focusing on the ears, cranial nerve function and temporomandibular joints. If the tinnitus has a pulsatile component, it is useful to ask the patient to tap out the rhythm while the clinician palpates the radial pulse to determine if the tinnitus is pulse-synchronous. If it is pulse-synchronous, a stethoscope should be used to listen for bruits. Bruits can be very quiet and very localised – listening should be carried out in a quiet environment and the stethoscope should be moved around multiple locations on the head and neck. Electronic stethoscopes that allow amplification of quiet sounds are available. If there is a history of non-pulse-synchronous pulsatile tinnitus the eardrums should be carefully observed under high magnification using an operating microscope and the palate should be examined, in both cases looking for involuntary movement. As opening the mouth sometimes abolishes myoclonic movements, using a fibreoptic endoscope passed through the nose to observe the palate from above may be helpful.

Healthcare questionnaires can help to quantify the degree of impact that the tinnitus is causing and whether there is associated psychological distress. Such tools are also useful for monitoring the patient's progress. As discussed in Chapter 5, there are many different questionnaires available, all with pros and cons. The Tinnitus Handicap Inventory (THI) and The Hospital Anxiety and Depression Scale (HADS) are probably the most widely used in UK tinnitus clinics. There is some debate as to how best to administer questionnaires and various methods have been tried: sending the questionnaires by post to the patient prior to the appointment; giving the questionnaires to the patient on arrival in clinic, to complete in the waiting room; completing the questionnaires in the consulting room with the clinician available to answer queries if required. One of the authors of this book gives the questionnaires out after he has taken the clinical history and examined the patient and asks them to fill in their responses in a quiet area of the clinic. This has the benefit of allowing the clinician time to write up his clinical notes and formulate an individual treatment plan for the patient. The exact method is probably unimportant and what matters is to be consistent and do the same for all patients. Other questionnaires are available but used less frequently. These include hyperacusis questionnaires, sleep questionnaires and the Nijmegen questionnaire for detecting chronic hyperventilation. These should only be used if the clinical history suggests they would be helpful. The results of the questionnaires should be calculated in the clinic and the findings fed back to the patient. It is important to note that a high score on a mental health questionnaire does not prove that the patient has depression or an anxiety state: these diagnoses can only be made by a suitably trained mental health professional. A high score would, however, suggest that a psychological assessment of that patient would be sensible.

Audiological assessment for the majority of the tinnitus and hyperacusis patients seen by the authors of this book comprises a pure tone audiogram and a tympanogram. If a diagnosis of middle ear muscle myoclonus or patulous Eustachian tube is suspected, a tympanometer may be used to indirectly observe changes in middle ear compliance that may be responsible for tinnitus. This is done by setting the tympanometric pressure to the point of maximum compliance with the tympanometer's probe tone turned on and observing spontaneous changes in static compliance synchronous with the patient's reported tinnitus. Other tests should only be utilised if they are going to alter the management of the patient. More investigation does not mean better investigation. Furthermore, some tests can be distressing for the patient and can make their clinical condition worse. In particular, stapedial reflex estimation and loudness discomfort levels (LDLs) risk exposing people who are sound intolerant to the very stimulus that they fear. LDLs can occasionally be helpful in the management of hyperacusis but the test is far from reliable and should only be undertaken after a detailed discussion with the patient. Measures of tinnitus pitch and loudness are difficult to perform and have poor test–retest reliability. Speech audiometry and otoacoustic emission testing rarely alter subsequent management.

A proportion of people with tinnitus require further investigation. For nonpulsatile tinnitus, the following guidelines can be used:

- Unilateral tinnitus
- Unilateral or asymmetrical hearing loss as indicated by a difference in the left/right bone conduction thresholds of 20 dB or greater at two or more of the following frequencies: 500, 1000, 2000 or 4000 Hz
- Unexplained persistent otalgia
- Other associated neurological symptoms or signs.

In addition, some patients volunteer that they are worried by the possibility of having intracranial pathology. Although there may not be any clinical reason for suspecting this, it is often very difficult to help this group of people until they have had their fears allayed. The most common investigation required in the investigation of idiopathic nonpulsatile tinnitus is MRI scanning (Fortnum et al., 2009). MRI scanners are noisy and this may distress those patients who have reduced sound tolerance. It is useful to forewarn patients that MRI is noisy and reassure them that ear defenders are available for them to wear during the scan. If the patient has an MRI contraindication or is unable to contemplate an MRI scan, CT may be useful. An occasional patient may decline all forms of imaging, in which case latency brainstem evoked audiometry still has a role. As discussed in Chapter 5, the investigation of pulsatile tinnitus depends on local availability and expertise. However, one possible approach is outlined below:

- Normal otoscopy, cervical bruit
  - Doppler ultrasound
- Normal otoscopy, no bruit
  - MRI, MRA or CT, CTA
  - If scan normal, no further test
- Normal otoscopy, cranial bruit
  - MRI, MRA or CT, CTA
  - If scan normal, angiography
- Abnormal otoscopy, middle ear mass
  - CT (may also need MR and angiography).

If the investigation throws up a causative diagnosis, a specific management strategy may be indicated. The majority of patients, however, will have no such diagnosis and can then progress to tinnitus management.

There is no 'correct' way of administering tinnitus management. It can be done as a one-to-one meeting or in a group session. With patients who live far from the clinician, portions may be undertaken by telephone or email. Similarly, there is no hard and fast rule about who undertakes the treatment: tinnitus therapy can be administered by an audiologist, hearing therapist, doctor or nurse. The following framework is useful:

- Education, explanation and reassurance
  - Why did tinnitus develop?
    - Mechanisms, ignition site, pathophysiology
  - Why is it bothersome?
    - Relationship with arousal
    - Sleep issues
    - Emotional impact
    - Association with depression/anxiety if relevant
- What is there that can be done about it?
  - Further information, including books (e.g. McKenna et al., 2010) and Internet sites.
  - Self-help literature, including tinnitus support groups.
  - Bedside environmental sound generator.
  - Other forms of environmental sound enrichment, such as apps for a smartphone that can then be played through a docking station.
  - Ear-level sound generator (used differently for tinnitus and hyperacusis).
  - Hearing aids. It can be useful to demonstrate the possible benefits of amplification using a personal listener (pocket amplifier) – this gives patients a good indication of what amplification might do for them and may help to prompt them to take this step.
  - Combination hearing aids with inbuilt sound generators, or use of an app for a smartphone to stream to a hearing aid using Bluetooth.
  - Relaxation therapy. Having a stock of relaxation CDs in clinic is helpful.

Where hearing aids are going to be fitted some of the normal best practices may need to be revisited and it is important that the audiologist fitting the aid understands that it is being used as part of a tinnitus management strategy. It has been suggested that it may be helpful to turn off some of the more sophisticated features of modern digital aids, disabling

Table A1.1   Appropriate activities for ENT/audiology involvement.

- Interviewing the patient/family
- Presenting the diagnosis
- Providing information about the diagnosis
- Discussing interventions for the diagnosis
- Dealing with the patient's reaction to the diagnosis
- Onward referral as appropriate
- Supporting the strengths of the person and their efforts to regain function
- Supporting the strengths of the family to help them interact optimally with the patient
- Creating supportive empowerment for the patient and family to develop the ability to manage their own problems and be independent of the clinician

directionality and noise suppression, together with using low knee point compression (Searchfield, 2005). Concurrent sound tolerance problems may require further modifications to the fitting protocol. Amplification must be within the patient's range of comfort so as not to aggravate tinnitus or produce discomfort or annoyance. The patient with sound tolerance issues may initially find the output of his hearing aids to be less than optimal for hearing purposes. Amplification can be gradually increased as sound tolerance permits. If the patient's hearing loss is sufficiently bad to be causing significant communication difficulties it is helpful to have a multiprogramme aid, set up with a 'tinnitus programme' and a 'hearing programme'.

Clearly not all of these therapeutic options will be relevant in each case and different emphases will need to be placed in different circumstances. There are some specific issues that arise when talking with tinnitus patients, and one of the most common is bereavement and unresolved grief: having the details of the local bereavement counselling service can be helpful.

Most tinnitus patients will require more than one clinic appointment: a common pattern would be to see the patient for a follow-up appointment in 6–8 weeks, at that point assessing compliance and progress, and then 3 months subsequently. It is possible to discharge many patients then. If questionnaires have been administered at the initial visit it is useful to repeat this, both from the patient's point of view to ensure progress has occurred and from the clinician's aspect as an internal audit of their service.

The suggested framework may be overly prescriptive for some clinicians, and specifically there may be some who prefer an open-ended counselling dialogue with the patient, though such an approach may best be sourced within formal counselling services rather than ENT/audiology.

The clientele of a tinnitus clinic include some very troubled individuals, and this brings two important implications. Firstly, the clinician should recognise their personal and professional boundaries. The boundaries for audiological practice have been described by Fogle and Flasher (2003) and are listed in Tables A1.1 and A1.2. When out-of-boundary issues arise, they should be acknowledged and agreed to be important, but the need for engagement with other appropriate professionals should be emphasised. The second implication derives from the first: tinnitus clinicians will encounter things they find distressing and where possible should embed themselves in formal clinical

Table A1.2 Issues that are beyond the boundaries for ENT/audiology involvement.

- Chemical dependence
- Child or elder abuse
- Chronic depression
- Marital problems
- Personality disorders
- Sexual abuse and sexual problems
- Suicidal ideation

supervision, wherein they can debrief and be supported. Although such arrangements are well established in mental health services they are rare within the ENT/audiology framework.

Details of any tinnitus session should be fed back to the primary care team in the form of a written report or letter. Many patients find it useful to receive a copy of such letters. Alternatively, some tinnitus clinicians give their patients audio recordings of their consultations.

Plainly, not every tinnitus patient will respond to the above programme and it is important to recognise when a therapeutic intervention is not working. Options then include referring the patient to a fellow ENT/audiology colleague for a second opinion or changing tack and using a different modality such as cognitive behavioural therapy.

Tertiary care

Patients seen within tertiary care include those whose tinnitus is associated with specific pathologies such as vestibular schwannomas, other skull base tumours, severe Ménière's disease or profound sensorineural hearing loss. The management of such patients has already been discussed in other chapters of this book and is beyond the scope of this appendix. However, there will also be referrals of patients with nonsyndromic tinnitus who have failed to progress with a previous clinician. The initial management of such patients is the same as previously described: taking a clinical history, performing an examination and arranging baseline audiometric investigations. It is very useful to ask two additional questions: firstly, what treatments, both conventional and complementary, have already been tried; secondly, what does the patient understand about tinnitus. Many patients at this stage of their journey will be embracing multiple different treatment modalities and may have received so many contradictory pieces of information that they have a very confused idea of tinnitus. Addressing any misconceptions is the first place to start. Reinvestigation may also be necessary – it should not be taken for granted that the patient has been given a correct diagnosis. Once these issues have been addressed, the same basic treatment structure described above can be utilised, but allowing more time and patient/clinician contact. If the patient has been through ENT/audiology management previously and appears to have a good grasp of the concepts, it may be sensible to consider an alternative treatment paradigm at this point, perhaps referring the person to a clinical psychologist (see Appendix 2).

Frequent questions

There are various topics that arise at various times during tinnitus consultations and it is important to have thought through these topics and formulated suitable responses.

Suicide

Patients sometimes confess suicidal ideation during a tinnitus consultation. This is not something that most ENT/audiology staff are comfortable dealing with but is something that should not be ignored. There is no evidence that by talking about suicide it will cause the patient to proceed with this action. Most people with tinnitus who mention suicide do so in a fairly abstract fashion using a phrase such as 'I wouldn't mind if I were hit by a bus on the way home'. Such people are at a relatively low risk of committing suicide. Factors that increase the risk include male gender, elderly, living alone, mental illness, lower social class, previous suicide attempts and developed plans of how to commit suicide. If any clinician encounters a patient who they feel is at immediate risk of suicide or other self-harm, they should obtain immediate telephone advice from their mental health team. If a tinnitus patient mentions suicide as one of their long-term tinnitus worries but has no immediate suicidal intention they can be reassured that it is extremely unlikely that tinnitus will drive them to this extreme. For further information please refer to the section on 'Tinnitus and suicide' in Chapter 7.

Flying

People with tinnitus and more especially hyperacusis often worry that travelling by airplane will exacerbate their symptoms. They then avoid flying, which restricts their life and adds to the overall tinnitus burden. Obviously, flying does carry a small risk of causing harm to the auditory system due to pressure changes. However, the risk of long-term damage is very small. By and large, if tympanometry suggests normal middle ear function tinnitus patients should be encouraged to fly if they wish. Advice regarding nasal decongestants and Eustachian tube exercises can be helpful if they are worried regarding pressure change. If their worry is the noise within the airplane they should be reassured that this does not exceed safe levels. Noise cancellation headphones or sound attenuating earplugs can be helpful.

Prescription drugs

A number of people with tinnitus attribute their symptom to starting or altering a course of medication. The vast majority of prescription drugs do not cause or exacerbate tinnitus directly. However, starting or altering medication can be worrying and can cause unpleasant effects on the body. This raises the overall anxiety levels, which in turn results in tinnitus. There are a few genuinely ototoxic drugs that are discussed in detail in Chapter 5. For other drugs, the patient should be reassured and encouraged to wait. If the problem persists there is usually an alternative drug that can be tried. Stopping drugs should be discouraged until the patient has discussed the matter with the clinician who initiated the prescription.

Recreational drugs

While not condoning the use of recreational drugs, ENT/audiology staff can reassure patients that the majority of recreational drugs do not cause tinnitus. The possible exceptions are LSD and solvents. Occasionally a patient may worry that they have brought tinnitus upon themselves by an activity such as smoking cannabis. They can then enter a downward spiral of self-blame and worsening tinnitus. Breaking this spiral by simple reassurance is helpful.

Complementary and alternative medicine

Just as there is no currently available prescription drug that cures tinnitus, there is no complementary and alternative medicine (CAM) modality that solves the problem. CAM can, however, be helpful: such treatments are generally pleasant and relaxing. They also involve a lot of contact between the patient and the practitioner. One pragmatic response to patients who seek advice regarding CAM for tinnitus is to explain that, while not curative, CAM can help them to relax more, which can benefit their tinnitus. They should ignore any advertising claims that CAM can eradicate their tinnitus and should try one rather than multiple modalities. One caveat here is a subgroup of patients who draw up a list of CAM treatments and then slowly progress down the list crossing off failed treatments as they go. Each failed treatment generally makes the problem worse and this 'endless quest' should be discouraged.

Recreational noise

Many tinnitus people restrict their social life because they are worried that going to the cinema, theatre, sporting or music event will expose them to excessive noise. Some of these events are genuinely excessively noisy but use of hearing protection devices can enable the person to attend something that they enjoy. Care should be taken to ensure that they understand not to overprotect their ears at other times.

Using the Internet and other media

Most clinicians who run tinnitus clinics will at some stage have been confronted with a patient bearing reams of newspaper clippings and information printed off the Internet. It is important not to be dismissive of this – it represents considerable time and hope on the patient's part. The main points contained in the patient's material should be sympathetically discussed. Often it will be a new treatment modality that is still very much at the experimental phase and the usual advice in this case is to wait for completion of the trial.

Diet and supplements

There is much information available on the Internet and other sources that suggests that certain foodstuffs cause or worsen tinnitus. If one avoided everything that has been mentioned, deficiency diseases or starvation would be real risks! Commonly suggested items include red meat, dairy products, wheat, alcoholic drinks and caffeine. There is no good experimental evidence to suggest that any of these are implicated in tinnitus causation. Removing items from the patient's diet can restrict their life and adds to the overall tinnitus burden. Tinnitus patients should be advised to consume a normal balanced diet with no specific restrictions. Altering caffeine dosage can result in headaches so patients should be advised to keep their intake reasonably constant. Alcohol can be consumed in moderation if the patient wishes. Conversely, some patients feel that their tinnitus is being caused or exacerbated by dietary deficiencies and take large quantities of vitamin and mineral supplements. By and large this does no harm though it is possible to overdose on some supplements. Patients should be advised that if they have a balanced diet they are unlikely to be deficient in most of these elements and compounds. If they are truly worried that they have a dietary deficiency they should be referred to a nutritionalist or dietician.

Appendix 2

Cognitive behaviour therapy

The elements of a CBT approach are outlined below. There are several component parts to a CBT programme. They are not always discrete or easily distinguished from one another. For example, sometimes answering an assessment question can prove therapeutic for a patient. Sometimes a response to a therapeutic intervention reveals new information that adds to the assessment. The order in which we have set things out below is therefore intuitive but is by no means set in stone; some components may be skipped and others repeated. Only the core elements of the CBT approach are described; the use of sound therapy and hearing tactics, which might be in the overall treatment package, are not described here. More detailed accounts of the various elements of CBT for tinnitus can be found in self-helps books such as *Living with tinnitus and hyperacusis* (McKenna et al., 2010); *Kognitiv beteendeterapi vid tinnitus* (*Cognitive behavioural treatment of tinnitus*) (Kaldo and Andersson, 2004) and *Tinnitus: a self management guide for the ringing in your ears* (Henry and Wilson, 2001).

Education

It is important to offer patients information about the nature of tinnitus, the process of habituation and the factors that influence habituation. Within this context the role of psychological factors is highlighted. The role of high levels of sympathetic autonomic nervous system (ANS) arousal (stress arousal) in impeding habituation is emphasised. The point is also made that habituation is slowed if the tinnitus acquires emotional significance, i.e. tinnitus takes on an unpleasant meaning.

Relaxation training

In order to increase patients' acceptance of relaxation as a useful tool in managing tinnitus it is helpful to provide specific education about the nature of relaxation and its role in the process of change. It is useful to highlight the role of the sympathetic ANS in bringing

Tinnitus: A Multidisciplinary Approach, Second Edition. David Baguley, Gerhard Andersson, Don McFerran and Laurence McKenna.
© 2013 David Baguley, Gerhard Andersson, Don McFerran and Laurence McKenna.
Published 2013 by Blackwell Publishing Ltd.

about bodily symptoms such as increased muscle tension, heart rate, respiration and sweating along with changes in gut motility. These processes account for many of the symptoms experienced as part of an aversive reaction to tinnitus. Increased sympathetic ANS may also bring about psychological changes such as feelings of emotional numbness or separateness from everyday life and difficulties in concentrating. Increased arousal in this way also leads to selective attention on to the perceived threat, i.e. tinnitus, so increasing the annoyance associated with tinnitus. The parasympathetic ANS operates to reduce arousal levels and activating this helps to reduce the physical and psychological symptoms. This can be achieved through the relaxation exercises. It is usual to start with muscle relaxation. When the muscles are relaxed other elements of the system (e.g. heart, lungs, perspiration, selective attention) follow suite.

Usually, there are four stages to learning relaxation skills:

• Progressive relaxation (tense and release body parts)
• Release-only relaxation without tension
• Cue-controlled relaxation (controlled breathing)
• Rapid relaxation in everyday situations.

Imagery techniques are taught in association with the relaxation training. There are many CDs available that contain detailed instructions for relaxation. Details can also be found in the tinnitus self-help books referred to above.

The cognitive component

This is the process of helping the patient understand the central role of thoughts in experience, and how to identify and change them in order to find a more helpful, less threatening, meaning of tinnitus.

Again, some education or 'socialising' about this approach is helpful. A key element in this is helping the patient understand that the way one thinks about, or interprets, an event is more important in determining the reaction than is the event itself. Another key element is helping the patient understand that the same event can be thought about in different ways. There are many ways in which this can be achieved. It is particularly useful to draw upon the patient's own experiences in this context, for example differences between initial thoughts about tinnitus and current ones. It is also common practice to use an illustrative exercise in which the patient is asked to consider their likely responses to variations of a particular situation. An example is to ask the patient about their likely response to someone poking them in the back while they are travelling on a crowded bus or metro. Most people say that they would feel annoyed. When asked what thoughts the imaginary situation provokes they usually say they think the person doing the poking is thoughtless or inconsiderate. The patient is then asked to consider their reaction when they discover that the person doing the poking is blind. Most people say they feel sympathetic towards the blind person and when asked about their thoughts say they believe the poking was accidental. The physical event remains the same but the reaction changes as the interpretation of the event changes.

It is also helpful at this stage to make the point that a person may think differently about the same event at different times. A key point is that thinking changes as stress levels change. With greater stress thinking can become more 'distorted'. Typical examples of *cognitive distortions* are:

- *All or none thinking*. Viewing situations in two categories rather than in shades of grey. 'My life is perfect/tinnitus ruins my life. Tinnitus is present/absent. If I can't go to noisy places then I will have nothing in my life/I will gradually habituate to it'.
- *Catastrophizing*. Predicting negative outcomes without looking at more likely ones. 'My tinnitus will get worse and drive me mad.'
- *Discounting positive information*. Telling yourself positive information doesn't count. 'OK, I am all right when I am with people (in spite of tinnitus) but that doesn't mean I am OK.'

McKenna et al. (2010) referred to cognitive distortions as 'middle of the night thinking'. Many people have had the experience of worrying about a problem in the middle of the night and understand that the way they think about things at that time has a different quality to it from when they think about things at, say, lunch time.

This 'socialisation' highlights the point that a person's thoughts or interpretation of events is more important in bringing about a reaction than the event itself. If there is sufficient information, this point is then reiterated by reference to the patient's thoughts about tinnitus; for example, the patient's anxiety is a result of the thought that tinnitus will stop her getting peace and quiet and therefore slowly drive her mad.

If the patient's thoughts about tinnitus are not evident from the information gathered in the routine assessment then the patient is asked to specifically monitor them. This can be done in the consultation by asking the patient to reflect on the last time he or she was very distressed by tinnitus. The situation is recalled in as much detail as possible and the person is asked 'What went through your mind at that time?' Alternatively, the patient is asked to monitor their reactions to tinnitus, particularly their thoughts, between consultations. It is considered helpful if the patient writes down the component parts of their reactions to tinnitus. For example, the patient is asked to note any provocations of tinnitus that may be present, to note their emotional feelings and then what went through their mind in that situation. Lastly, the patient is asked to note what they did in response to the situation.

Typical NATs about tinnitus are:

- My quality of life has gone.
- I can't do normal things anymore.
- I will always feel like this.
- I'll have a nervous breakdown.
- I will go deaf.
- I will never get any peace and quiet.
- I must avoid loud sounds/silence.
- It's not fair.
- Other people don't understand.

Such thoughts are referred to as *negative automatic thoughts* (NATs). They are referred to as automatic because they are uninvited and they can be difficult to switch off. These thoughts have a 'middle of the night quality' and they are unhelpful in that they keep the person feeling bad and make it difficult to change. These thoughts are plausible; they seem right and may contain a grain of truth. The therapeutic task, however, is to consider the extent to which these thoughts are accurate and the extent to which they are a reflection of cognitive distortion or 'middle of the night thinking'.

It is important to highlight the link between the NATs and the emotional response. It is good practice to develop *a formulation* of the patient's problems at this stage, if not earlier. A formulation is simply a way of structuring the information concerning the patient's problems. It is a hypothesis about the causes and maintaining factors for the patient's problems that is guided, in this case, by CBT theory. Making the links between the various factors within a person's problems, and in particular highlighting the link between thoughts and emotions and between thoughts and behaviour, can help develop the patient's insight and suggest ways to resolve the problems. The formulation should be developed in collaboration with the patient and revised if necessary. Its job is to help the patient and therapist make sense of the problem. Formulations are often summarised as flow diagrams; very often feedback loops within the diagram represent points for intervention.

There is no set method for *evaluating* NATs. There are, however, some tried and trusted methods and an enquiry based on the following questions is among the most commonly used:

- What tells you that the thought is true – what evidence supports it?
- Is there anything that tells you it is not true – what evidence do you have against it?
- Is there any other explanation for what is happening?
- If a friend asked you for advice about the same problem what would you say?

These questions form only the basis of the enquiry. How they are addressed and answered may require creativity and ingenuity. For example, a detailed diary may be needed to address NATs such as 'tinnitus has ruined my life' or 'I can't enjoy things anymore'. Similarly, the use of relaxation exercises may help provide information about the NAT 'I always feel stressed' as well as offering a therapeutic intervention in its own right.

The approach to evaluating NATs should be one of collaboration with the patient and curiosity. The aim is not to prove the patient wrong but to help the patient discover a new perspective that takes into account all the information, both positive and negative, that is available. The result may not be one that completely removes a belief. Rather, it is often the case that the strength of thoughts are weakened and as a result negative emotions are less strong.

The *behavioural element* of CBT needs to be addressed carefully. Some tinnitus patients become depressed and as a result withdraw from many aspects of life. As there is a relationship between wellbeing and activity such patients are likely to benefit from increasing the amount and variety of things that they do. The behavioural component, however, is generally more sophisticated than a simple encouragement to do more and is set in the context of the patient's NATs and the formulation of their problems.

A careful consideration of NATs using the approach suggested above is usually helpful in weakening thoughts that are of mild to moderate strength. It is usually necessary, however, to combine the questioning approach with changes in behaviour in order to tackle more strongly held negative thoughts. In this context changes in behaviour are not made simply to increase a person's activity level. Rather, changes in behaviour are used as a further means of evaluating NATs. The function of the patient's current behaviour must therefore be understood in terms of their current NATs. In other words, an understanding is needed of what behaviour is being provoked by the NATs and, in turn, how that behaviour is maintaining or strengthening the NATs. In this context a person who believes that tinnitus might drive him mad, and as a consequence continually distracts himself through activity, may be asked to reduce his activity levels in order to evaluate this NAT. A patient who is suffering from tinnitus-related insomnia might believe that a poor night's sleep will lead to poor performance during the day and as a consequence takes things easy, with the result that he achieves little and is constantly aware of tinnitus; that patient may be asked to test the belief by taking a more active approach to the day. The patient who believes that constant background noise is necessary to prevent tinnitus from becoming overwhelming may be asked to experiment with periods of quiet or even silence. The behavioural component of CBT is therefore one in which the patient tests unhelpful NATs by experimenting with different ways of doing things. In the best traditions of experimentation it is good practice to clearly state the NAT, or 'hypothesis', to be tested and then to carefully work out the changes in behaviour that will effectively test this. Predictions are made about what might happen when the change is made and then the behavioural change is implemented, with whatever support the patient needs. The outcome is noted and, in order to facilitate learning, the process is reflected upon. The information gathered is used in a reconsideration of the NAT and the formulation.

It is good practice to evaluate the CBT through the use of *measures* of tinnitus complaint and possibly through the use of questionnaire measures of emotional wellbeing. The strength of NATs and of accompanying emotions should also be rated, usually on a simple 0–100 scale. These ratings should be repeated after each cognitive evaluation or behavioural experiment.

References

Aazh, H., El Refaie, A. and Humphriss, R. (2011) Gabapentin for tinnitus: a systematic review. *American Journal of Audiology*, **20**, 151–118.

Abbott, J. M., Kaldo, V., Klein, B., Austin, D., Hamilton, C., Piterman, L. and Andersson, G. (2009) A cluster randomised controlled trial of an Internet-based intervention program for tinnitus distress in an industrial setting. *Cognitive Behaviour Therapy*, **38**, 162–173.

Abdul-Baqi, K. J. (2004) Objective high-frequency tinnitus of middle-ear myoclonus. *Journal of Laryngology and Otology*, **118**, 231–233.

Abel, S. M. (1990) The extra-auditory effects of noise and annoyance: an overview of research. *Journal of Otolaryngology*, Suppl. 1, 1–13.

Adjamian, P., Sereda, M. and Hall, D. A. (2009) The mechanisms of tinnitus: perspectives from human functional neuroimaging. *Hearing Research*, **253**, 15–31.

Adoga, A. A., Adoga, A. S. and Obindo, J. T. (2008) Tinnitus and the prevalence of co-morbid psychological stress. *Nigerian Journal of Medicine*, **17**, 95–97.

Agarwal, L. and Pothier, D. D. (2009) Vasodilators and vasoactive substances for idiopathic sudden sensorineural hearing loss. *Cochrane Database of Systematic Reviews*, CD003422.

Agrawal, Y., Clark, J., Limb, C., Niparko, J. and Francis, H. (2010) Predictors of vestibular schwannoma growth and clinical implications. *Otology and Neurootology*, **31**, 807–812.

Akkuzu, B., I, Y., Cakmak, O. and Ozluoglu, L. (2004) Efficacy of misoprostol in the treatment of tinnitus in patients with diabetes and/or hypertension. *Auris Nasus Larynx*, **31**, 226–232.

Aksoy, S., Akdogan, O., Gedikli, Y. and Belgin, E. (2007a) The extent and levels of tinnitus in children of central Ankara. *International Journal of Pediatric Otorhinolaryngology*, **71**, 263–268.

Aksoy, S., Firat, Y. and Alpar, R. (2007b) The Tinnitus Handicap Inventory: a study of validity and reliability. *International Tinnitus Journal*, **13**, 94–98.

Alexander, R. W., Koenig, A. H., Cohen, H. S. and Lebo, C. P. (1979) The effects of noise on telephone operators. *Journal of Occupational Medicine*, **21**, 21–25.

Alhammadi, M., Jonsson, R., Olbers, T. and Yassin, O. (2009) Patulous Eustachian tube complicating gastric bypass surgery. *Journal of Laryngology and Otology*, **123**, 1058–1060.

Allan, C. L., Herrmann, L. L. and Ebmeier, K. P. (2011) Transcranial magnetic stimulation in the management of mood disorders. *Neuropsychobiology*, **64**, 163–169.

Allen, R. E. (1990) *Concise Oxford dictionary of current English*, Oxford: Clarendon Press.

Alster, J., Shemesh, Z., Ornan, M. and Attias, J. (1993) Sleep disturbance associated with chronic tinnitus. *Biological Psychiatry*, **34**, 84–90.

Altschuler, R. and Shore, S. (2010) Central auditory neurotransmitters. *The Oxford handbook of auditory science*, Volume 2, *The auditory brain* (eds A. Rees and A. Palmer), Oxford: Oxford University Press.

American Psychiatric Association (2000) *Diagnostic and statistical manual of mental disorders*, Washington, DC: American Psychiatric Press.

Anari, M., Axelsson, A., Eliasson, A. and Magnusson, L. (1999) Hypersensitivity to sound. Questionnaire data, audiometry and classification. *Scandinavian Audiology*, **28**, 219–230.

Andersson, G. (1996) The role of optimism in patients with tinnitus and in patients with hearing impairment. *Psychology and Health*, **11**, 697–707.

Andersson, G. (1997) Prior treatments in a group of tinnitus sufferers seeking treatment. *Psychotherapy and Psychosomatics*, **66**, 107–110.

Andersson, G. (2000a) Longitudinal follow-up of occupational status in tinnitus patients. *International Tinnitus Journal*, **6**, 127–129.

Andersson, G. (2000b) *Tinnitus: orsaker, teorier och behandlingsmöjligheter (Tinnitus. Theories, causes, and treatment options)*, Lund: Studentlitteratur.

Andersson, G. (2000c) Hearing impairment. In *Cognitive-behavioral interventions for persons with disabilities* (ed. C. Radnitz), Northvale, NJ: Jason Aronson.

Andersson, G. (2001) The role of psychology in managing tinnitus: a cognitive behavioural approach. *Seminars in Hearing*, **22**, 65–76.

Andersson, G. (2002a) A cognitive-affective theory for tinnitus: experiments and theoretical implications. In *Proceedings of the Seventh International Tinnitus Seminar* (ed. R. Patuzzi), Freemantle, Australia, University of Western Australia.

Andersson, G. (2002b) Psychological aspects of tinnitus and the application of cognitive-behavioral therapy. *Clinical Psychology Review*, **22**, 977–990.

Andersson, G. (2003) Tinnitus loudness matchings in relation to annoyance and grading of severity. *Auris Nasus Larynx*, **30**, 129–133.

Andersson, G. (2009) Using the Internet to provide cognitive behaviour therapy. *Behaviour Research and Therapy*, **47**, 175–180.

Andersson, G. and Kaldo, V. (2006) Cognitive-behavioral therapy with applied relaxation. In *Tinnitus treatment. Clinical protocols* (ed. R. S. Tyler), New York: Thieme.

Andersson, G. and Kaldo-Sandström, V. (2004) Internet-based cognitive behavioral therapy for tinnitus. *Journal of Clinical Psychology*, **60**, 171–178.

Andersson, G. and Lyttkens, L. (1996) Acupuncture for tinnitus: time to stop? *Scandinavian Audiology*, **25**, 273–275.

Andersson, G. and Lyttkens, L. (1999) A meta-analytic review of psychological treatments for tinnitus. *British Journal of Audiology*, **33**, 201–210.

Andersson, G. and McKenna, L. (1998) Tinnitus masking and depression. *Audiology*, **37**, 174–182.

Andersson, G. and McKenna, L. (2006) The role of cognition in tinnitus. *Acta Otolaryngologica*, **126**, 39–43.

Andersson, G. and Vretblad, P. (2000) Tinnitus and anxiety sensitivity. *Scandinavian Journal of Behaviour Therapy*, **29**, 57–64.

Andersson, G. and Westin, V. (2008) Understanding tinnitus distress: introducing the concepts of moderators and mediators. *International Journal of Audiology*, **47**(Suppl. 2), S178–S183.

Andersson, G., Melin, L., Lindberg, P. and Scott, B. (1995a) Development of a short scale for self-assessment of experiences of hearing impairment: the Hearing Coping Assessment. *Scandinavian Audiology*, **24**, 147–154.

Andersson, G., Melin, L., Scott, B. and Lindberg, P. (1995b) An evaluation of a behavioural treatment approach to hearing impairment. *Behaviour Research and Therapy*, **33**, 283–292.

Andersson, G., Kinnefors, A., Ekvall, L. and Rask-Andersen, H. (1997) Tinnitus and translabyrinthine acoustic neuroma surgery. *Audiology and Neurootology*, **2**, 403–409.

Andersson, G., Lyttkens, L. and Larsen, H. C. (1999) Distinguishing levels of tinnitus distress. *Clinical Otolaryngology*, **24**, 404–410.

Andersson, G., Eriksson, J., Lundh, L.-G. and Lyttkens, L. (2000a) Tinnitus and cognitive interference: a Stroop paradigm study. *Journal of Speech, Hearing, and Language Research*, **43**, 1168–1173.

Andersson, G., Lyttkens, L., Hirvelä, C., Furmark, T., Tillfors, M. and Fredrikson, M. (2000b) Regional cerebral blood flow during tinnitus: a PET case-study with lidocaine and auditory stimulation. *Acta Oto-Laryngologica*, **120**, 967–972.

Andersson, G., Olsson, E., Rydell, A.-M. and Larsen, H. C. (2000c) Social competence and behaviour problems in children with hearing impairment. *Audiology*, **39**, 88–92.

Andersson, G., Vretblad, P., Larsen, H.-C. and LyttkenS, L. (2001) Longitudinal follow-up of tinnitus complaints. *Archives of Otolaryngology, Head and Neck Surgery*, **127**, 175–179.

Andersson, G., Khakpoor, A. and Lyttkens, L. (2002a) Masking of tinnitus and mental activity. *Clinical Otolaryngology*, **27**, 270–274.

Andersson, G., Lindvall, N., Hursti, T. and Carlbring, P. (2002b) Hypersensitivity to sound (hyperacusis). A prevalence study conducted via the Internet and post. *International Journal of Audiology*, **41**, 545–554.

Andersson, G., Strömgren, T., Ström, L. and Lyttkens, L. (2002c) Randomised controlled trial of Internet based cognitive behavior therapy for distress associated with tinnitus. *Psychosomatic Medicine*, **64**, 810–816.

Andersson, G., Ingerholt, C. and Jansson, M. (2003a) Autobiographical memory in patients with tinnitus. *Psychology and Health*, **18**, 667–675.

Andersson, G., Kaldo-Sandström, V., Ström, L. and Strömgren, T. (2003b) Internet administration of the Hospital Anxiety and Depression Scale (HADS) in a sample of tinnitus patients. *Journal of Psychosomatic Research*, **55**, 259–262.

Andersson, G., Carlbring, P., Kaldo, V. and Ström, L. (2004a) Screening of psychiatric disorders via the Internet. A pilot study with tinnitus patients. *Nordic Journal of Psychiatry*, **58**, 287–291.

Andersson, G., Kaldo, V., Strömgren, T. and Ström, L. (2004b) Are coping strategies really useful for the tinnitus patient? An investigation conducted via the Internet. *Audiological Medicine*, **2**, 54–59.

Andersson, G., Airikka, M.-L., Buhrman, M. and Kaldo, V. (2005a) Dimensions of perfectionism and tinnitus distress. *Psychology, Health and Medicine*, **10**, 78–87.

Andersson, G., Bakhsh, R., Johansson, L., Kaldo, V. and Carlbring, P. (2005b) Stroop facilitation in tinnitus patients: an experiment conducted via the world wide web. *Cyberpsychology and Behavior*, **8**, 32–38.

Andersson, G., Jüris, L., Classon, E., Fredrikson, M. and Furmark, T. (2006) Consequences of suppressing thoughts about tinnitus and the effects of cognitive distraction on brain activity in tinnitus patients. *Audiology and Neurootology*, **11**, 301–309.

Andersson, G., Edsjö, L., Kaldo, V. and Westin, V. (2009a) Tinnitus and short-term serial recall in stable versus intermittent masking conditions. *Scandinavian Journal of Psychology*, **50**, 517–522.

Andersson, G., Freijd, A., Baguley, D. M. and Idrizbegovic, E. (2009b) Tinnitus distress, anxiety, depression, and hearing problems among cochlear implant patients with tinnitus. *Journal of the American Academy of Audiology*, **20**, 315–319.

Andersson, G., Keshishi, A. and Baguley, D. M. (2011) Benefit from hearing aids in users with and without tinnitus. *Audiological Medicine*, **9**, 73–78.

Andersson, G., Sandström, S., Lindström, M., Baguley, D. M. and Hesser, H. (2012) Prevalence of tinnitus in the general population in relation to psychological characteristics. Unpublished manuscript.

Araújo, M. F., Oliveira, C. A. and Bahmad Jr, F. (2005) Intratympanic dexamethasone injections as a treatment for severe, disabling tinnitus: does it work? *Archives of Otolaryngology, Head and Neck Surgery*, **131**, 113–117.

Arda, H. N., TunceL, U., Akdogan, O. and Ozluoglu, L. N. (2003) The role of zinc in the treatment of tinnitus. *Otology Neurotology*, **24**, 86–89.

Armony, J. L. and LeDoux, J. (2010) Emotional resonses to auditory stimuli. In *The Oxford handbook of auditory science*, Volume 2, *The auditory brain* (eds A. Rees and A. Palmer), Oxford: Oxford University Press.

Arndt, S., Aschendorff, A., Laszig, R., Beck, R., Schild, C., Kroeger, S., Ihorst, G. and Wesarg, T. (2011) Comparison of pseudobinaural hearing to real binaural hearing rehabilitation after cochlear implantation in patients with unilateral deafness and tinnitus. *Otology and Neurootology*, **32**, 39–47.

Arnesen, A. R. (1984) Fibre population of the vestibulocochlear anastomosis in humans. *Acta Otolaryngology*, **98**, 501–518.

Arnold, W. and Friedmann, I. (1988) Otosclerosis – an inflammatory disease of the otic capsule of viral aetiology. *Journal of Laryngology and Otology*, **102**, 865–871.

Arnold, W., Bartenstein, P., Oesstreicher, E., Römer, W. and Schwaiger, M. (1996) Focal metabolic activation in the predominant left auditory cortex in patients with tinnitus: a PET study with [18F] deoxyclucose. *ORL Journal of Otorhinolaryngology and Related Specialities*, **58**, 195–199.

Arts, H. (1998) Differential diagnosis of sensorineural hearing loss. In *Otolaryngology head and neck surgery*, Volume 4, *Ear and cranial base* (eds C. Cummings, J. Fredrickson and L. Harker), St Louis: Mosby.

Ash, C. M. and Pinto, O. F. (1991) The TMJ and the middle ear: structural and functional correlates for aural symptoms associated with temporomandibular joint dysfunction. *International Journal of Prosthodontics*, **4**, 51–57.

Ashmore, J. and Gale, J. (2000) The cochlea: a primer. *Current Biology*, **10**, 325–327.

Ashton, H., Reid, K., Marsh, R., Johnson, I., Alter, K. and Griffiths, T. (2007) High frequency localised 'hot spots' in temporal lobes of patients with intractable tinnitus: a quantitative electro-encephalographic (QEEG) study. *Neuroscience Letters*, **426**, 23–28.

Asplund, R. (2003) Sleepiness and sleep in elderly persons with tinnitus. *Archives of Gerontology and Geriatrics*, **37**, 139–145.

Attias, J., Shemsh, Z., Shoam, C., Shahar, A. and Sohmer, H. (1990) Efficacy of self-hypnosis for tinnitus relief. *Scandinavian Audiology*, **19**, 245–249.

Attias, J., Urbach, D., Gold, S. and Shemsh, Z. (1993a) Auditory event related potentials in chronic tinnitus patients with noise induced hearing loss. *Hearing Research*, **71**, 106–113.

Attias, J., Shemsh, Z., Sohmer, H., Gold, S., Shoam, C. and Faraggi, D. (1993b) Comparison between self-hypnosis, masking and attentiveness for alleviation of chronic tinnitus. *Audiology*, **32**, 302–212.

Attias, J., Weisa, G. and Almog, S. (1994) Oral magnesium intake reduces permanent hearing loss induced by noise exposure. *American Journal of Otolaryngology*, **15**, 26–32.

Attias, J., Shemsh, Z., Bleich, A., Solomon, Z., Bar-Or, G., Alster, J. and Sohmer, H. (1995) Psychological profile of help-seeking and non-help-seeking tinnitus patients. *Scandinavian Audiology*, **24**, 13–18.

Attias, J., Furman, V., Shemsh, Z. and Bresloff, I. (1996a) Impaired brain processing in noise-induced tinnitus patients as measured by auditory and visual event-related potentials. *Ear and Hearing*, **17**, 327–333.

Attias, J., Pratt, H., Bresloff, I., Horowitz, G., Polyakov, A. and Shemsh, Z. (1996b) Detailed analysis of auditory brainstem responses in patients with noise-induced tinnitus. *Audiology*, **35**, 259–270.

Attias, J., Raveh, E., Ben-Naftali, N. F., Zarchi, O. and Gothelf, D. (2008) Hyperactive auditory efferent system and lack of acoustic reflexes in Williams syndrome. *Journal of Basic and Clinical Physiology and Pharmacology*, **19**, 193–207.

Aust, G. (2002) Tinnitus in childhood. *International Tinnitus Journal*, **8**, 20–26.

Austen, S. and Lynch, C. (2004) Non-organic hearing loss redefined: understanding, categorizing and managing non-organic behaviour. *International Journal of Audiology*, **43**, 449–457.

Axelsson, A. and Ringdahl, A. (1989) Tinnitus – a study of its prevalence and characteristics. *British Journal of Audiology*, **23**, 53–62.

Axelsson, A., Coles, R., Erlandsson, S., Meikle, M. and Vernon, J. (1993) Evaluation of tinnitus treatment: methodological aspects. *Journal of Audiological Medicine*, **2**, 141–150.

Axelsson, A., Andersson, S. and Gu, L.-D. (1994) Acupuncture in the management of tinnitus: a placebo controlled study. *Audiology*, **33**, 351–360.

Axelsson, A., Anari, M. and Eliasson, A. (1995) *Överkänslighet för Ljud (ÖFL)*, Stockholm: Socialstyrelsen.

Ayache, D., Earally, F. and Elbaz, P. (2003) Characteristics and postoperative course of tinnitus in otosclerosis. *Otology and Neurotology*, **24**, 48–51.

Aydin, O., Iseri, M. and Ozturk, M. (2006) Radiofrequency ablation in the treatment of idiopathic bilateral palatal myoclonus: a new indication. *Annals of Otology, Rhinology and Laryngology*, **115**, 824–826.

Azevedo, A. and Figueiredo, R. (2005) Tinnitus treatment with acamprosate: double-blind study. *Brazilian Journal of Otorhinolaryngology*, **71**, 618–623.

Baddeley, A. D. (1986) *Working memory*, Oxford: Oxford University Press.

Badia, L., Parikh, A. and Brookes, G. (1994) Management of middle ear myoclonus. *Journal of Laryngology and Otology*, **108**, 380–382.

Baguley, D. M. (1997) Neurophysiological approach to tinnitus patients (Letter to the Editor). *American Journal of Otology*, **18**, 265.

Baguley, D. M. (2002) Mechanisms of tinnitus. *British Medical Bulletin*, **63**, 195–212.

Baguley, D. M. (2003) Hyperacusis. *Journal of the Royal Society of Medicine*, **96**, 582–585.

Baguley, D. M. (2006) What progress have we made with tinnitus? The Tonndorf Lecture 2005. *Acta Oto-Laryngologica*, **126**, 4–8.

Baguley, D. M. (2010) Cochlear implants in unilateral hearing loss and tinnitus. *Seminars in Hearing*, **31**, 410–413.

Baguley, D. M. and Andersson, G. (2002) Comment on Howard. *Otology and Neurotology*, **23**, 411–412.

Baguley, D. M. and Andersson, G. (2003) Factor analysis of the Tinnitus Handicap Inventory. *American Journal of Audiology*, **12**, 31–34.

Baguley, D. M. and Andersson, G. (2007) *Hyperacusis: Mechanisms, diagnosis, and therapies*, San Diego, CA: Plural Publishing Inc.

Baguley, D. M. and Atlas, M. D. (2007) Cochlear implants and tinnitus. *Progress in Brain Research*, **166**, 347–355.

Baguley, D. M. and McFerran, D. J. (1999) Tinnitus in childhood. *International Journal of Pediatric Otorhinolaryngology*, **49**, 99–105.

Baguley, D. M. and McFerran, D. J. (2002) Current perspectives on tinnitus. *Archives in Diseases in Children*, **86**(3), March, 141–143.

Baguley, D. M. and McFerran, D. J. (2011) Hyperacusis and disorders of loudness perception. In *Textbook of tinnitus* (eds A. R. Møller, B. Langguth, D. De Ridder and T. Kleinjung), New York: Springer.

Baguley, D. M., Moffat, D. A. and Hardy, D. G. (1992) What is the effect of translabyrinthine acoustic schwannoma removal upon tinnitus? *Journal of Laryngology and Otology*, **106**, 329–331.

Baguley, D. M., Beynon, G. J. and Thornton, F. (1997) A consideration of the effect of ear canal resonance and hearing loss upon white noise generators for tinnitus retraining therapy. *Journal of Laryngolgy and Otology*, **111**, 810–813.

Baguley, D. M., Stoddart, R. L. and Hodgson, C. A. (2000) Convergent validity of the Tinnitus Handicap Inventory and the Tinnitus Questionnaire. *Journal of Laryngology and Otology*, **114**, 840–843.

Baguley, D. M., Chang, P. and Moffat, D. A. (2001) Tinnitus in vestibular schwannoma. *Seminars in Hearing*, **22**, 77–88.

Baguley, D. M., Axon, P., Winter, I. M. and Moffat, D. A. (2002) The effect of vestibular nerve section upon tinnitus. *Clinical Otolaryngology*, **27**, 219–226.

Baguley, D. M., Davies, E. and Hazell, J. W. P. (2003) A vision for tinnitus research. *International Journal of Audiology*, **42**, 2–3.

Baguley, D., Jones, S., Wilkins, I., Axon, P. and Moffat, D. (2005) The inhibitory effect of intravenous lidocaine infusion upon tinnitus following translabyrinthine removal of vestibular schwannoma: a double blind placebo control crossover study. *Otology Neurotology*, **26**, 169–176.

Baguley, D. M., Bird, J., Humphriss, R. L. and Prevost, A. T. (2006a) The evidence base for the application of contralateral bone anchored hearing aids in acquired unilateral sensorineural hearing loss in adults. *Clinical Otolaryngology*, **31**, 6–14.

Baguley, D. M., Phillips, J., Humphriss, R. L., Jones, S., Axon, P. R. and Moffat, D. A. (2006b) The prevalence and onset of gaze modulation of tinnitus and increased sensitivity to noise after translabyrinthine vestibular schwannoma excision. *Otology and Neurootology*, **27**, 220–224.

Baguley, D. M., Plydoropulou, V. and Prevost, A. T. (2009) Bone anchored hearing aids for single-sided deafness. *Clinical Otolaryngology*, **34**, 176–177.

Baguley, D. M., Knight, R. and Bradshaw, L. (2011) Does caloric vestibular stimulation modulate tinnitus? *Neuroscience Letters*, **492**, 52–54.

Baguley, D. M., Bartnik, G., Kleinjung, T., Savastano, M. and Hough, E. (in press) Troublesome tinnitus in children: data from expert centres. *International Journal of Paediatric Otorhinolaryngology*.

Bahmad Jr, F. M., Venosa, A. R. and Oliveira, C. A. (2006) Benzodiazepines and GABAergics in treating severe disabling tinnitus of predominantly cochlear origin. *International Tinnitus Journal*, **12**, 140–144.

Bakhshaee, M., Ghasemi, M., Azarpazhooh, M., Khadivi, E., Rezaei, S., Shakeri, M. and Tale, M. (2008) Gabapentin effectiveness on the sensation of subjective idiopathic tinnitus: a pilot study. *European Archives of Oto-Rhino-Laryngology*, **265**, 525–530.

Baldo, P., Doree, C., Lazzarini, R., Molin, P. and McFerran, D. J. (2006) Antidepressants for patients with tinnitus. *Cochrane Database of Systematic Reviews*, CD003853.

Baldwin, T. M. (2009) Tinnitus, a military epidemic: is hyperbaric oxygen therapy the answer? *Journal of Special Operations Medicine*, **9**, 33–43.

Banbury, S. P., Macken, W. J., Tremblay, S. and Jones, D. M. (2001) Auditory distraction and short-term memory: phenomena and practical implications. *Human Factors*, **43**, 12–29.

Bárány, R. (1935) Die Beeinflussung des Ohrensausens durch Intravenös Injizierte Lokalanästhetica. *Acta Otolaryngologica*, **23**, 201–203.

Barlow, D. H. (2001) *Clinical handbook of psychological disorders. A step-by-step treatment manual*, New York: Guilford Press.

Barnea, G., Attias, J., Gold, S. and Shahar, A. (1990) Tinnitus with normal hearing sensitivity: extended high-frequency audiometry and auditory-nerve brain-stem-evoked responses. *Audiology*, **29**, 36–45.

Barnes, P., Powell-Griner, E., McFann, K. and Nahin, R. (2004) Complementary and alternative medicine use among adults: United States, 2002. Advance Data from vital and health statistics 343.

Baron, R. M. and Kenny, D. A. (1986) The moderator–mediator variable distinction in social psychological research: conceptual, strategic, and statistical considerations. *Journal of Personality and Social Psychology*, **51**, 1173–1182.

Barratt, S. and Pool, M. (2008) *Principles of clinical medicine for space flight*, New York, Springer.

Bartels, H., Pedersen, S. S., van der Laan, B. F., Staal, M. J., Albers, F. W. and Middel, B. (2010) The impact of Type D personality on health-related quality of life in tinnitus patients is mainly mediated by anxiety and depression. *Otology and Neurootology*, **31**, 11–18.

Bartlett, C., Pennings, R., Ho, A., Kirkpatrick, D., van Wijhe, R. and Bance, M. (2010) Simple mass loading of the tympanic membrane to alleviate symptoms of patulous Eustachian tube. *Journal of Otolaryngology – Head and Neck Surgery*, **39**, 259–268.

Bartnik, G., Fabijanska, A. and Rogowski, M. (1999) Our experience in treatment of patients with tinnitus and/or hyperacusis using the habituation method. In *Proceedings of the Sixth International Tinnitus Seminar* (ed. J. Hazell), Cambridge, UK, The Tinnitus and Hyperacusis Centre.

Bartnik, G., Stepien, A., Raj-Koziak, D., Fabijanska, A., Niedzialek, I. and Skarzynski, H. (2012) Troublesome tinnitus in children: epidemiology, audiological profile, and preliminary results of treatment. *International Journal of Paediatric Otorhinolaryngology*, **2012**, 945356.

Baskill, J. L., Bradley, P. J. M., Coles, R. R. A., Graham, R. L., Grimes, S., Handscomb, L., Hazell, J. W. P. and Sheldrake, J. B. (1999) Effects of publicity on tinnitus. In *Proceedings of the Sixth International Tinnitus Seminar* (ed. J. Hazell), Cambridge, UK, The Tinnitus and Hyperacusis Centre, pp. 229–231.

Basmajian, J. V. (1999) Debonafide effects vs 'placebo effects'. *Proceedings of the Royal College of Physicians Edinburgh*, **29**, 243–244.

Bastien, C. H., Vallières, A. and Morin, C. M. 2001. Validation of the Insomnia Severity Index as an outcome measure for insomnia research. *Sleep Medicine*, **2**, 297–307.

Bauer, C. A. and Brozoski, T. J. (2006) Effect of gabapentin on the sensation and impact of tinnitus. *Laryngoscope*, **116**, 675–681.

Bauer, C. A. and Brozoski, T. J. (2011) Effect of tinnitus retraining therapy on the loudness and annoyance of tinnitus: a controlled trial. *Ear and Hearing*, **32**, 145–155.

Bauer, C. A., Brozoski, T. J. and Myers, K. (2007) Primary afferent dendrite degeneration as a cause of tinnitus. *Journal of Neuroscience Research*, **85**, 1489–1498.

Baum, W. M. (1994) *Understanding behaviorism*, New York: HarperCollins College Publishers.

Bayar, N., Boke, B., Turan, E. and Belgin, E. (2001) Efficacy of amitriptyline in the treatment of subjective tinnitus. *Journal of Otolaryngology*, **30**, 300–303.

Bayay, N., Oguzturk, O. and Koc, C. (2002) Minnesota Multiphasic Personality Inventory profile of patients with subjective tinnitus. *Journal of Otolaryngology*, **31**, 317–322.

Beard, A. W. (1965) Results of leucotomy operations for tinnitus. *Journal of Psychosomatic Research*, **9**(1), September, 29–32.

Beck, A. T., Rush, A. J., Shaw, B. F. & Emery, G. 1979. *Cognitive therapy of depression*, New York, Guilford press.

Beck, J. G., Stanley, M. A. and Zebb, B. J. (1996) Characteristics of generalized anxiety disorder in older adults: a descriptive study. *Behaviour Research and Therapy*, **34**, 225–234.

Bedeschi, M. F., Bianchi, V., Colli, A., Natacci, F., Cereda, A., Milani, D., Maitz, S., Lalatta, F. and Selicomi, A. (2011) Clinical follow-up of young adults affected by Williams syndrome: experience of 45 Italian patients. *American Journal of Medical Genetics A*, **155A**, 353–359.

Been, G., Ngo, T. T., Miller, S. M. and Fitzgerald, P. B. (2007) The use of tDCS and CVS as methods of non-invasive brain stimulation. *Brain Research Reviews*, **56**, 346–361.

Belli, S., Belli, H., Bahcebasi, T., Ozcetin, A., Alpay, E. and Ertem, U. (2008) Assessment of psychopathological aspects and psychiatric comorbidities in patients affected by tinnitus. *European Archives of Oto-Rhino-Laryngology*, **265**, 279–285.

Bennett, M. H., Kertesz, T. and Yeung, P. (2007) Hyperbaric oxygen for idiopathic sudden sensorineural hearing loss and tinnitus. *Cochrane Database of Systematic Reviews*, Issue 1, Article CD004739. DOI: 10.1002/14651858.CD004739.pub3.

Bento, R. F., Sanchez, T. G., Miniti, A. and Tedesco-Marchesi, A. J. (1998) Continuous, high-frequency objective tinnitus caused by middle ear myoclonus. *Ear, Nose and Throat Journal*, **77**, 814–818.

Bernard, P. (1981) Freedom from ototoxicity in aminoglycoside treated neonates: a mistaken notion. *Laryngoscope*, **91**, 1985–1994.

Bernhardt, O., Mundt, T., Welk, A., Koppl, N., Kocher, T., Meyer, G. and Schwahn, C. (2011) Signs and symptoms of temporomandibular disorders and the incidence of tinnitus. *Journal of Oral Rehabilitation*, **38**, 891–901.

Berninger, E., Nordmark, J., Alvan, G., Karlsson, K. K., Idrizbegovic, E., Meurling, L. and Al-Shurbaji, A. (2006) The effect of intravenously administered mexiletine on tinnitus – a pilot study. *International Journal of Audiology*, **45**, 689–696.

Bhatnagar, S. (2002) *Neuroscience for the study of communicative disorders*, Philadelphia, PA, Lippincott Williams & Wilkins.

Bhimrao, S. K., Masterson, L. and Baguley, D. M. (2012) Systematic review of management strategies for middle ear myoclonus. *Otolaryngology, Head and Neck Surgery*, **146**(5), May, 698–706.

Biggs, N. D. W. and Ramsden, R. T. (2002) Gaze-evoked tinnitus following acoustic neuroma resection: A de-afferentation plasticity phenomenon? *Clinical Otolaryngology*, **27**, 338–343.

Bjelland, I., Dahl, A. A., Haug, T. T. and Neckelman, D. (2002). The validity of the hospital anxiety and depression scale. An updated literature review. *Journal of Psychosomatic Research*, **52**, 69–77.

Blasing, L., Goebel, G., Flotzinger, U., Berthold, A. and Kroner-Herwig, B. (2010) Hypersensitivity to sound in tinnitus patients: an analysis of a construct based on questionnaire and audiological data. *International Journal of Audiology*, **49**, 518–526.

Blaustein, M. P. (1988) Cellular calcium: nervous system. In *Calcium in human biology* (ed. B. E. C. Nordin), London: Springer-Verlag.

Blayney, A. W., Phillips, M. S., Guy, A. M. and Colman, B. H. (1985) A sequential double blind cross-over trial of tocainide hydrochloride in tinnitus. *Clinical Otolaryngology*, **10**, 97–101.

Blomberg, S., Rosander, M. and Andersson, G. (2006) Fears, hyperacusis and musicality in Williams syndrome. *Research in Developmental Disabilities*, **27**, 668–680.

Blood, A. J., Zatorre, R. J., Bermudex, P. and Evans, A. C. (1999) Emotional responses to pleasant and unpleasant music correlate with activity in paralimbic brain regions. *Nature Neuroscience*, **2**, 382–387.

Bohlmeijer, E., Prenger, R., Taal, E. and Cuijpers, P. (2010) The effects of mindfulness-based stress reduction therapy on mental health of adults with a chronic medical disease: a meta-analysis. *Journal of Psychosomatic Research*, **68**, 539–544.

Bonneville, F., Savatovsky, J. and Chiras, J. (2007) Imaging of cerebellopontine angle lesions: an update. Part 2: intra-axial lesions, skull base lesions that may invade the CPA region, and non-enhancing extra-axial lesions. *European Radiology*, **17**, 2908–2920.

Bornstein, S. P. and Musiek, F. E. (1993) Loudness discomfort level and reliability as a function of instructional set. *Scandinavian Audiology*, **22**, 125–131.

Bouscau-Faure, F., Keller, P. and Dauman, R. (2003) Further validation of the Iowa tinnitus handicap questionnair. *Acta Otolaryngology*, **123**, 227–231.

Brattberg, G. (1983) An alternative method of treating tinnitus: relaxation-hypnotherapy primarily through the home use of a recorded audio cassette. *International Journal of Clinical and Experimental Hypnosis*, **31**, 90–97.

Breivik, C. N., Varughese, J. K., Wentzel-Larsen, T., Vassbotn, F. & Lund-Johansen, M. (2012) Conservative management of vestibular schwannoma – a prospective cohort study: treatment, symptoms and quality of life. *Neurosurgery*, **70**(5), May, 1072–1080.

Briner, W., Risey, J., Guth, P. and Noris, C. (1990) Use of the million clinical multiaxial inventory in evaluating patients with severe tinnitus. *American Journal of Otolaryngology*, **11**, 334–337.

Broadbent, D., Cooper, P. F., Fitzgerald, P. and Parkes, K. R. (1982) The cognitive failures questionnaire and its correlates. *British Journal of Clinical Psychology*, **21**, 1–16.

Brodel M. (1946) *Three unpublished drawings of the anatomy of the human ear*, WB Saunders.

Brookes, G. (1996) Vascular decompression surgery for severe tinnitus. *American Journal of Otolology*, **17**, 569–576.

Brookes, G. B., Maw, A. R. and Coleman, M. J. (1980) 'Costen's syndrome' – correlation or coincidence: a review of 45 patients with temporomandibular joint dysfunction, otalgia and other aural symptoms. *Clinical Otolaryngology*, **5**, 23–36.

Brooks, D. N. (1989) *Adult Aural Rehabilitation*, London: Chapman & Hall.

Brooks, D. N. and Chalmers, P. (1991) Training in audiology. *British Journal of Audiology*, **25**, 73–75.

Brown, S. C. (1990) Older Americans and tinnitus: a demographic study and chartbook. In R. C. Johnson and S. A. Hotto (eds.), Gallaudet Research Institute, Gallaudet University.

Browning, G. and Gatehouse, S. 1992. The prevalence of middle ear disease in the adult British population. *Clinical Otolaryngology*, **17**, 317–321.

Budd, R. J. and Pugh, R. (1995) The relationship between locus of control, tinnitus severity, and emotional distress in a group of tinnitus sufferers. *Journal of Psychosomatic Research*, **39**, 1015–1018.

Budd, R. J. and Pugh, R. (1996a) The relationship between coping style, tinnitus severity and emotional distress in a group of tinnitus sufferers. *British Journal of Health Psychology*, **1**, 219–229.

Budd, R. J. & Pugh, R. (1996b) Tinnitus coping style and its relationship to tinnitus severity and emotional distress. *Journal of Psychosomatic Research*, **40**, 327–335.

Burgess, A. and Kundu, S. (2006) Diuretics for Ménière's disease or syndrome. *Cochrane Database of Systematic Reviews*, Issue 3, Article CD003599. DOI: 10.1002/14651858.CD003599.pub2.

Burns, E. M. (1984) A comparison of variability among measurements of subjective tinnitus and objective stimuli. *Audiology*, **23**, 426–440.

Buysse, D., Reynolds, C., Monk, T., Berman, S. and Kupfer, D. 1989. The Pittsburgh Sleep Quality Index: a new instrument for psychiatric practice and research. *Psychiatry Research*, **28**, 193–213.

Cacace, A. T. (1999) Delineating tinnitus-related activity in the nervous system: application of functional imaging at the fin de siècle. In *Proceedings of the Sixth International Tinnitus Seminar* (ed. J. Hazell), Cambridge, UK, The Tinnitus and Hyperacusis Centre, pp. 39–44.

Cacace, A. T. (2003) Expanding the biological basis of tinnitus: cross-modal origins and the role of neuroplasticity. *Hearing Research*, **175**, 112–132.

Cacace, A. T., Lovely, T. J., McFarland, D. J., M, P. S.and Winter, D. F. (1994) Anomalous cross-modal plasticity following posterior fossa surgery: some speculations on gaze-evoked tinnitus. *Hearing Research*, **81**, 22–32.

Cacace, A. T., Cousins, J. P., Moonen, C. T. W., van Gelderen, P., Miller, D., Parnes, S. M. and Lovely, T. J. (1996) *In-vivo* localization of phantom auditory perceptions during functional magnetic resonance imaging of the human brain. In *Proceedings of the Fifth International Tinnitus Seminar* (eds G. E. Reich and J. A. Vernon), Portland, OR, American Tinnitus Association, pp. 397–401.

Cacace, A. T., Cousins, J. C., Pames, S., Semenoff, D., Holmes, T., McFarland, D. J., Davenport, C., Stegbauer, K. and Lovely, T. J. (1999a). Cutaneous-evoked tinnitus. I. Phenomenology, psychophysics, and functional imaging. *Audiology and Neurootology*, **4**, 247–257.

Cacace, A. T., Cousins, J. C., Pames, S., McFarland, D. J., Semenoff, D., Holmes, T., Davenport, C., Stegbauer, K. and Lovely, T. J. (1999b). Cutaneous-evoked tinnitus . II. Review of neuroanatomical, physiological, and functional imaging studies. *Audiology and Neurootology*, **4**, 258–268.

Cahani, M., Paul, G. and Shahar, A. (1984) Tinnitus assymetry. *Audiology*, **23**, 127–135.

Campbell, K. (1993) Tinnitus and vertigo. *Archives of Otolaryngology, Head and Neck Surgery*, **119**, 474.

Campbell, K., Meech, R., Klemens, J., Gerberi, M., Dyrstad, S., Larsen, D., Mitchell, D., El-Azizi, M., Verhulst, S. and Hughes, L. (2007) Prevention of noise- and drug-induced hearing loss with D-methionine. *Hearing Research*, **226**, 92–103.

Campbell, K., Claussen, A., Meech, R., Verhulst, S., Fox, D. and Hughes, L. (2011) D-methionine (D-met) significantly rescues noise-induced hearing loss: timing studies. *Hearing Research*, **282**, 138–144.

Caperton, K. and Thompson, A. (2011) Activation of serotonergic neurons during salicylate-induced tinnitus. *Otology and Neurotology*, **32**, 301–307.

Carlsson, S. G. and Erlandsson, S. I. (1991) Habituation and tinnitus: an experimental study. *Journal of Psychosomatic Research*, **35**, 509–514.

Carman, J. S. (1973) Imipramine in hyperacusic depression. *American Journal of Psychiatry*, **130**, 937.

Carmen, R. and Svihovec, D. (1984) Relaxation-biofeedback in the treatment of tinnitus. *American Journal of Otology*, **5**, 376–381.

Carrick, D. G., Davies, W. M., Fielder, C. P. and Bihari, J. (1986) Low-powered ultrasound in the treatment of tinnitus: a pilot study. *British Journal of Audiology*, **20**, 153–155.

Cassileth, B. R. and Deng, G. (2004) Complementary and alternative therapies for cancer. *Oncologist*, **9**, 80–89.

Catalano, P. and Post, K. (1996) Elimination of tinnitus following hearing preservation surgery for acoustic neuromas. *American Journal of Otology*, **17**, 443–445.

Cawthorne, T. and Hewlett, A. (1954) Ménière's disease. *Proceedings of the Royal Society of Medicine*, **47**, 663–670.

Cesarani, A., Capobianco, S., Soi, D., Giuliano, D. A. and Alpini, D. (2002) Intratympanic dexamethasone treatment for control of subjective idiopathic tinnitus: our clinical experience. *International Tinnitus Journal*, **8**, 111–114.

Chan, C. and Palaniappan, R. (2010) Middle ear myoclonus: a new technique for suppression of spontaneous clicking tinnitus. *International Tinnitus Journal*, **16**, 51–54.

Chan, S. W. Y. and Reade, P. C. (1994) Tinnitus and temporomandibular pain-dysfunction disorder. *Clinical Otolaryngology*, **19**, 370–380.

Chen, G. and Jastreboff, P. J. (1995) Salicylate induced abnormal activity in the inferior colliculus of rats. *Hearing Research*, **82**, 158–178.

Chen, D. A. and Luxford, W. M. (1990) Myringotomy and tube for relief of patulous Eustachian tube symptoms. *American Journal of Otology*, **11**, 272–273.

Chen, P. W., Young, Y. H. and Lou, P. J. (1999) Patulous Eustachian tube in long-term survivors of nasopharyngeal carcinoma. *Annals of Otology, Rhinology and Laryngology*, **108**, 201–204.

Chien, W. W., Carey, J. P. and Minor, L. B. (2011) Canal dehiscence. *Current Opinion in Neurology*, **24**, 25–31.

Chiossoine-Kerdel, J. A., Baguley, D. M., Stoddart, R. L. and Moffat, D. A. (2000) An investigation of the audiologic handicap associated with unilateral sudden sensorineural hearing loss. *American Journal of Otology*, **21**, 645–651.

Chouard, C. H., Meyer, B. and Maridat, D. (1981) Transcutaneous electrotherapy for severe tinnitus. *Acta Otolaryngology*, **91**, 415–422.

Choy, D. S., Lipman, R. A. and Tassi, G. P. (2010) Worldwide experience with sequential phase-shift sound cancellation treatment of predominant tone tinnitus. *Journal of Laryngology and Otology*, **124**, 366–369.

Cima, R. F., Crombez, G. and Vlaeyen, J. W. (2011) Catastrophizing and fear of tinnitus predict quality of life in patients with chronic tinnitus. *Ear and Hearing*, **32**, 634–641.

Clark, W. W., Kim, D. O., Zurek, P. M. and Bohne, B. A. (1984) Spontaneous otoacoustic emissions in chinchilla ear canals: correlation with histopathology and suppression by external tones. *Hearing Research*, **16**, 299–314.

Coelho, C. B., Sanchez, T. G. and Tyler, R. S. (2007a) Tinnitus in children and associated risk factors. *Progress in Brain Research*, **166**, 179–191.

Coelho, C. B., Sanchez, T. G. and Tyler, R. S. (2007b) Hyperacusis, sound annoyance, and loudness hypersensitivity in children. *Progress in Brain Research*, **166**, 169–178.

Coelho, D., Roland, J. J., Rush, S., Narayana, A., St Clair, E., Chung, W. and Golfinos, J. (2008) Small vestibular schwannomas with no hearing: comparison of functional outcomes in stereotactic radiosurgery and microsurgery. *Laryngoscope*, **118**, 1909–1916.

Cohen, J. (1988) *Statistical power analysis for the behavioral sciences*, Hillsdale, NJ: Lawrence Erlbaum Associates.

Cohen, D. and Perez, R. (2003) Bilateral myoclonus of the tensor tympani: a case report. *Otolaryngology, Head and Neck Surgery*, **128**, 441.

Colding-Jørgensen, E., Lauritzen, M., Johnsen, N. J., Mikkelsen, K. B. and Særmark, K. (1992) On the evidence of auditory evoked magnetic fields as an objective measure of tinnitus. *Electroencephalography and Clinical Neurophysiology*, **83**, 322–327.

Coles, R. R. A. (1984) Epidemiology of tinnitus: (2) Demographics and clinical features. *Journal of Laryngology and Otology*, Suppl. 9, 195–202.

Coles, R. R. A. (1987) Tinnitus and its management. In *Adult audiology. Scott Brown's otolaryngology* (ed. D. Stephens), fifth edition, London: Butterworths, pp. 368–414.

Coles, R. R. A. (1992) A survey of tinnitus management in National Health Service hospitals. *Clinical Otolaryngology and Allied Sciences*, **17**, 313–316.

Coles, R. R. A. and Hallam, R. S. (1987) Tinnitus and its management. *British Medical Bulletin*, **43**, 983–998.

Coles, R., Bradley, P., Donaldson, I. and Dingle, A. (1991) A trial of tinnitus therapy with ear-canal magnets. *Clinical Otolaryngology*, **16**, 371–372.

Coles, R. R. A., Thompson, A. C. and O'Donoghue, G. M. (1992) Intra-tympanic injections in the treatment of tinnitus. *Clinical Otolaryngology*, **17**, 240–242.

Collet, L., Moussu, M. F., Disant, F., Ahami, T. and Morgon, A. (1990) Minnesota multiphasic personality inventory in tinnitus disorders. *Audiology*, **29**, 101–106.

Collins, W. (1860) *The woman in white*, London: Penguin Classics.

Committee on Hearing and Equilibrium (1995) Guidelines for the diagnosis and evaluation of therapy in Menière's disease. *Otolaryngology, Head and Neck Surgery*, **113**, 181–185.

Cooper, J. C. (1994) Health and nutrition examination survey of 1971–75: Part II. Tinnitus, subjective hearing loss, and well-being. *Journal of the American Academy of Audiology*, **5**, 37–43.

Cope, T. E. (2008) Clinical hypnosis for the alleviation of tinnitus. *International Journal of Tinnitus*, **14**, 135–138.

Cope, T. E. and Baguley, D. M. (2009) Is musical hallucination an otological phenomenon? A review of the literature. *Clinical Otolaryngology*, **34**, 423–430.

Cope, T., Baguley, D. and Moore, B. (2011) Tinnitus loudness in quiet and noise after resection of vestibular schwannoma. *Otology and Neurootology*, **32**, 488–496.

Cortopassi, G. & Hutchin, T. 1994. A molecular and cellular hypothesis for aminoglycoside induced deafness. *Hearing Research*, **78**, 27–30.

Costen, J. B. (1934) A syndrome of ear and sinus symptoms dependent upon disturbed function of the temporomandibular joint. *Annals of Otology, Rhinology and Laryngology*, **43**, 1–15.

Cotanche, D. A. (2008) Genetic and pharmacological intervention for treatment/prevention of hearing loss. *Journal of Communication Disorders*, **41**, 421–443.

Coyle, P. K. and Schutzer, S. E. (2002) Neurological aspects of Lyme disease. *Medical Clinics of North America*, **86**, 261–284.

Crippa, A., Lanting, C. P., van Dijk, P. and Roerdink, J. B. (2010) A diffusion tensor imaging study on the auditory system and tinnitus. *The Open Neuroimaging Journal*, **4**, 16–25.

Crocetti, A., Forti, S. and Del Bo, L. (2011) Neurofeedback for subjective tinnitus patients. *Auris Nasus Larynx*, **38**, 735–738.

Cronlein, T., Langguth, B., Geisler, P. and Hajak, G. (2007) Tinnitus and insomnia. *Progress in Brain Research*, **166**, 227–233.

Cuijpers, P., Donker, T., van Straten, A. and Andersson, G. (2010) Is guided self-help as effective as face-to-face psychotherapy for depression and anxiety disorders? A meta-analysis of comparative outcome studies. *Psychological Medicine*, **40**, 1943–1957.

Cuny, C., Norena, A., El Massious, F. and Chéry-Croze, S. (2004) Reduced attention shift in response to auditory changes in subjects with tinnitus. *Audiology and Neuro-otology*, **9**, 294–302.

Damgaard-Morch, N. L., Nielsen, L. J. and Uldall, S. W. (2008) Kobenhavnsje medicinstuderendes kendskab og holdininger til komplementaer og alternativ medicin. www.vifab.dk/uk.

Dan, B. (2005) Titus's tinnitus. *Journal of the History of the Neurosciences*, **14**, 210–213.

Darlington, C. and Smith, P. (2007) Drug treatments for tinnitus. *Progress in Brain Research*, **166**, 249–262.

Datzov, E., Danev, S., Haralanov, H., Naidenova, V., Sachanska, T. and Savov, A. (1999) Tinnitus, heart rate variability, and some biochemical indicators. *International Tinnitus Journal*, **5**, 20–23.

Dauman, R. (2000) Electrical stimulation for tinnitus suppression. In *Tinnitus handbook* (ed. R. S. Tyler), San Diego, CA: Singular, Thomson Learning.

Dauman, R. and Bouscau-Faure, F. (2005) Assessment and amelioration of hyperacusis in tinnitus patients. *Acta Oto-Laryngologica*, **125**, 503–509.

Dauman, R. and Tyler, R. S. (1992) Some considerations on the classification of tinnitus. In *Tinnitus 91. Proceedings of the Fourth International Tinnitus Seminar* (eds J.-M. Aran and R. Dauman), Amsterdam/New York: Kugler Publications.

Dauman, R. and Tyler, R. S. (1993) Tinnitus suppression in cochlear implant users. *Advances in Otorhinolaryngology*, **48**, 168–173.

Dauman, R., Tyler, R. and Aran, J.-M. (1993) Intracochlear electrical tinnitus suppression. *Acta Oto-Laryngologica*, **113**, 291–295.

Dauman, R., Cuny, E., Bonnard, D. and Dauman, N. (2011) Double-blind assessment of tinnitus relief produced by chronic electrical stimulation of audtory cortex. Abstract book, 5th International Tinnitus Research Initiative Conference.

Davies, E., Knox, E. and Donaldson, I. (1994) The usefulness of nimodipine, an L-calcium channel antagonist, in the treatment of tinnitus. *British Journal of Audiology*, **28**, 125–129.

Davies, S., McKenna, L. and Hallam, R. S. (1995) Relaxation and cognitive therapy: a controlled trial in chronic tinnitus. *Psychology and Health*, **10**, 129–143.

Davis, A. C. (1989) The prevalence of hearing impairment and reported hearing disability among adults in Great Britain. *International Journal of Epidemiology*, **18**, 911–917.

Davis, A. (1995) *Hearing in adults*, London: Whurr.

Davis, A. and El Rafaie, A. (2000) Epidemiology of tinnitus. In *Tinnitus handbook* (ed. R. S. Tyler), San Diego, CA: Singular, Thomson Learning.

Davis, M., Astrachan, D. I. and Kass, E. (1980) Excitatory and inhibitory effects of serotonin on sensorimotor reactivity measured with acoustic startle. *Science*, **209**, 521–523.

Davis, P., Paki, B. and Hanley, P. (2007) Neuromonics tinnitus treatment: third clinical trial. *Ear and Hearing*, **28**, 242–250.

de Azevedo, A. A., Langguth, B., De Oliveira, P. M. and Rodrigues Figueiredo, R. (2009) Tinnitus treatment with piribedil guided by electrocochleography and acoustic otoemissions. *Otology & Neurootology*, **30**, 676–680.

de Azevedo, R. F., Chiari, B. M., Okada, D. M. and Onishi, E. T. (2007) Impact of acupuncture on otoacoustic emissions in patients with tinnitus. *Brazilian Journal of Otorhinolaryngology*, **73**, 599–607.

DeBartolo, H. M. (1989) Zinc and diet for tinnitus. *American Journal of Otology*, **10**, 256.

Declau, F., van Spaendonck, M., Timmermans, J. P., Michaels, L., Liang, J., Qiu, J. P., van der Heyning, P. (2001) Prevalence of otosclerosis in an unselected series of temporal bones. *Otology and Neurotology*, **22**(5), September, 596–602.

de Houwer, J., Thomas, S. and Baeyens, F. (2001) Associative learning of likes and dislikes: a review of 25 years of research on human evaluative conditioning. *Psychological Bulletin*, **127**, 853–869.

de Klaver, M. J., van Rijn, M. A., Marinus, J., Soede, W., de Laat, J. A. and van Hilten, J. J. (2007) Hyperacusis in patients with complex regional pain syndrome related dystonia. *Journal of Neurology, Neurosurgery and Psychiatry*, **78**, 1310–1313.

Delb, W., Strauss, D. J., Low, Y. F., Seidler, H., Rheinschmitt, A., Wobrock, T. and D'Amelio, R. (2008) Alterations in event related potentials (ERP) associated with tinnitus distress and attention. *Applied Psychophysiology and Biofeedback*, **33**, 211–221.

Del Bo, L., Forti, S., Ambrosetti, U., Costanzo, S., Mauro, D., Ugazio, G., Langguth, B. and Mancuso, A. (2008) Tinnitus aurium in persons with normal hearing: 55 years later. *Otolaryngology, Head and Neck Surgery*, **139**, 391–394.

DeLucchi, E. (2000) Transtympanic pilocarpine in tinnitus. *International Tinnitus Journal*, **6**, 37–40.

den Hartigh, J., Hilders, C. G. J. M., Schoemaker, R. C., Hulsohof, J. H., Cohen, A. F. and Vermeij, P. (1993) Tinnitus suppression by intravenous lidocaine in relation to its plasma concentration. *Clinical Pharmacology and Therapeutics*, **54**, 415–420.

Denk, D., H, H., Franz, P. and Ehrenberger, K. (1997) Caroverine in tinnitus treatment. *Acta Otolaryngologica*, **117**, 825–830.

Department of Health (2009) *Provision of services for adults with tinnitus. A good practice guide*, London: DH Publications. http://www.dh.gov.uk/en/Publicationsandstatistics/Publications/PublicationsPolicyAndGuidance/DH_093844.

De Ridder, D. and Møller, A. (2011) Microvascular compression of the vestibulocochlear nerve. In *Textbook of tinnitus* (eds A. R. Møller, B. Langguth, D. De Ridder, and T. Kleinjung), New York: Springer.

De Ridder, D. and Vanneste, S. (2011) Auditory cortex stimulation for tinnitus. In *Textbook of tinnitus* (eds A. R. Møller, B. Langguth, D. De Ridder, and T. Kleinjung), New York: Springer.

De Ridder, D., De Ridder, L., Nowé, V., Thierens, H., van der Heyning, P. and Møller, A. (2005) Pulsatile tinnitus and the intrameatal vascular loop: why do we not hear our carotids? *Neurosurgery*, **57**(6), December, 1213–1217.

Dib, G. C., Kasse, C. A., Alves de Andrade, T., Gurgel Testa, J. R. and Cruz, O. L. (2007) Tinnitus treatment with Trazodone. *Brazilian Journal of Otorhinolaryngology*, **73**, 390–397.

Diesch, E., Andermann, M., Flor, H. and Rupp, A. (2010) Functional and structural aspects of tinnitus-related enhancement and suppression of auditory cortex activity. *NeuroImage*, **50**, 1545–1559.

Di Nardo, W., Cantore, I., Cianfrone, F., Melillo, P., ScorpeccI, A. and Paludetti, G. (2007) Tinnitus modifications after cochlear implantation. *European Archives of Otorhinolaryngology*, **264**, 1145–1149.

Dineen, R., Doyle, J. and Bench, J. (1997a) Audiological and psychological characteristics of a group of tinnitus sufferers, prior to tinnitus management training. *British Journal of Audiology*, **31**, 27–38.

Dineen, R., Doyle, J. and Bench, J. (1997b) Managing tinnitus: a comparison of different approaches to tinnitus management training. *British Journal of Audiology*, **31**, 331–344.

Dobie, R. A. (1999) A review of randomized clinical trials of tinnitus. *Laryngoscope*, **109**, 1202–1211.

Dobie, R. A. (2004) Clinical trials and drug therapy for tinnitus. In *Tinnitus: theory and management* (ed. J. B. Snow), Hamilton, BC: Decker.

Dobie, R. A., Hoberg, K. E. and Rees, T. S. (1986) Electrical tinnitus suppression: a double-blind crossover study. *Otolaryngology, Head and Neck Surgery*, **95**, 319–323.

Doherty, J. K. and Slattery III, W. H. (2003) Autologous fat grafting for the refractory patulous Eustachian tube. *Otolaryngology, Head and Neck Surgery*, **128**, 88–91.

Dohrmann, K., Weisz, N., Schlee, W., Hartmann, T. and Elbert, T. (2007) Neurofeedback for treating tinnitus. *Progress in Brain Research*, **166**, 473–485.

Donaldson, I. (1981) Tegretol: a double blind trial in tinnitus. *Journal of Laryngology and Otology*, **95**, 947–951.

Douek, E. (1981) Classification of tinnitus. In *Tinnitus, Ciba Foundation Symposium 85* (eds D. Evered and G. Lawrenson), London: Pitman Books.

Douek, E. and Reid, J. (1968) The diagnostic value of tinnitus pitch. *Journal of Laryngology and Otology*, **82**, 1039–1042.

Dressler, D., Saberi, F. A. and Barbosa, E. R. (2005) Botulinum toxin: mechanisms of action. *Arquivos de Neuro-Psiquiatria*, **63**, 180–185.

Drew, S. and Davies, E. 2001. Effectiveness of Ginkgo biloba in treating tinnitus: double blind, placebo controlled trial. *British Medical Journal*, **322**, 1–6.

Drukier, G. S. (1989) The prevalence and characteristics of tinnitus with profound sensori-neural hearing impairment. *American Annals of the Deaf*, **134**, 260–264.

Dubal, S. and Viaud-Delmon, I. (2008) Magical ideation and hyperacusis. *Cortex*, **44**, 1379–1386.

Duckert, L. G. and Rees, T. S. (1983) Treatment of tinnitus with intravenous lidocaine: a double-blind randomized trial. *Otolaryngology, Head and Neck Surgery*, **91**, 550–555.

Duckert, L. G. and Rees, T. S. (1984) Placebo effect in tinnitus management. *Otolaryngology, Head and Neck Surgery*, **92**, 697–699.

DuVerney, J. G. (1683) *Traité de l'Organe de l'Ouie*, Paris: Michallet.

East, C. A. and Hazell, J. W. (1987) The suppression of palatal (or intra-tympanic) myoclonus by tinnitus masking devices. A preliminary report. *Jounal of Laryngoloy and Otology*, **101**, 1230–1234.

Edwards, L. and Crocker, S. (2008) *Psychological processes in deaf children with complex needs. An evidence based practical guide*, London: Jessica Kingsley Publishers.

Eggermont, J. J. (1990) On the pathophysiology of tinnitus; a review and a peripheral model. *Hearing Research*, **48**, 111–124.

Eggermont, J. J. 2000 Physiological mechanisms and neural models. In *Tinnitus handbook* (ed. R. S. Tyler), San Diego, CA: Singular, Thomson Learning.

Eggermont, J. J. (2006) Cortical tonotopic map reorganization and its implications for treatment of tinnitus. *Acta Otolaryngologica*, **126**, 9–12.

Eggermont, J. J. (2010) Tinnitus. In *The Oxford handbook of auditory science*, Volume 2, *The auditory brain* (eds A. Rees and A. Palmer), Oxford Oxford University Press.

Eichhammer, P., Kleinjung, T., Landgrebe, M., Hajak, G. and Langguth, B. (2007) TMS for treatment of chronic tinnitus: neurobiological effects. *Progress in Brain Research*, **166**, 369–375.

Eisenberg, D. M., Davis, R. B., L, E. S., Appel, S., Wilkey, S., M, V. R. and Kessler, R. C. (1998) Trends in alternative medicine use in the United States, 1990–1997: results of a follow-up national survey. *Journal of the American Medical Association*, **280**, 1569–1575.

El Rafaie, A., Davis, A., Baskill, J., Lovell, E., Taylor, A. and Spencer, H. (1999) Quality of family life of people who report tinnitus. In *Proceedings of the Sixth International Tinnitus Seminar* (ed. J. Hazell), Cambridge, UK, The Tinnitus and Hyperacusis Centre.

Englesson, S., Larsson, B., Lindquist, N. G., Lyttkens, L. and Stahle, J. (1976) Accumulation of ^{14}C-lidocaine in the inner ear. *Acta Oto-Laryngologica*, **82**, 297–300.

Epstein, M. and Marozeau, J. (2010) Loudness and intensity coding. In *The Oxford handbook of auditory science*, Volume 3, *Hearing* (ed. C. Plack), Oxford: Oxford University Press.

Erlandsson, S. I. (1990) *Tinnitus: tolerance or threat? Psychological and psychophysiological perspectives*, Doctoral Dissertation, Department of Psychology, University of Göteborg.

Erlandsson, S. I. (1992) Assessment of tinnitus. In *Tinnitus 91. Proceedings of the Fourth International Tinnitus Seminar* (eds J.-M. Aran and R. Dauman), Amsterdam/New York: Kugler Publications.

Erlandsson, S. (2000) Psychological profile of tinnitus patients. In *Tinnitus handbook* (ed. R. S. Tyler), San Diego, CA: Singular, Thomson Learning.

Erlandsson, S. I. and Hallberg, L. R.-M. (2000) Prediction of quality of life in patients with tinnitus. *British Journal of Audiology*, **34**, 11–20.

Erlandsson, S. and Persson, M.-L. (2006) A longitudinal study investigating the contribution of mental illness in chronic tinnitus patients. *Audiological Medicine*, **4**, 124–133.

Erlandsson, S., Ringdahl, A., Hutchins, T. and Carlsson, S. G. (1987) Treatment of tinnitus: a controlled comparison of masking and placebo, *British Journal of Audiology*, **21**, 37–44.

Erlandsson, S., Rubenstein, B. and Carlsson, S. G. (1991) Tinnitus: evaluation of biofeedback and stomatognatic treatment. *British Journal of Audiology*, **25**, 151–161.

Erlandsson, S. I., Hallberg, L. R.-M. and Axelsson, A. (1992) Psychological and audiological correlates of perceived tinnitus severity. *Audiology*, **31**, 168–179.

Erlandsson, S. I., Eriksson-Mangold, M. and Wiberg, A. (1996) Ménière's disease: trauma, distress and adaption studied through focus interview analyses. *Scandinavian Audiology*, **25** (Suppl. 43), 45–56.

Ernst, E. (2002) The risk-benefit profile of commonly used herbal therapies: ginkgo, St John's wort, gingseng, echinacea, saw palmetto, and kava. *Annals of Internal Medicine*, **136**, 42–53.

Ernst, E. (2004) Ear candles: a triumph of ignorance over science. *Journal of Laryngology and Otology*, **118**, 1–2.

Ernst, E. and Stevinson, C. (1999) Ginkgo biloba for tinnitus: a review. *Clinical Otolaryngology*, **24**, 164–167.

EuroQol Group (1990) EuroQoL: a new facility for the measurement of health related quality in life. *Health Policy*, **16**, 199–208.

Evans, D. (2003) *Placebo. The belief effect*, London: Harper Collins.

Evans, D. G. (2009) Neurofibromatosis type 2 (NF2): a clinical and molecular review. *Orphanet Journal of Rare Diseases*, **4**, 16.

Evans, E. F., Wilson, J. P. and Borerwe, T. A. (1981) Animal models of tinnitus. *Tinnitus. Ciba Foundation Symposium 85* (eds D. Evered and G. Lawrenson), London: Pitman Books, pp. 108–138.

Eysel-Gosepath, K. and Selivanova, O. (2005) Characterization of sleep disturbance in patients with tinnitus. *Laryngorhinootologie*, **84**, 323–327.

Eysenck, H. and Eysenck, S. (1975) *Manual of the Eysenck Personality Questionnaire*, London: Hodder & Stoughton.

Fabijanska, A., Rogowski, M., Bartnik, G. and Skarzynski, H. (1999) Epidemiology of tinnitus and hyperacusis in Poland. In *Proceedings of the Sixth International Tinnitus Seminar* (ed. J. Hazell), Cambridge, UK, The Tinnitus and Hyperacusis Centre.

Fagelson, M. (2007) The association between tinnitus and post traumatic stress disorder. *American Journal of Audiology*, **16**, 107–117.

Fausti, S. A., Wilmington, D. J., Gallun, F. J., Myers, P. J. and Henry, J. A. (2009) Auditory and vestibular dysfunction associated with blast-related traumatic brain injury. *Journal of Rehabilitation Research and Development*, **46**, 797–810.

Feeny, D., Furlong, W., Boyle, M. and Torrence, G. (1995) Multi-attribute health status classification sysyems. Health Utilities Index. *Pharmacoeconomics*, **7**, 490–502.

Feldmann, H. (1971) Homolateral and contralateral masking of tinnitus by noise-bands and pure tones. *Audiology*, **10**, 138–144.

Feldmann, H. 1997. A history of tinnitus research. In *Tinnitus: diagnosis/treatment* (ed. S. A), San Diego, CA: Singular.

Figueiredo, R., Langguth, B., Mello de Oliveira, P. and Aparecida de Azevedo, A. (2008) Tinnitus treatment with memantine. *Otolaryngology, Head and Neck Surgery*, **138**, 492–496.

Filipo, R., Barbara, M., Cordier, A., Mafera, B., Romeo, R., Attanasio, G., Manchini, P. and Marzetti, A. (1997) Osmotic drugs in the treatment of cochlear disorders: a clinical and experimental study. *Acta Otolaryngology*, **117**, 229–231.

First, M. B., Gibbon, M., Spitzer, R. L. and Williams, J. B. W. (1997) *Structured clinical interview for DSM-IV Axis I Disorders (SCID-I)*, Washington, DC: American Psychiatric Press.

Fishman, R. 1980. *Benign intracranial hypertension. Cerebrospinal fluid in disease of the nervous system*, Philadelphia, PA: WB Saunders.

Fitzgerald, M. and Folan-Curran, J. (2002) *Clinical neuroanatomy and related neuroscience*, Edinburgh: WB Saunders.

Florentine, M. (2011) Loudness. In *Loudness* (eds M. Florentine, A. Popper and R. Fay), New York: Springer.

Fogle, P. and Flasher L. V. (2003) *Counselling skills for speech–langauage pathologists and audiologists*, New York: Delmar.

Folkman, S. and Lazarus, R. S. (1988) Coping as a mediator of emotion. *Journal of Personality and Social Psychology*, **54**, 466–475.

Folmer, R. L. (2002) Long-term reductions in tinnitus severity. *BMC Ear, Nose and Throat Disorders*, **2**, http://www.biomedcentral.com/1472-6815/2/3.

Folmer, R. L. and Griest, S. E. (2000) Tinnitus and insomnia. *American Journal of Otolaryngology*, **21**, 287–293.

Folmer, R., Griest, S., Bonaduce, A. and Edlefsen, L. (2002) Use of serotonin reuptake inhibitors (SSRIs) by patients with chronic tinnitus. In *Proceedings of the Seventh International Tinnitus Seminar* (ed. R. Patuzzi), Freemantle, Australia, University of Western Australia.

Folmer, R. L., McMillan, G. P., Austin, D. F. and Henry, J. A. (2011) Audiometric thresholds and prevalence of tinnitus among male veterans in the United States: data from the National Health and Nutrition Examination Survey, 1999–2006. *Journal of Rehabilitation Research and Development*, **48**, 503–516.

Fonagy, P. (2005) The outcome of psychodynamic psychotherapy for psychological disorders. *Clinical Neuroscience Reviews*, **4**, 367–377.

Fordyce, W. E., Shelton, J. L. and Dundore, D. E. (1982) The modification of avoidance learning pain behaviors. *Journal of Behavioral Medicine*, **5**, 405–414.

Formby, C., Sherlock, L. P. and Gold, S. L. (2003) Adaptive plasticity of loudness induced by chronic attenuation and enhancement of the acoustic background. *Journal of the Acoustical Society of America*, **114**, 55–58.

Fortnum, H., O'Neill, C., Taylor, R., Lenthall, R., Nikolopoulous, T., O'Donoghue, G., Mason, S., Baguley, D., Jones, H. and Mulvaney, C. (2009) The role of magnetic resonance imaging in the identification of suspected acoustic neuroma: asystematic review of clinical and cost effectiveness and natural history. *Health Technology Assessment*, **13**, 1–154.

Fowler, E. P. (1936) A method for the early detection of otosclerosis. *Archives of Otolaryngology*, **24**, 731–734.

Fowler, E. P. (1941) Tinnitus aurium in the light of recent research. *Annals of Otology*, **50**, 139–158.

Fowler, E. P. (1942) The 'illusion of loudness' of tinnitus – its etiology and treatment. *Laryngoscope*, **52**, 275–285.

Fowler, E. P. (1943) Control of head noises. Their illusion of loudness and timbre. *Archives of Otolaryngology*, **37**, 391–398.

Fowler, E. P. (1944) Head noises in normal and disordered ears. Significance, measurement, differentiation and treatment. *Archives of Otolaryngology*, **39**, 498–503.

Fowler, E. P. (1948) The emotional factor in tinnitus aurium. *Laryngoscope*, **58**, 145–154.

Fowler, E. P. (1953) Intravenous procaine in the treatment of Ménière's disease. *Annals of Otology, Rhinology and Laryngology*, **62**, 1186–1200.

Fowler, E. P. and Fowler, E. P. J. (1955) Somatopsychic and psychosomatic factors in tinnitus, deafness and vertigo. *Annals of Otology, Rhinology and Laryngology*, **64**, 29–37.

Frank, G., Kleinjung, T., Landgrebe, M., Vielsmeier, V., Steffenhagen, C., Burger, J., Frank, E., Vollberg, G., Hajak, G. and Langguth, B. (2010) Left temporal low-frequency rTMS for the treatment of tinnitus: clinical predictors of treatment outcome – a retrospective study. *European Journal of Neurology*, **17**, 951–956.

Frank, E., Schecklmann, M., Landgrebe, M., Burger, J., Kreuzer, P., Poeppl, T. B., Kleinjung, T., Hajak, G. and Langguth, B. (2012) Treatment of chronic tinnitus with repeated sessions of prefrontal transcranial direct current stimulation: outcomes from an open-label pilot study. *Journal of Neurology*, **259**, 327–333.

Frankenburg, F. R. and Hegarty, J. D. (1994) Tinnitus, psychosis and suicide. *Archives of Internal Medicine*, **154**, 2371–2375.

Fredrikson, M. and Furmark, T. (2003) Amygdaloid regional cerebral blood flow and subjective fear during symptom provocation in anxiety disorders. *Annals of the New York Academy of Science*, **985**, 341–347.

Fregni, F., Marcondes, R., Boggio, P. S., Marcolin, M. A., Rigonatti, S. P., Sanchez, T. G., Nitsche, M. A. and Pascual-Leone, A. (2006) Transient tinnitus suppression induced by repetitive transcranial magnetic stimulation and transcranial direct current stimulation. *European Journal of Neurology*, **13**, 996–1001.

Friedland, D. R., Gaggl, W., Runge-Samuelson, C., Ulmer, J. L. and Kopell, B. H. (2007) Feasibility of auditory cortical stimulation for the treatment of tinnitus. *Otology and Neurootology*, **28**, 1005–1012.

Fritsch, M. H., Wynne, M. K., Matt, B. H., Smith, W. L. and Smith, C. M. (2001) Objective tinnitus in children. *Otology and Neurotology*, **22**, 644–649.

Fuchs, P. A. (2010) Introduction and overview. In *The Oxford Handbook of Auditory Science* Volume 1, *The Ear* (ed. P. A. Fuchs), Oxford: Oxford University Press.

Furmark, T., Tillfors, M., Marteinsdottir, I., Fischer, H., Pissiota, A., Langstrom, B. and Fredrikson, M. (2002) Common changes in cerebral blood flow in patients with social phobia treated with citalopram or cognitive-behavioral therapy. *Archives of General Psychiatry*, **59**, 425–433.

Furugård, S., Hedin, P.-J., Eggertz, A. and Laurent, C. (1998) Akupunktur värt att pröva vid svår tinnitus. *Läkartidningen*, **95**, 1922–1928.

Gabriels, P. 1993. Hyperacusis – can we help? *Australian Journal of Audiology*, **15**, 1–4.

Gabriels, P. (1996) Children with tinnitus. In *Proceedings of the Fifth International Tinnitus Seminar 1995* (eds G. Reich and J. Vernon), Portland, OR, The American Tinnitus Association.

Gananca, M. M., Caovilla, H. H., Gananca, F. F., Gananca, C. F., Munhoz, M. S., Da Silva, M. L. and Serafini, F. (2002) Clonazepam in the pharmacological treatment of vertigo and tinnitus. *International Tinnitus Journal*, **8**, 50–53.

Gander, P. E., Hoare, D. J., Collins, L., Smith, S. and Hall, D. A. (2011) Tinnitus referral pathways within the National Health Service in England: a survey of their perceived effectiveness among audiology staff. *BMC Health Services Research*, **11**, 162.

Gardner, A., Pagani, M., Jacobsson, H., Lindberg, G., Larsson, S. A., Wägner, A. and Hällström, T. (2002) Differences in resting state regional cerebral blood flow assessed with 99mTc-HMPAO SPECT and brain atlas matching between depressed patients with or without tinnitus. *Nuclear Medicine Communications*, **23**, 429–439.

Garduno-Anaya, M. A., Couthino de Toledo, H., Hinojosa-Gonzalez, R., Pane-Pianese, C. and Rios-Castaneda, L. C. (2005) Dexamethasone inner ear perfusion by intratympanic injection in unilateral Meniere's disease: a two-year prospective, placebo-controlled, double-blind, randomized trial. *Otolaryngology, Head and Neck Surgery*, **133**, 285–294.

Garin, P., Gilain, C., van Damme, J. P., de Fays, K., Jamart, J., Ossemann, M. and Vandermeeren, Y. (2011) Short- and long-lasting tinnitus relief induced by transcranial direct current stimulation. *Journal of Neurology*, **258**, 1940–1948.

Gatehouse, S. and Noble, W. (2004) The Speech, Spatial and Qualities of Hearing Scale (SSQ). *International Journal of Audiology*, **43**, 85–99.

Geisser, M., Glass, J., Rajcevska, L., Clauw, D., Williams, D., Kileny, P. and Gracely, R. (2008) A psychophysical study of auditory and pressure sensitivity in patients with fibromyalgia and healthy controls. *Journal of Pain*, **9**, 417–422.

Gelb, H. and Bernstein, I. (1983) Clinical evaluation of two hundred patients with temporomandibular joint syndrome. *Journal of Prosthetic Dentistry*, **49**, 234–243.

George, M. S. 2010. Transcranial magnetic stimulation for the treatment of depression. *Expert Reviews in Neurotherapeutics*, **10**, 1761–1772.

George, R. N. and Kemp, S. (1991) A survey of New Zealanders with tinnitus. *British Journal of Audiology*, **25**, 331–336.

Gerken, G. M. (1996) Central tinnitus and lateral inhibition: an auditory brainstem model. *Hearing Research*, **97**, 75–83.

Gerken, G. M., Hesse, P. S. and Wiorkowski, J. J. (2001) Auditory evoked responses in control subjects and in patients with problem-tinnitus. *Hearing Research*, **157**, 52–64.

Gersdorff, M., Robinillard, T., Steinm, F., Declaye, X. and Vanderbemden, S. (1987) A clinical correlation between hypozincemia and tinnitus. *Archives of Otorhinolaryngology*, **244**, 190–193.

Gersdorff, M., Nouwen, J., Gilain, C., Decat, M. and Betsch, C. (2000) Tinnitus and otosclerosis. *European Archives of Otorhinolaryngology*, **257**, 314–316.

Geven, L., De Kliene, E., Free, R. and van Dijk, P. (2011) Contralateral suppression of otoacoustic emissions in tinnitus patients. *Otology and Neurotology*, **32**, 315–321.

Ghatan, P., Ingvar, D. H., Stone-Elander, S. and Ingvar, M. (1996) Serial seven, an arithmetical test of working memory and attention: a PET study. *NeuroImage*, **3**, S179.

Ghatan, P. H., Hsieh, J. C., Petersson, K. M., Stone-Elander, S. and Ingvar, M. (1998) Coexistence of attention-based facilitation and inhibition in the human cortex. *Neuroimage*, **7**, 23–29.

Ghulyan-Bedikian, V., Paolino, M., Giorgetti-D'Esclercs, F. and Paolino, F. (2010) Propriétés psychométriques d'une version française du Tinnitus Handicap Inventory (Psychometric properties of a French adaptation of the Tinnitus Handicap Inventory). *L'Encephale*, **36**, 390–396.

Gibson, R. (1973) Paget's disease of the temporal bone. *Acta Otolaryngologica*, **87**, 299–301.

Gibson, W. and Arenberg, I. (1997) Pathophysiologic theories in the etiology of Ménière's disease. *Otolaryngologic Clinics of North America*, **30**, 961–967.

Giraud, A. L., Chéry-Croze, S., Fischer, G., Fischer, C., Vighetto, A., Grégoire, M.-C., Lavenne, F. and Collet, L. (1999) A selective imaging of tinnitus. *NeuroReport*, **10**, 1–5.

Goebel, G. and Floetzinger, U. (2008) Pilot study to evaluate psychiatric co-morbidity in tinnitus patients with and without hyperacusis. *Audiological Medicine*, **6**, 78–84.

Goebel, G. and Hiller, W. (1999) Quality management in the therapy of chronic tinnitus. In *Proceedings of the Sixth International Tinnitus Seminar* (ed. J. Hazell), Cambridge, UK, The Tinnitus and Hyperacusis Centre, pp. 357–363.

Gold, T. (1948) Hearing II. The physical basis of the action of the cochlea. *Proceedings of the Royal Society of Edinburgh (Biological Sciences)*, **135**, 492–498.

Gold, S., Formby, C., Frederick, E. A. and Suter, C. (2002) Shifts in loudness discomfort level in tinnitus patients with or without hyperacusis. In: PATUZZI, R. (ed.) *Proceedings of the Seventh International Tinnitus Seminar* (ed. R. Patuzzi), Freemantle, Australia, University of Western Australia.

Goldberg, D. (1978) *Manual of the General Health Questionnaire*, Slough: National Foundation for Educational Research.

Gomot, M., Belmote, M., Bullmore, E., Bernard, F. and Baron-Cohen, S. (2008) Brain hyper-reactivity to auditory novel targets in children with high-functioning autism. *Brain*, **131**, 2479–2488.

Goodey, R. J. (1981) Drugs in the treatment of tinnitus. In *Tinnitus, Ciba Foundation Symposium 85* (eds D. Evered and G. Lawrenson), London: Pitman Books.

Goodwin, P. E. and Johnson, R. M. (1980a) A comparison of reaction times to tinnitus and nontinnitus frequencies. *Ear and Hearing*, **1**, 148–155.

Goodwin, P. E. and Johnson, R. M. (1980b) The loudness of tinnitus. *Acta Otolaryngology*, **90**, 353–359.

Gopinath, B., McMahon, C. M., Rochtchina, E., Karpa, M. J. and Mitchell, P. (2010) Risk factors and impacts of incident tinnitus in older adults. *Annals of Epidemiology*, **20**(2), February, 129–135.

Gothelf, D., Farber, N., Raveh, E., Apter, A. and Attias, J. (2006) Hyperacusis in Williams syndrome: characteristics and associated neuroaudiologic abnormalities. *Neurology*, **66**, 390–395.

Graham, J. M. (1981) Tinnitus in children with hearing loss. In *Tinnitus, Ciba Foundation Symposium 85* (eds D. Evered and G. Lawrenson), London: Pitman Books.

Graham, J. M. (1987) Tinnitus in hearing impaired children. In *Tinnitus* (ed. J. W. P. Hazell), London: Churchill Livingstone.

Graham, J. T. and Newby, H. A. (1962) Acoustical characteristics of tinnitus. *Archives of Otolaryngology*, **75**, 162–167.

Graham, R. E., Ghandi, T. K., Borus, J., Segar, A. C., E, B., Bates, D. W., Philips, R. S. and Weingart, S. N. (2008) Advances in patient safety: new directions and alternative approaches. In

Technology and medication safety (eds K. Henriksen, J. B. Battles, M. A. Keyes and M. L. Grady), Rockville: Agency for Healthcare Research and Quality.

Granqvist, P., Lantto, S., Ortiz, L. and Andersson, G. (2001) Adult attachment, perceived family support, and problems experienced by tinnitus patients. *Psychology and Health*, **16**, 357–366.

Grauvogel, J., Kaminsky, J. and Rosahl, S. (2010) The impact of tinnitus and vertigo on patient-perceived quality of life after cerebellopontine angle surgery. *Neurosurgery*, **67**, 601–609.

Grayeli, A. B., Sterkers, O. and Toupet, M. (2009) Audiovestibular function in patients with otosclerosis and balance disorders. *Otology and Neurootology*, **30**(8), December, 1085–1091.

Green, J. D., Blum, D. J. and Harner, S. G. (1991) Longitudinal followup of patients with Meniere's disease. *Otolaryngology, Head and Neck Surgery*, **104**, 783–788.

Griffiths, T. D. (2000) Musical hallucinosis in acquired deafness. Phenomenology and brain substrate. *Brain*, **123**, 2065–2076.

Gross, J. J. (2002) Emotion regulation: affective, cognitive, and social consequences. *Psychophysiology*, **39**, 281–291.

Groves, P. M. and Thompson, R. F. (1970) Habituation: a dual process theory. *Psychological Review*, **77**, 419–450.

Gryczyńska, D., Drobik-Wasiewicz, K., Malicka, M. and Kotecki, M. (2007) Therapy of tinnitus in children (in Polish). *Otolaryngologia Polska*, **61**, 784–788.

Gu, L.-D. and Axelsson, A. (1996) Acupuncture for tinnitus: a review from five years of clinical investigations. In *Proceedings of the Fifth International Tinnitus Seminar 1995* (eds G. E. Reich and J. A. Vernon), Portland, OR, American Tinnitus Association, pp. 84–89.

Guitton, M., Caston, J., Johnson, R., Pujol, R. and Puel, J. (2003) Salicylate induces tinnitus through activation of cochlear NMDA receptors. *Journal of Neuroscience*, **23**, 3944–3952.

Gultekin, S., Celik, H., Akpek, S., Oner, Y., Gumus, T. and Tokgoz, N. (2008) Vascular loops at the cerebellopontine angle: is there a correlation with tinnitus? *American Journal of Neuroradiology*, **29**, 1746–1749.

Gulya, A. J. and Schuknecht, H. F. (1995) *Anatomy of the temporal bone with surgical implications*, New York: Parthenon.

Ha, C. 2007. Objective ear click of middle-ear myoclonus induced by a welding flux into ear canal. *Parkinsonism and Related Disorders*, **13**, S78.

Halford, J. B. S. and Anderson, S. D. (1991a) Tinnitus severity measured by a subjective scale, audiometry and clinical judgement. *Journal of Laryngology and Otology*, **105**, 89–93.

Halford, J. B. S. and Anderson, S. D. (1991b) Anxiety and depression in tinnitus sufferers. *Journal of Psychosomatic Research*, **35**, 383–390.

Hall, D. A., Haggard, M. P., Akeroyd, M. A., Palmer, A. R., Summerfield, A. Q., Elliott, M. R., Gurney, E. M. & Bowtell, R. W. 1999. "Sparse" temporal sampling in auditory fMRI. *Human Brain Mapping*, **7**, 213–223.

Hall, J. W. I. 2000. *Handbook of otoacoustic emissions*, San Diego, Singular.

Hallam, R. S. (1987) Psychological approaches to the evaluation and management of tinnitus distress. In *Tinnitus* (ed. J. Hazell), London: Churchill-Livingstone.

Hallam, R. S. (1989) *Living with tinnitus: dealing with the ringing in your ears*, Wellingborough: Thorsons.

Hallam, R. S. (1996a) Correlates of sleep disturbances in chronic distressing tinnitus. *Scandinavian Audiology*, **25**, 263–266.

Hallam, R. S. (1996b) *Manual of the Tinnitus Questionnaire*, London: The Psychological Corporation, Brace & Co.

Hallam, R. S., Rachman, S. and Hinchcliffe, R. (1984) Psychological aspects of tinnitus. In *Contributions to medical psychology* (ed. S. Rachman), Oxford: Pergamon Press.

Hallam, R. S., Jakes, S. C. and Hinchcliffe, R. (1988) Cognitive variables in tinnitus annoyance. *British Journal of Clinical Psychology*, **27**, 213–222.

Hallam, R. S., McKenna, L. and Shurlock, L. (2004) Tinnitus impairs cognitive efficiency. *International Journal of Audiology*, **43**, 218–226.

Hallberg, L. R.-M. and Erlandsson, S. I. (1993) Tinnitus characteristics in tinnitus complainers and noncomplainers. *British Journal of Audiology*, **27**, 19–27.

Hallberg, L. R.-M., Erlandsson, S. I. and Carlsson, S. G. (1992) Coping strategies used by middle-aged males with noise-induced hearing loss, with and without tinnitus. *Psychology and Health*, **7**, 273–288.

Haller, S., Birbaumer, N. and Veit, R. (2010) Real-time fMRI feedback training may improve chronic tinnitus. *European Radiology*, **20**, 696–703.

Hallpike, C. and Cairns, H. (1938) Observations on the pathology of Ménière's syndrome. *Journal of Laryngology and Otology*, **53**, 625.

Hamilton, A. and Munro, K. (2010) Uncomfortable loudness levels in experienced unilateral and bilateral hearing aid users: evidence of adaptive plasticity following asymmetrical sensory input? *International Journal of Audiology*, **49**, 667–671.

Han, B., Gfroerer, J. and Colliver, J. (2010) Associations between duration of illicit drug use and health conditions: results from the 2005–2007 national surveys on drug use and health. *Annals of Epidemiology*, **20**, 289–297.

Handscomb, L. (2006) Use of bedside sound generators by patients with tinnitus-related sleeping difficulty: Which sounds are preferred and why? *Acta Oto-Laryngologica*, **126**, 59–63.

Hannaford, P. C., Simpson, J. A., Bisset, A. F., Davis, A., McKerrow, W. and Mills, R. (2005) The prevalence of ear, nose and throat problems in the community: results from a national cross-sectional postal survey in Scotland. *Family Practice*, **22**, 227–233.

Hannula, S., Blogiu, R., Majamaa, K., Sorri, M. and Mäki-Torkko, E. (2011) Self-reported hearing problems among older adults: prevalence and comparison to measured hearing impairment. *Journal of the American Academy of Audiology*, **22**, 550–559.

Hansen, P. E., Hansen, J. H. and Bentzen, O. (1982) Acupuncture treatment of chronic unilateral tinnitus – a double-blind cross-over trial. *Clinical Otolaryngology*, **7**, 325–329.

Haralambous, G., Wilson, P. H., Platt-Hepworth, S., Tonkin, J. P., Hensley, V. R. and Kavanagh, D. (1987) EMG biofeedback in the treatment of tinnitus: an experimental evaluation. *Behaviour Research and Therapy*, **25**, 49–55.

Hardy, T. 1873. *A pair of blue eyes*, London: Penguin.

Harrop-Griffiths, J., Katon, W., Dobie, R., Sakai, C. and Russo, J. (1987) Chronic tinnitus: association with psychiatric diagnoses. *Journal of Psychosomatic Research*, **31**, 613–621.

Hartmann, T., Lorenz, I. and Wiesz, N. (2011) Neurobiofeedback. In *Textbook of tinnitus* (eds A. R. Møller, B. Langguth, D. DeRidder and T. Kleinjung), New York: Springer.

Harvey, A. and Schmidt, D. (2000) Clock monitoring in the maintenance of insomnia. *Sleep*, **24** (Suppl.), 334–335.

Hathaway, S. and McKinley, J. (1940) A multiphasic personality schedule (Minnesota). I. Construction of the schedule. *Journal of Psychology*, **10**, 249–254.

Hauptmann, C. and Tass, P. A. (2010) Restoration of segregated, physiological neuronal connectivity by desynchronizing stimulation. *Journal of Neural Engineering*, **7**, 056008.

Hauri, P. J. (1993) Consulting about insomnia: a method and some preliminary data. *Sleep*, **16**, 344–350.

Hausler, R., Toupet, M., Guidetti, G., Basseres, F. and Montandon, P. (1987) Meniere's disease in children. *Amerian Journal of Otolaryngology*, **8**, 187–193.

Hawthorne, G., Osborne, R., Taylor, A. and Sansomi, J. (2007) The SF36 version 2: critical analyses of population weights, scoring algorithms and population norms. *Quality of Life Research*, **16**, 661–673.

Hayes, S. C. (2003) Acceptance. In *Cognitive behavior therapy. Applying empirically supported techniques in your practice* (eds W. O'Donohue, J. E. Fisher and S. C. Hayes). New Jersey: John Wiley & Sons, Inc.

Hayes, S. C., Wilson, K. G., Strosahl, K., Gifford, E. V. and Follette, V. M. (1996) Experiental avoidance and behavioral disorders: a functional dimensional approach to diagnosis and treatment. *Journal of Consulting and Clinical Psychology*, **64**, 1152–1168.

Hayes, S. C., Strosahl, K. D. and Wilson, K. G. (1999) *Acceptance and commitment therapy*, New York: Guilford Press.

Hayes, S. C., Barnet-Holmes, D. and Roche, B. (eds) (2001) *Relational frame theory. A post-Skinnerian account of human language and cognition*, New York: Kluwer.

Hayes, S. C., Villatte, M., Levin, M. and Hildebrandt, M. (2011) Open, aware, and active: contextual approaches as emerging trends in the behavioral and cognitive therapies. *Annual Review of Clinical Psychology*, **7**, 141–168.

Hazell, J. W. P. (1987) A cochlear model for tinnitus. In *Proceedings of the Third International Tinnitus Seminar* (ed. F. H), Karlsruhe: Harsch Verlag.

Hazell, J. W. P. (1990a) Tinnitus II: surgical management of conditions associated with tinnitus and somatosounds. *Journal of Otolaryngology*, **19**, 6–10.

Hazell, J. W. P. (1990b) Tinnitus III: the practical management of sensorineural tinnitus. *Journal of Otolaryngology*, **19**, 11–18.

Hazell, J. (1991) Tinnitus and disability in ageing. *Acta Oto-Laryngologica*, **476** (Suppl.), 202–208.

Hazell, J. W. P. (1996) Support for a neurophysiological model of tinnitus. In *Proceedings of the Fifth International Tinnitus Seminar 1995* (eds G. E. Reich and J. A. Vernon), Portland, OR, American Tinnitus Association, pp. 51–57.

Hazell, J. W. P. and Jastreboff, P. J. (1990) Tinnitus I: auditory mechanisms: a model for tinnitus and hearing impairment. *Journal of Otolaryngology*, **19**, 1–5.

Hazell, J. W. P. and Sheldrake, J. B. (1992) Hyperacusis and tinnitus. In *Tinnitus 91. Proceedings of the Fourth International Tinnitus Seminar* (eds J.-M. Aran and R. Dauman), Amsterdam/New York: Kugler Publications.

Hazell, J. W. P., Wood, S. M., Cooper, H. R., Stephens, S. D. G., Corcoran, A. L., Coles, R. R. A., Baskill, J. L. and Sheldrake, J. B. (1985) A clinical study of tinnitus maskers. *British Journal of Audiology*, **19**, 65–146.

Hazell, J. W. P., Sheldrake, J. B. and Graham, R. L. (2002) Decreased sound tolerance: predisposing factors, triggers and outcomes after TRT. In *Proceedings of the Seventh International Tinnitus Seminar* (ed. R. Patuzzi), Freemantle, Australia, University of Western Australia.

Hébert, S. and Lupien, S. J. 2007. The sound of stress: blunted cortisol reactivity to psychosocial stress in tinnitus sufferers. *Neuroscience Letters*, **411**, 138–142.

Hébert, S., Paiement, P. and Lupien, S. J. (2004) A physiological correlate for the intolerance to both internal and external sounds. *Hearing Research*, **190**, 1–9.

Hedges, L. V. and Olkin, I. (1985) *Statistical methods for meta-analysis*, San Diego, CA, Academic Press.

Heidary, G. and Rizzo, J. R. (2010) Use of optical coherence tomography to evaluate papilledema and pseudopapilledema. *Seminars in Ophthalmology*, **25**, 198–205.

Heimer, L. (1995) *The human brain and apinal cord: functional neuroanatomy and dissection guide*, second edition, New York: Springer-Verlag.

Heinecke, K., Weise, C., Schwarz, K. and Rief, W. (2008) Physiological and psychological stress reactivity in chronic tinnitus. *Journal of Behavioral Medicine*, **31**, 179–188.

Helfer, T. M. (2011) Noise-induced hearing injuries, active component, U.S. Armed Forces, 2007–2010. *Medical Surveillance Monthly Report*, **18**, 7–10.

Helfer, T. M., Jordan, N. N., Lee, R. B., Pietrusiak, P., Cave, K. and Schairer, K. (2011) Noise-induced hearing injury and comorbidities among postdeployment U.S. Army soldiers: April 2003–June 2009. *American Journal of Audiology*, **20**, 33–41.

Heller, M. F. and Bergman, M. (1953) Tinnitus aurium in normally hearing persons. *Annals of Otology, Rhinology and Laryngology*, **62**, 73–83.

Helm, J. (1981) Tympanoplastik und ohrgerausche. *Laryngology, Rhinology and Otology*, **60**, 99–100.

Henry, J. A. and Meikle, M. B. (2000) Psychoacoustic measures of tinnitus. *Journal of the American Academy of Audiology*, **11**, 138–155.

Henry, J. L. and Wilson, P. H. (1995) Coping with tinnitus: two studies of psychological and audiological characteristics of patients with high and low tinnitus-related distress. *International Tinnitus Journal*, **1**, 85–92.

Henry, J. L. and Wilson, P. H. (1998) Psychological treatments for tinnitus. In *Tinnitus. Treatment and relief* (ed. J. A. Vernon), Boston, MA: Allyn & Bacon.

Henry, J. L. and Wilson, P. H. (2001) *Psychological management of chronic tinnitus. A cognitive-behavioral approach*, Boston, MA: Allyn & Bacon.

Henry, J. and Wilson, P. (2002) *Tinnitus. A self-management guide for the ringing in your ears*, Boston, MA: Allyn & Bacon.

Henry, J. A., Flick, C. L., Gilbert, A., Ellingson, R. M. and Fausti, S. A. (1999) Reliability of tinnitus loudness matches under procedural variation. *Journal of the American Academy of Audiology*, **10**, 502–520.

Henry, J. A., Schechter, M. A., Nagler, S. M. and Fausti, S. A. (2002a) Comparison of tinnitus masking and tinnitus retraining therapy. *Journal of the American Academy of Audiology*, **13**, 559–581.

Henry, J. A., Jastreboff, M. M., Jastreboff, P. J., Schechter, M. A. and Fausti, S. A. (2002b) Assessment of patients for treatment with tinnitus retraining therapy. *Journal of the American Academy of Audiology*, **13**, 523–544.

Henry, J. A., Jastreboff, M. M., Jastreboff, P. J., Schechter, M. A. and Fausti, S. A. (2002c) Assessment of patients for treatment with tinnitus retraining therapy. *Journal of the American Academy of Audiology*, **13**, 523–544.

Henry, J. A., Zaugg, T. L. and Schechter, M. A. (2005a) Clinical guide for audiologic tinnitus management I: assessment. *American Journal of Audiology*, **14**, 21–48.

Henry, J. A., Zaugg, T. L. and Schechter, M. A. (2005b) Clinical guide for audiologic tinnitus management II: treatment. *American Journal of Audiology*, **14**, 49–70.

Henry, J. A., Dennis, K. C. and Schechter, M. A. (2005c) General review of tinnitus: prevalence, mechanisms, effects, and management. *Journal of Speech, Language, and Hearing Research*, **48**, 1204–1235.

Henry, J. A., Rheinsburg, B., Owens, K. K. and Ellingson, R. M. (2006a) New instrumentation for automated tinnitus psychoacoustic assessment. *Acta Oto-Laryngologica*, 34–38.

Henry, J. A., Schechter, M. A., Zaugg, T. L., Griest, S., Jastreboff, P. J., Vernon, J. A., Kaelin, C., Meikle, M. B., Lyons, K. S. and Stewart, B. J. (2006b) Clinical trial to compare tinnitus masking and tinnitus retraining therapy. *Acta Otolaryngology Supplement*, **126**, 64–69.

Henry, J. A., Schechter, M. A., Zaugg, T. L., Griest, S., Jastreboff, P., Vernon, J. A., Kaelin, C., Meikle, M. B., Lyons, K. S. and Stewart, B. J. (2006c) Outcomes of clinical trial: tinnitus masking versus tinnitus retraining therapy. *Journal of the American Academy of Audiology*, **17**, 104–132.

Henry, J. A., Zaugg, T. L., Myers, P. and Schechter, M. A. (2010) Using therapeutic sound with progressive audiologic tinnitus management. *Trends in Amplification*, **12**, 188–209.

Henry, J. A., Galvez, G., Turbin, M. B., Thielman, E. J., McMillan, G. P. and Istvan, J. A. 2012. Pilot study to evaluate ecological momentary assessment of tinnitus. *Ear and Hearing*, **32**, 179–290.

Herraiz, C., Hernandez Calvin, J., Plaza, G., Tapia, M. and De los Santos, G. (2001) Evaluacion de la incapacidad en los pacientes con acufenos. *Acta Otorrinolaringologica Espanol*, **52**, 534–538.

Herraiz, C., Miguel Aparicio, J. and Plaza, G. (2010) Intratympanic drug delivery for the treatment of inner ear diseases. *Acta Otorrinolaringologica Espanola*, **61**, 225–232.

Hesser, H. (2010) Methodological considerations in treatment evaluations of tinnitus distress: a call for guidelines. *Journal of Psychosomatic Research*, **69**, 305–307.

Hesser, H. and Andersson, G. (2009) The role of anxiety sensitivity and behavioral avoidance in tinnitus disability. *International Journal of Audiology*, **48**, 295–299.

Hesser, H., Westin, V., Hayes, S. C. and Andersson, G. (2009) Clients' in-session acceptance and cognitive defusion behaviors in acceptance-based treatment of tinnitus distress. *Behaviour Research and Therapy*, **47**, 523–528.

Hesser, H., Weise, C., Zetterqvist-Westin, V. and Andersson, G. (2011a) A systematic review and meta-analysis of randomized controlled trials of cognitive-behavioral therapy for tinnitus distress. *Clinical Psychology Review*, **31**, 545–553.

Hesser, H., Weise, C., Rief, W. and Andersson, G. (2011b) The effect of waiting: a meta-analysis of wait-list control groups in trials for tinnitus distress. *Journal of Psychosomatic Research*, **70**, 378–384.

Hesser, H., Gustafsson, T., Lundén, C., Henriksson, O., Fattahi, K., Johnsson, E., Zetterqvist-Westin, V., Carlbring, P., Mäki-Torkko, E., Kaldo, V. and Andersson, G. (2012) A randomized controlled trial of Internet-delivered cognitive behavior therapy and acceptance and commitment therapy in the treatment of tinnitus. *Journal of Consulting and Clinical Psychology*, **16**, January (Epub ahead of print).

Hiller, W. and Goebel, G. (1992) A psychometric study of complaints in chronic tinnitus. *Journal of Psychosomatic Research*, **36**, 337–348.

Hiller, W. and Goebel, G. (1999) Assessing audiological, pathophysiological, and psychological variables in chronic tinnitus: a study of reliability and search for prognostic factors. *International Journal of Behavioral Medicine*, **6**, 312–330.

Hiller, W. and Goebel, G. (2004) Rapid assessment of tinnitus-related psychological distress using the Mini-TQ. *International Journal of Audiology*, **43**, 600–604.

Hiller, W. and Goebel, G. (2007) When tinnitus loudness and annoyance are discrepant: audiological characteristics and psychological profile. *Audiology and Neurootology*, **12**, 391–400.

Hiller, W. and Haerkötter, C. (2005) Does sound stimulation have additive effects on cognitive-behavioral treatment of chronic tinnitus? *Behaviour Research and Therapy*, **43**, 595–612.

Hilton, M. and Stuart, E. (2004) Ginkgo biloba for tinnitus. *Cochrane Database of Systematic Reviews* (2).

Hinchcliffe, R. (1961) Prevalence of the commoner ear, nose, and throat conditions in the adult rural population of Great Britain. *British Journal of Preventive and Social Medicine*, **15**, 128–140.

Hinchcliffe, R. and Chambers, C. (1983) Loudness of tinnitus: an approach to measurement. *Advances in Oto-Rhino-Laryngology*, **29**, 163–173.

Hinchcliffe, R. and King, P. F. (1992) Medicolegal aspects of tinnitus. 1: medicolegal position and current state of knowledge. *Journal of Audiological Medicine*, **1**, 38–58.

Hinke, K. and Brask, K. (1999) *An investigation of the telephone services of the call centre of Tele Danmark in Aabenraa*, Haderslev: Milijomedicinsk Klinik.

Hinton, D. E., Chhean, D., Pich, V., Hofmann, S. G. and Barlow, D. H. (2006) Tinnitus among Cambodian refugees: relationship to PTSD severity. *Journal of Traumatic Stress*, **19**, 541–546.

Hoare, D., Kowalkowski, V., Kang, S. and Hall, D. (2011) Systematic review and meta-analyses of randomized controlled trials examining tinnitus management. *Laryngoscope*, **121**, 1555–1564.

Hobson, J., Chisholm, E. and El Rafaie, A. (2010) Sound therapy (masking) in the management of tinnitus in adults. *Cochrane Database of Systematic Reviews*, CD006371.

Hofmann, S. G., Sawyer, A. T., Witt, A. A. and Oh, D. (2010) The effect of mindfulness-based therapy on anxiety and depression: a meta-analytic review. *Journal of Consulting and Clinical Psychology*, **78**, 169–183.

Hoke, M., Feldmann, H., Pantev, C., Lütkenhöner, B. and Lehnertz, K. (1989) Objective evidence of tinnitus in auditory evoked magnetic fields. *Hearing Research*, **37**, 281–286.

Hoke, E. S., Mühlnickel, W., Ross, B. and Hoke, M. (1998) Tinnitus and event-related activity of the auditory cortex. *Audiology and Neurootology*, **3**, 300–331.

Holgers, K.-M. (2003) Tinnitus in 7-year-old children. *European Journal of Pediatrics*, **162**, 276–278.

Holgers, K. M. and Juul, J. (2006) The suffering of tinnitus in childhood and adolescence. *International Journal of Audiology*, **45**, 267–272.

Holgers, K.-M., Axelsson, A. and Pringle, I. (1994) Ginkgo biloba for the treatment of tinnitus. *Audiology*, **33**, 85–92.

Holgers, K.-M., Erlandsson, S. I. and Barrenäs, M.-L. (2000) Predictive factors for the severity of tinnitus. *Audiology*, **39**, 284–291.

Holley, M. C. (1996) Outer hair cell motility. In *The Cochlea* (eds P. Dallos, A. N. Popper and R. R. Fay), New York: Springer.

Horvath, T. (1980) Arousal and anxiety. In *Handbook of studies in anxiety* (eds G. D. Burrows and D. B), North Holland: Elsevier.

House, J. W. (1978) Treatment of severe tinnitus with biofeedback training. *Laryngoscope*, **88**, 406–412.

House, J. (1981) Panel on tinnitus control: management of the tinnitus patient. *Annals of Otorynolaryngology*, **90**, 597–601.

House, J. W., Miller, L. and House, P. R. (1977) Severe tinnitus: treatment with biofeedback training (results in 41 cases). *Transactions of the American Academy of Ophthalmology and Otology*, **84**, 697–703.

Howard, M. L. (2001) Myths in neurotology, revisited: smoke and mirrors in tinnitus therapy. *Otology and Neurotology*, **22**, 711–714.

Howsam, G. D., Sharma, A., Lambden, S. P., Fitzgerald, J. and Prinsley, P. R. (2005) Bilateral objective tinnitus secondary to congenital middle-ear myoclonus. *Journal of Laryngology and Otology*, **119**, 489–491.

Hueb, M. M., Goycoolea, M. V., Paparella, M. M. and Oliveira, J. A. (1991) Otosclerosis: the University of Minnesota temporal bone collection. *Otolaryngology, Head and Neck Surgery*, **105**, 396–405.

Hughes, G. (1998) Sudden hearing loss. In *Current therapy in otolaryngology – head and neck surgery* (ed. G. Gates), sixth edition, St Louis: Mosby.

Humphriss, R., Baguley, D., Axon, P. and Moffat, D. (2006) Preoperative audiovestibular handicap in patients with vestibular schwannoma. *Skull Base*, **16**, 193–199.

Hurley, L. M., Thompson, A. M. and Pollack, G. D. (2002) Serotonin in the inferior colliculus. *Hearing Research*, **168**, 1–11.

Hurtuk, A., Dome, C., Holloman, C. H., Wolfe, K., Welling, D. B., Dodson, E. E. and Jacob, A. (2011) Melatonin: can it stop the ringing? *Annals of Otology, Rhinology and Laryngology*, **120**, 433–440.

Husain, F. T., Medina, R. E., Davis, C. W., Szymko-Bennett, Y., Simonyan, K., Pajor, N. M. and Horwitz, B. (2011a) Neuroanatomical changes due to hearing loss and chronic tinnitus: a combined VBM and DTI study. *Brain Research*, **1369**, 74–88.

Husain, F. T., Pajor, N. M., Smith, J. F., Kim, H. J., Rudy, S., Zalewski, C., Brewer, C. and Horwitz, B. (2011b) Discrimination task reveals differences in neural bases of tinnitus and hearing impairment. *PloS one*, **6**, e26639.

Huth, M. E., Ricci, A. J. and Cheng, A. G. (2011) Mechanisms of aminoglycoside ototoxicity and targets if hair vell protection. *International Journal of Otolaryngology*, Article ID 937861.

Ikeda, R., Oshima, T., Oshima, H., Miyazaki, M., Kikuchi, T., Kawase, T. and Kobayashi, T. (2011) Management of patulous Eustachian tube with habitual sniffing. *Otology and Neurotology*, **32**, 790–793.

Ikner, C. L. and Hassen, A. H. (1990) The effect of tinnitus on ABR latencies. *Ear and Hearing*, **11**, 16–20.

Ince, L. P., Greene, R. Y., Alba, A. and Zaretsky, H. H. (1987) A matching-to-sample feedback technique for training self-control of tinnitus. *Health Psychology*, **6**, 173–182.

International Statistical Classification of Diseases and Related Health Problems, 10th Revision (ICD-10), Version for 2010. http://apps.who.int/classifications/icd10/browse/2010

Ireland, C. E., Wilson, P. H., Tonkin, J. P. and Platt-Hepworth, S. (1985) An evaluation of relaxation training in the treatment of tinnitus. *Behaviour Research and Therapy*, **23**, 423–430.

Irvine, D. (2010) Plasticity in the auditory pathway. In *The Oxford handbook of auditory science*, Volume 2, *The auditory brain* (eds A. Rees and A. Palmer), Oxford: Oxford University Press.

Israel, J. M., Connelly, J. S., McTigue, S. T., Brummett, R. E. and Brown, J. (1982) Lidocaine in the treatment of tinnitus aurium. *Archives of Otolaryngology*, **108**, 471–473.

Iversen, S., Kupfermann, I. and Kandel, E. R. (2000) Emotional states and feelings. In *Principles of Neural Science* (eds E. R. Kandel, J. H. Schwartz and T. M. Jessel), New York: McGraw-Hill.

Jackson, A., MacPherson, H. and Hahn, S. (2006) Acupuncture for tinnitus: a series of six $n = 1$ controlled trials. *Complementray Therapies in Medicine*, **14**, 39–46.

Jacobson, G. P. and McCaslin, D. L. (2001) A search for evidence of direct relationship between tinnitus and suicide. *Journal of the American Academy of Audiology*, **12**, 493–496.

Jacobson, N. S. and Truax, P. (1991) Clinical significance: a statistical approach to defining meaningful change in psychotherapy research. *Journal of Consulting and Clinical Psychology*, **59**, 12–19.

Jacobson, G. P., Ahmad, B. K., Moran, J., Newman, C. W., Tepley, N. and Wharton, J. (1991) Auditory evoked cortical magnetic field (M100–M200) measurements in tinnitus and normal groups. *Hearing Research*, **56**, 44–52.

Jacobson, G. P., Calder, J. A., Newman, C. W., Peterson, E. L., Wharton, J. A. and Ahmad, B. K. (1996) Electrophysiological indices of selective auditory attention in subjects with and without tinnitus. *Hearing Research*, **97**, 66–74.

Jakes, S. C., Hallam, R. S., Chambers, C. and Hinchcliffe, R. (1985) A factor analytical study of tinnitus complaint behaviour. *Audiology*, **24**, 195–206.

Jakes, S. C., Hallam, R. S., McKenna, L. and Hinchcliffe, R. (1992) Group therapy for medical patients: an application to tinnitus. *Cognitive Therapy and Research*, **16**, 67–82.

Jalali, M. M., Kousha, A., Naghavi, S. E., Soleimani, R. and Banan, R. (2009) The effects of alprazolam on tinnitus: a cross-over randomized clinical trial. *Medical Science Monitor*, **15**, PI55–PI60.

James, W. (1890) *Principles of psychology*, Cambridge, MA: Harvard University Press.

James, A. and Burton, M. J. (2001) Betahistine for Ménière's disease or syndrome. *Cochrane Database of Systematic Reviews*, Issue 1, Article CD001873. DOI: 10.1002/14651858. CD001873.

Jannetta, P. J. (1998) Microvascular decompression surgery for tinnitus. In *Tinnitus. Treatment and relief* (ed. J. A. Vernon), Boston, MA: Allyn & Bacon.

Jastreboff, P. J. (1990) Phantom auditory perception (tinnitus): mechanisms of generation and perception. *Neuroscience Research*, **8**, 221–254.

Jastreboff, P. J. (1995) Tinnitus as a phantom perception: theories and clinical implications. In *Mechanisms of tinnitus* (eds J. A. Vernon and A. R. Møller), London: Allyn & Bacon.

Jastreboff, P. J. (1998) Tinnitus. In *Current therapy in otorhinolaryngology – head and neck surgery* (ed. G. Gates), St Louis, MO: Mosby, pp. 90–95.

Jastreboff, P. J. (1999) The neurophysiological model of tinnitus and hyperacusis. In *Proceedings of the Sixth International Tinnitus Seminar* (ed. J. Hazell), Cambridge, UK, The Tinnitus and Hyperacusis Centre, pp. 32–38.

Jastreboff, P. J. (2000) Tinnitus habituation therapy (THT) and tinnitus retraining therapy (TRT). In *Tinnitus handbook* (ed. R. S. Tyler), San Diego: Singular, Thomson Learning.

Jastreboff, P. J. (2007) Tinnitus retraining therapy. *Progress in Brain Research*, **166**, 415–424.

Jastreboff, P. J. and Hazell, J. W. P. (1993) A neurophysiological approach to tinnitus: clinical implications. *British Journal of Audiology*, **27**, 7–17.

Jastreboff, P. J. and Hazell, J. (2004) *Tinnitus retraining therapy: implementing the neurophysiological model*, Cambridge: Cambridge University Press.

Jastreboff, P. J. and Jastreboff, M. M. (2000) Tinnitus retraining therapy (TRT) as a method for treatment of tinnitus and hyperacusis patients. *Journal of the American Academy of Audiology*, **11**, 162–177.

Jastreboff, P. J. and Jastreboff, M. M. (2003) Tinnitus retraining treatment for patients with tinnitus and decreased sound tolerance. *Otolaryngologic Clinics of North America*, **36**, 321–336.

Jastreboff, P. J. and Sasaki, C. T. (1986) Salicylate induced changes in spontaneous activity of single units in the inferior colliculus of the guinea pig. *Journal of the Acoustic Society of America*, **50**, 1384–1391.

Jastreboff, P. J., Brennan, J. F., Coleman, J. K. and Sasaki, C. T. (1988) Phantom auditory sensation in rats: an animal model for tinnitus. *Behavioral Neuroscience*, **102**, 811–822.

Jastreboff, P. J., Brennan, J. F. and Sasaki, C. T. (1991) Quinine-induced tinnitus in rats. *Archives of Otolaryngology, Head and Neck Surgery*, **117**, 1162–1166.

Jastreboff, P. J., Hazell, J. W. P. and Graham, R. L. (1994) Neurophysiological model of tinnitus: dependence of the minimal masking level on treatment outcome. *Hearing Research*, **80**, 216–232.

Jastreboff, P. J., Gray, W. C. and Gold, S. L. (1996) Neurophysiological approach to tinnitus patients. *American Journal of Otology*, **17**, 236–240.

Jayarajan, V. and Coles, R. (1993) Treatment of tinnitus with frusemide. *Journal of Audiological Medicine*, **2**, 114–119.

Jensen, I. and Nygren, Å., Gamberale, F., Goldie, I., Westerholm, P. and Jonsson, E. (1995) The role of the psychologist in multidisciplinary treatments for chronic neck and shoulder pain: a controlled cost-effectiveness study. *Scandinavian Journal of Rehabilitation Medicine*, **27**.

Job, R. F. S. (1996) The influence of subjective reactions to noise on health effects of the noise. *Environmental International*, **22**, 93–104.

Johansson, M. S. K. and Arlinger, S. D. (2003) Prevalence of hearing impairments in a population in Sweden. *International Journal of Audiology*, **42**, 18–28.

Johnson, R. M., Brummett, R. and Schleuning, A. (1993) Use of alprazolam for relief of tinnitus. A double-blind study. *Archives of Otolaryngology, Head and Neck Surgery*, **119**, 842–845.

Johnsrude, I. S., Giraud, A. L. and Frackowiak, R. S. J. (2002) Functional imaging of the auditory system: the use of positron emission tomography. *Audiology and Neurootology*, **7**, 251–276.

Johnston, M. and Walker, M. (1996) Suicide in the elderly. Recognizing the signs. *General Hospital Psychiatry*, **18**, 257–260.

Jones, I. H. and Knudsen, V. O. (1928) Certain aspects of tinnitus, particularly treatment. *Laryngoscope*, **38**, 597–611.

Jones, D. M. and Macken, W. J. (1993) Irrelevant tones produce an irrelevant speech effect. *Journal of Experimental Psychology: Learning, Memory, and Cognition*, **19**, 369–381.

Josephson, E. M. (1931) A method of measurement of tinnitus. *Archives of Otolaryngology*, **14**, 282–283.

Josephson, I. (1988) Lidocaine blocks Na, Ca and K currents of chick ventricular myocytes. *Journal of Molecular and Cell Cardiology*, **20**, 593–604.

Jung, T., Rhee, C., Lee, C., Park, Y. and Choi, D. (1993) Ototoxicity of salicylate, nonsteroidal anti-inflammatory drugs, and quinine. *Otolaryngolic Clinics of North America*, **26**, 791–810.

Jung, T., Kim, J., Bumme, J., Davamony, D., Duncan, J. and Fletcher, W. (1997) Effect of leukotrine inhibitor on salicylate induced morphological changes of isolated cochlear outer hair cells. *Acta Otolaryngologica*, **117**, 258–264.

Juul, J., Barrenäs, M. L. and Holgers, K. M. (2012) Tinnitus and hearing in 7-year-old children. *Archives of Disability in Children*, **97**, 28–30.

Kaada, B., Hognestad, S. and Havstad, J. (1989) Transcutaneous nerve stimulation (TNS) in tinnitus. *Scandinavian Audiology*, **18**, 211–217.

Kabat-Zinn, J. (1990) *Full catastrophe living*, New York: Delacorte.

Kadner, A., Viirre, E., Wester, D. C., Walsh, S. F., Hestenes, J., Vankov, A. and Pineda, J. A. (2002) Lateral inhibition in the auditory cortex: an EEG index of tinnitus? *Neuroreport*, **13**, 443–446.

Kahneman, D. (1973) *Attention and effort*, Englewood Cliffs, NJ: Prentice Hall.

Kaldo, V. and Andersson, G. (2004) *Kognitiv beteendeterapi vid tinnitus (Cognitive-behavioral treatment of tinnitus)*, Lund, Studentlitteratur.

Kaldo, V., Renn, S., Rahnert, M., Larsen, H.-C. and Andersson, G. (2007) Use of a self-help book with weekly therapist contact to reduce tinnitus distress: a randomized controlled trial. *Journal of Psychosomatic Research*, **63**, 195–202.

Kaldo, V., Levin, S., Widarsson, J., Buhrman, M., Larsen, H. C. and Andersson, G. (2008) Internet versus group cognitive-behavioral treatment of distress associated with tinnitus. A randomised controlled trial. *Behavior Therapy*, **39**, 348–359.

Kaldo-Sandström, V., Larsen, H. C. and Andersson, G. (2004) Internet-based cognitive-behavioral self-help treatment of tinnitus: clinical effectiveness and predictors of outcome. *American Journal of Audiology*, **13**, 185–192.

Kaltenbach, J. A. and McAslin, D. L. (1996) Increases in spontaneous activity in the dorsal cochlearnucleus following exposure to high intensity sound: a possible neural correlate of tinnitus. *Auditory Neuroscience*, **3**, 57–78.

Kaltenbach, J. A., Godfrey, D. A., McCaslin, D. L. and Squire, A. B. (1996) Changes in spontaneous activity and chemistry of the cochlear nucleus following intense sound exposure. In *Proceedings of the Fifth International Tinnitus Seminar 1995* (eds G. E. Reich and J. A. Vernon), American Tinnitus Association, Portland, pp. 429–440.

Kaltenbach, J. A., Heffner, H. E. and Afman, C. E. (1999) Effects of intense sound on spontaneous activity in the dorsal cochlear nucleus and its relation to tinnitus. In *Proceedings of the Sixth International Tinnitus Seminar* (ed. J. Hazell), Cambridge, The Tinnitus and Hyperacusis Centre, pp. 133–138.

Kam, A. C., Cheung, A. P., Chan, P. Y., Leung, E. K., Wong, T. K., van Hasselt, C. A. and Tong, M. C. (2009) Psychometric properties of the Chinese (Cantonese) Tinnitus Handicap Inventory. *Clinical Otolaryngology*, **34**, 309–15.

Kameda, K., Shono, T., Hashiguchi, K., Yoshida, F. and Sasaki, T. (2010) Effect of tumor removal on tinnitus in patients with vestibular schwannoma. *Journal of Neurosurgery*, **112**, 152–157.

Kandel, E. R. (2000) Cellular mechanisms of learning and the biological basis of individuality. In: *Principles of neural science* (eds E. R. Kandel, J. H. Schwartz and T. M. Jessel). New York: McGraw-Hill.

Kandel, E. R., Schwartz, J. H. and Jessel, T. (eds) (2000) *Principles of neural science*, New York: McGraw-Hill.

Karwautz, A., Hafferl, A., Ungar, D. and Sailer, H. (1999) Patulous Eustachian tube in a case of adolescent anorexia nervosa. *International Journal of Eating Disorders*, **25**, 353–355.

Katzenell, U. and Segal, S. (2001) Hyperacusis: review and clinical guidelines. *Otology and Neurotology*, **22**, 321–327.

Kay, N. (1981) Oral chemotherapy in tinnitus. *British Journal of Audiology*, **15**, 123–124.

Kaye, J. M., Marlowe, F. I., Ramchandani, D., Berman, S., Schindler, B. and Loscalzo, G. (1994) Hypnosis as an aid for tinnitus patients. *Ear, Nose and Throat Journal*, **73**, 309–315.

Kehrle, H. M., Granjeiro, R. C., Sampaio, A. L., Bezerra, R., Almeida, V. F. and Oliveira, C. A. (2008) Comparison of auditory brainstem response results in normal-hearing patients with and without tinnitus. *Archives of Otolaryngology, Head and Neck Surgery*, **134**, 647–651.

Kemp, D. T. (1978) Stimulated acoustic emissions from within the hunan auditory system. *Journal of the Acoustic Society of America*, **64**, 1386–1391.

Kemp, D. T. (2010) Otoacoustic emissions and evoked potentials. In: FUCHS, P. A. (ed.) *The Oxford handbook of auditory science*, Volume 1, *The ear*, Oxford: Oxford University Press.

Kemp, S. and George, R. N. (1992) Diaries of tinnitus sufferers. *British Journal of Audiology*, **26**, 381–386.

Kentish, R. C. and Crocker, S. R. (2006) Scary monsters and waterfalls: tinnitus narrative therapy for children. In *Tinnitus treatment. Clinical protocols* (ed. R. S. Tyler), New York: Thieme.

Kentish, R. C., Crocker, S. R. and McKenna, L. (2000) Children's experience of tinnitus: a preliminary survey of children presenting to a psychology department. *British Journal of Audiology*, **34**, 335–340.

Kerns, R. D., Turk, D. C. and Rudy, T. E. (1985) The West Haven Yale Multidimensional Pain Inventory (WHYMPI). *Pain*, **23**, 345–356.

Kessler, R. C., Andrews, G., Mroczek, D., Ustun, B. and Wittchen, H.-U. (1998) The World Health Organization composite international diagnostic interview short-form (CIDI). *International Journal of Methods in Psychiatric Research*, **7**, 171–185.

Khalfa, S., Dubal, S., Veuillet, E., Perez-Sdiaz, F., Jouvent, R. and Collet, L. (2002) Psychometric normalisation of a Hyperacusis Questionnaire. *ORL: Journal for Oto-Rhino-Laryngology and Its Related Specialties*, **64**, 436–442.

Khalfa, S., Bruneau, N., Roge, B., Georgieff, N., Veuillet, E., Adrien, J. L., Barthelemy, C. and Collet, L. (2004) Increased perception of loudness in autism. *Hearing Research*, **198**, 87–92.

KhaliL, S., Ogunyemi, L. and Osbourne, J. (2002) Middle cerebral artery aneurysm presenting as isolated hyperacusis. *Journal of Laryngology and Otology*, **116**, 376–378.

Khedr, E. M., Rothwell, J. C. and El-Atar, A. (2009) One-year follow up of patients with chronic tinnitus treated with left temporoparietal rTMS. *European Journal of Neurology*, **16**, 404–408.

Khedr, E. M., Ahmed, M. A., Shawky, O. A., Mohamed, E. S., El Attar, G. S. and Mohammad, K. A. (2010) Epidemiological study of chronic tinnitus in Assiut, Egypt. *Neuroepidemiology*, **35**, 45–52.

Kiang, N. Y. S., Moxon, E. C., Levine, R. A. (1970) Auditory-nerve activity in cats with normal and abnormal cochleas. In *Sensorineural hearing loss* (eds G. E. Wolstenholme and J. Knight), London: Churchill Livingstone, pp. 241 –276.

Kihlstrom, J. F. (1985) Hypnosis. *Annual Review of Psychology*, **36**, 385–418.

Killion, M. C., Monroe, T. and Drambarean, V. (2011) Better protection from blasts without sacrificing situational awareness. *International Journal of Audiology*, **50** (Suppl. 1), S38–S45.

Kim, D. K., Park, S. N., Kim, H. M., Son, H. R., Kim, N. G., Park, K. H. and Yeo, S. W. (2011) Prevalence and significance of high-frequency hearing loss in subjectively normal-hearing patients with tinnitus. *Annals of Otology, Rhinology and Laryngology*, **120**, 523–528.

Kirk, K., McGuire, A., Nielsen, L., Cosgrove, T., McClintock, C., Nasveld, P. E. and Treloar, S. A. (2011) Self-reported tinnitus and ototoxic exposures among deployed Australian Defence Force personnel. *Military Medicine*, **176**, 461–467.

Kirsch, C. A., Blanchard, E. B. and Parnes, S. M. (1989) Psychological characteristics of individuals high and low in their ability to cope with tinnitus. *Psychosomatic Medicine*, **51**, 209–217.

Klein, A. J., Armstrong, B. L., Greer, M. K. and Brown III, F. R. (1990) Hyperacusis and otitis media in individuals with Williams syndrome. *Journal of Speech and Hearing Disorders*, **55**, 339–344.

Kleinjung, T. (2011) Low-level laser therapy. In *Textbook of tinnitus* (eds A. R. Møller, B. Langguth, D. DeRidder and T. Kleinjung), New York: Springer.

Kleinjung, T., Eichhammer, P., Langguth, B., Jacob, P., Marienhagen, J., Hajak, G., Wolf, S. R. and Strutz, J. (2005) Long-term effects of repetitive transcranial magnetic stimulation (rTMS) in patients with chronic tinnitus. *Otolaryngology, Head and Neck Surgery*, **132**, 566–569.

Kleinjung, T., Fischer, B., Langguth, B., Sand, P. G., Hajak, G., Dvorakova, J. and Eichhammer, P. (2007) Validation of the German-Version Tinnitus Handicap Inventory (THI). *Psychiatrische Praxis*, **34**, 140–142.

Kleinjung, T., Steffens, T., Landgrebe, M., Vielsmeier, V., Frank, E., Hajak, G., Strutz, J. and Langguth, B. (2009) Levodopa does not enhance the effect of low-frequency repetitive transcranial magnetic stimulation in tinnitus treatment. *Otolaryngology, Head and Neck Surgery*, **140**, 92–95.

Kleinjung, T., Langguth, B. and Khedr, E. (2011) Transcranial magnetic stimulation. In *Textbook of tinnitus* (eds A. R. Møller, B. Langguth, D. DeRidder and T. Kleinjung), New York: Springer.

Klockhoff, I. and Lindblom, U. (1967) Ménière's disease and hydrochlorothiazide (Dichlotride®) – a critical analysis of symptoms and therapeutic effects. *Acta Oto-Laryngologica*, **63**, 347–365.

Klockhoff, I., Lindholm, L. and Westerberg, C. E. (1971) Spontaneous impedance fluctuation – a 'tensor tympani syndrome' with special reference to tension headache. *Nordisk Medicin*, **85**, 577.

Knauer, S., Heinrich, U., Bier, C., Habtemichael, N., Docter, D., Helling, K., Mann, W. and Stauber, R. (2010) An otoprotective role for the apoptosis inhibitor protein survivin. *Cell Death Disorders*, **1**, e51.

Knobel, K. A. B. and Sanchez, T. (2008) Influence of silence and attention on tinnitus perception. *Otolaryngology, Head and Neck Surgery*, **138**, 18–22.

Kong, S. K., Lee, I. W., Goh, E. K. and Park, S. H. (2010) Autologous cartilage injection for the patulous Eustachian tube. *American Journal of Otolaryngology*, **32**, 346–348.

Konig, O., Schaette, R., Kempter, R. and Gross, M. (2006) Course of hearing loss and occurrence of tinnitus. *Hearing Research*, **221**, 59–64.

Korres, S., Mountricha, A., Balatsouras, D., Maroudias, N., Riga, M. and Xenelis, I. (2010) Tinnitus Retraining Therapy (TRT): outcomes after one-year treatment. *International Tinnitus Journal*, **16**, 55–59.

Kotimaki, J., Sorri, M., Aantaa, E. and Nuutinen, J. (1999) Prevalence of Ménière disease in Finland. *Laryngoscope*, **109**, 748–753.

Kröner-Herwig, B., Hebing, G., van Rijn-Kalkmann, U., Frenzel, A., Schilkowsky, G. and Esser, G. (1995) The management of chronic tinnitus. Comparison of a cognitive-behavioural group training with yoga. *Journal of Psychosomatic Research*, **39**, 153–165.

Kröner-Herwig, B., Biesinger, E., Goebel, G., Greimel, K. V. and Hiller, W. (2000) Retraining therapy for chronic tinnitus. *Scandinavian Audiology*, **29**, 67–78.

Kröner-Herwig, B., Frenzel, A., Fritsche, G., Schilkowsky, G. and Esser, G. (2003) The management of chronic tinnitus. Comparison of an outpatient cognitive-behavioral group training to minimal-contact interventions. *Journal of Psychosomatic Research*, **54**, 381–389.

Kuk, F. K., Tyler, R. S., Russell, D. and Jordan, H. (1990) The psychometric properties of a tinnitus handicap questionnaire. *Ear and Hearing*, **11**, 434–445.

Kvestad, E., Czajkowski, N., Engdahl, B., Hoffman, H. J. and Tambs, K. (2010) Low heritability of tinnitus: results from the second Nord-Trondelag health study. *Archives of Otolaryngology, Head and Neck Surgery*, **136**, 178–182.

Landgrebe, M., Langguth, B., Rosengarth, K., Braun, S., Koch, A., Kleinjung, T., May, A., De Ridder, D. and Hajak, G. (2009) Structural brain changes in tinnitus: grey matter decrease in auditory and non-auditory brain areas. *NeuroImage*, **46**, 213–218.

Langenbach, M., Olderog, M., Michel, O., Albus, C. and Kohle, K. (2005) Psychosocial and personality predictors of tinnitus-related distress. *General Hospital Psychiatry*, **27**, 73–77.

Langguth, B. (2011) The psychiatrist. In *Textbook of tinnitus* (eds A. R. Møller, B. Langguth, D. DeRidder and T. Kleinjung), New York: Springer.

Langguth, B. and Elgoyhen, A. (2011) Emerging pharmacotherapy of tinnitus. *Expert Opinon in Emerging Drugs*, **16**, 603–606.

Langguth, B., Eichhammer, P., Kreutzer, A., Maenner, P., Marienhagen, J., Kleinjung, T., Sand, P. and Hajak, G. (2006) The impact of auditory cortex activity on characterizing and treating patients with chronic tinnitus – first results from a PET study. *Acta Oto-Laryngologica*, **126**, 84–88.

Langguth, B., Kleinjung, T., Fischer, B., Hajak, G., Eichhhammer, P. and Sand, P. (2007) Tinnitus severity, depression, and the big five personality traits. *Progress in Brain Research*, **166**, 221–226.

Langguth, B., Kleinjung, T., Frank, E., Landgrebe, M., Sand, P., Dvorakova, J., Frick, U., Eichhammer, P. and Hajak, G. (2008) High-frequency priming stimulation does not enhance the effect of low-frequency rTMS in the treatment of tinnitus. *Experimental Brain Research*, **184**, 587–591.

Langguth, B., Salvi, D. and Elgoyhen, A. (2009) Emerging pharmacotherapy of tinnitus. *Expert Opinon in Emerging Drugs*, **14**, 687–702.

Langguth, B., Kleinjung, T., Landgrebe, M., De Ridder, D. and Hajak, G. (2010) rTMS for the treatment of tinnitus: the role of neuronavigation for coil positioning. *Clinical Neurophysiology*, **40**, 45–58.

Langner, G. and Wallhäusser-Franke, E. (1999) Computer simulation of a tinnitus model based on labelling of tinnitus activity in the auditory cortex. In *Proceedings of the Sixth International Tinnitus Seminar* (ed. J. Hazell), Cambridge, The Tinnitus and Hyperacusis Centre, pp. 20–25.

Lanting, C. P., De Kleine, E., Bartels, H. and van Dijk, P. (2008) Functional imaging of unilateral tinnitus using fMRI. *Acta Oto-Laryngologica*, **128**, 415–421.

Lanting, C. P., De Kleine, E. and van Dijk, P. (2009) Neural activity underlying tinnitus generation: results from PET and fMRI. *Hearing Research*, **255**.

Lanting, C. P., De Kleine, E., Eppinga, R. N. and van Dijk, P. (2010) Neural correlates of human somatosensory integration in tinnitus. *Hearing Research*, **267**, 78–88.

Lasisi, A. O., Abiona, T. and Gureje, O. (2010) Tinnitus in the elderly: profile, correlates, and impact in the Nigerian Study of Ageing. *Otolaryngology, Head and Neck Surgery*, **143**, 510–515.

Lazarus, R. S. and Folkman, S. (1984) Coping and adaption. In *Handbook of behavioral medicine* (ed. W. D. Gentry), New York: The Guilford Press.

Leaver, A. M., Renier, L., Chevillet, M. A., Morgan, S., Kim, H. J. and Rauschecker, J. P. (2011) Dysregulation of limbic and auditory networks in tinnitus. *Neuron*, **69**, 33–43.

LeDoux, J. E. 1998. *The emotional brain*, London, Weidenfeld and Nicholson.

Lee, H., Whitman, G., Lim, J., Yi, S., Cho, Y., Ying, S. and Baloh, R. (2003) Hearing symptoms in migraneous infarction. *Archives of Neurology*, **60**, 113–116.

Lempert, J. (1938) Improvement in hearing in cases of otosclerosis. A new one-stage surgical technique. *Archives of Otolaryngology*, **28**, 42–97.

Le Prell, C., Ac, J., Lindblad, A., Skjönsberg, A., UlfendahL, M., Guire, K., Green, G., Campbell, K. and Miller, J. (2011) Increased vitamin plasma levels in Swedish military personnel treated with nutrients prior to automatic weapon training. *Noise and Health*, **13**, 432–443.

Leske, M. C. (1981) Prevalence estimates of communicative disorders in the U.S.: language, hearing and vestibular disorders. *American Speech and Hearing Association*, **23**, 229–237.

Lethem, J., Slade, P. D., Troup, J. D. G. and Bentley, G. (1983) Outline of a fear-avoidance model of exaggerated pain perception – I. *Behaviour Research and Therapy*, **21**, 401–408.

Lew, H. L., Jerger, J. F., Guillory, S. B. and Henry, J. A. (2007) Auditory dysfunction in traumatic brain injury. *Journal of Rehabilitation Research and Development*, **44**, 921–928.

Leventhall, H. G. (2003) *A review of published research on low frequency noise and its effects*, London: Defra Publications. http://archive.defra.gov.uk/environment/quality/noise/research/lowfrequency/documents/lowfreqnoise.pdf.

Leventhall, G., Benton, S. and Robertson, D. (2008) Coping strategies for low frequency noise. *Low Frequency Noise, Vibration and Active Control*, **27**, 35–52.

Levin, G., Fabian, P. and Stahle, J. (1988) Incidence of otosclerosis. *American Journal of Otology*, **9**, 299–301.

Levine, R. (1999) Somatic modulation appears to be a fundamental attribute of tinnitus. In *Proceedings of the Sixth International Tinnitus Seminar* (ed. J. Hazell), Cambridge, The Tinnitus and Hyperacusis Centre.

Levine, R. A. (2001) Diagnostic issues in tinnitus: a neuro-otological perspective. *Seminars in Hearing*, **22**, 23–36.

Levine, R. A. (2006) Typewriter tinnitus: a carbamazepine-responsive syndrome related to auditory nerve vascular compression. *ORL: Journal for Oto-Rhino-Laryngology and Its Related Specialties*, **68**, 43–46.

Levine, R. and Kiang, N. (1995) A conversation about tinnitus. In *Mechanisms of tinnitus* (ed. J. A. Vernon and A. R. Møller), Boston: Allyn & Bacon.

Lewis, J. E. and Stephens, S. D. G. (1995) Parasuicide and tinnitus. *Journal of Audiological Medicine*, **4**, 34–43.

Lewis, J., Stephens, D. and Huws, D. (1992) Suicide in tinnitus. *Journal of Audiological Medicine*, **1**, 30–37.

Lewis, J. E., Stephens, S. D. G. and McKenna, L. (1994) Tinnitus and suicide. *Clinical Otolaryngology*, **19**, 50–54.

Levitin, D. J., Menon, V., Schmitt, J. E., Eliez, S., White, C. D., Glover, G. H., Kadis, J., Korenberg, J. R., Bellugi, U. and Reiss, A. L. (2003) Neural correlates of auditory perception in Williams syndrome: an FMRI study. *Neuroimage*, **18**, 74–82.

Levitin, D. J., Cole, K., Lincoln, A. and Bellugi, U. (2005) Aversion, awareness, and attraction: investigating claims of hyperacusis in the Williams syndrome phenotype. *Journal of Child Psychology and Psychiatry*, **46**, 514–523.

Lewy, R. B. (1937) Treatment of tinnitus aurium by the intravenous use of local anestethic agents. *Archives of Otolaryngology*, **25**, 178–183.

Liedgren, S. R., Ödkvist, L. M., Davis, E. R. and Fredrickson, J. M. (1976) Effect of marihuana on hearing. *Journal of Otolaryngology*, **5**, 233–237.

Lima A. S., Sanchez, T., Marcondes, R. and Bento, R. (2005) The effect of stapedotomy on tinnitus in patients with otospongiosis. *Ear, Nose and Throat Journal*, **84**, 412–414.

Lima, A. S., Sanchez, T., Bonadia Moraes, M., Batezati Alves, S. and Bento, R. (2007) The effect of timpanoplasty on tinnitus in patients with conductive hearing loss: a six month follow-up. *Brazlian Journal of Otorhinolaryngology*, **73**, 384–389.

Lind, O. (1996) Transient evoked otoacoustic emissions and contralateral suppression in patients with unilateral tinnitus. *Scandinavian Audiology*, **25**, 167–172.

Lindberg, P. (1989) *Assessment of tinnitus aurium. A behavioural approach to the evaluation of symtoms and the effects of intervention.* Acta Universitas Upsaliensis, Comprehensive Summaries of Uppsala Dissertations from the Faculty of Social Sciences, 12 (Dissertation), 52 pp.

Lindberg, P., Lyttkens, L., Melin, L. and Scott, B. (1984) Tinnitus-incidence and handicap. *Scandinavian Audiology*, **13**, 287–291.

Lindblad, A. C., Hagerman, B. and Rosenhall, U. (2011) Noise-induced tinnitus: a comparison between four clinical groups without apparent hearing loss. *Noise and Health*, **13**, 423–431.

Linde, K., Hondras, M., Vickers, A., Ter Riet, G. and Melchart, D. (2001) Systematic reviews of complementary therapies – an annotated bibliography. Part 3: homeopathy. *BMC Complementary and Alternative Medicine*, **1**, 4.

Linton, S. J., Overmeer, T., Jansson, M., Vlaeyen, J. W. S. and De Jong, J. R. (2002) Graded *in-vivo* exposure treatment for fear-avoidant pain patients with functional disability: a case study. *Cognitive Behaviour Therapy*, **31**, 49–58.

Liu, H., Fan, J., Lin, S., Zhao, S. and Lin, Z. (2011) Botox transient treatment of tinnitus due to stapedius myoclonus: case report. *Clinical Neurology and Neurosurgery*, **113**, 57–58.

Lloyd, S., Kasbekar, A., Baguley, D. and Moffat, D. (2010) Audiovestibular factors influencing quality of life in patients with conservatively managed sporadic vestibular schwannoma. *Otology and Neurootology*, **31**, 968–976.

Lockwood, A. H., Salvi, R. J., Coad, M. L., Towsley, M. L., Wack, D. S. and Murphy, B. W. (1998) The functional neuroanatomy of tinnitus. Evidence for limbic system links and neural plasticity. *Neurology*, **50**, 114–120.

Lockwood, A. H., Wack, D. S., Burkard, R. F., Coad, M. L., Reyes, S. A., Arnold, S. A. and Salvi, R. J. (2001) The functional anatomy of gaze-evoked tinnitus and sustained lateral gaze. *Neurology*, **56**, 472–480.

Londero, A., Peignard, P., Malinvaud, D., Avan, P. and Bonfils, P. (2006) Tinnitus and cognitive-behavioral therapy: results after 1 year. *La Presse Médicale*, **35**, 1213–1221.

Long, G. R. and Tubis, A. (1988) Modification of spontaneous and evoked otoacoustic emissions and associated psychoacoustic microstructure by aspirin consumption. *Journal of the Acoustical Society of America*, **84**, 1343–1353.

Lopez-Gonzalez, M. A. and Esteban-Ortega, F. (2005) Tinnitus Dopaminergic Pathway. Ear noises treatment by dopamine modulation. *Medical Hypotheses*, **65**, 349–352.

Lopez-Gonzalez, M., Muratori Leon, M. and Vaquera, J. (2003) Sulpirida como tratamiento de inicio en la terapia de rehabilitaciòn del acùfeno (Sulpiride as initial treatment in the Tinnitus Retraining Therapy). *Acta Otorrinolaringologica Espanola*, **54**, 237–241.

Lopez-Gonzalez, M., Santiago, A. and Esteban-Ortega, F. (2007) Sulpiride and melatonin decrease tinnitus perception modulating the auditolimbic dopaminergic pathway. *Journal of Otolaryngology*, **36**, 213–219.

Lorenz, I., Muller, N., Schlee, W., Langguth, B. and Weisz, N. (2010) Short-term effects of single repetitive TMS sessions on auditory evoked activity in patients with chronic tinnitus. *Journal of Neurophysiology*, **104**, 1497–1505.

Lorito, G., Hatzopoulos, S., Laurell, G., Campbell, K., Petruccelli, J., Giordano, P., Kochanek, K., L, S., Martini, A. and Skarzynski, H. (2011) Dose-dependent protection on cisplatin-induced ototoxicity – an electrophysiological study on the effect of three antioxidants in the Sprague-Dawley rat animal model. *Medical Science Monitor*, **17**, 179–186.

Lysyansky, B., Popovych, O. V. and Tass, P. A. (2011) Search for the optimal strength of coordinated reset stimulation. *Conference Proceedings of the Medical Biological Society*, pp. 667–670.

Lyttkens, L., Lindberg, P., Scott, B. and Melin, L. (1986) Treatment of tinnitus by external electrical stimulation. *Scandinavian Audiology*, **15**, 157–164.

MacLean, P. D. (1955) The limbic system ('visceral brain') and emotional behavior. *Archives of Neurology and Psychiatry*, **73**, 130–134.

MacLeod-Morgan, C., Court, J. and Roberts, R. (1982) Cognitive restructuring: a technique for the relief of chronic tinnitus. *Australian Journal of Clinical and Experimental Hypnosis*, **10**, 27–33.

MacNaughton Jones, H. (1891) *Subjective noises in the head and ears*, London: Ballière, Tindall & Cox.

Madani, G. and Connor, S. (2009) Imaging in pulsatile tinnitus. *Clinical Radiology*, **64**, 319–328.

Mahoney, C. J., Rohrer, J. D., Goll, J. C., Fox, N. C., Rossor, M. N. and Warren, J. D. (2011) Structural neuroanatomy of tinnitus and hyperacusis in semantic dementia. *Journal of Neurology, Neurosurgery and Psychiatry*, **82**, 1274–1278.

Malouff, J. M., Noble, W., Schutte, N. S. and Bhullar, N. (2010) The effectiveness of bibliotherapy in alleviating tinnitus-related distress. *Journal of Psychosomatic Research*, **68**, 245–251.

Mammano, F. and Ashmore, J. (1993) Reverse transduction measured in the isolated cochlea by laser Michelson interferometry. *Nature*, **365**, 838–841.

Marciano, E., Carrabba, L., Giannini, P., Sementina, C., Verde, P., Bruno, C., Di Petro, G. and Ponsillo, N. G. (2003) Psychiatric comorbidity in a population of outpatients affected by tinnitus. *International Journal of Audiology*, **42**, 4–9.

Marcus, D. C. and Wangemann, P. (2010) Inner ear homeostasis. In *The Oxford handbook of auditory science*, Volume 1, *The ear* (ed. P. A. Fuchs), Oxford: Oxford University Press.

Marks, N. J., Emery, P. and Onisphorou, C. (1984) A controlled trial of acupuncture in tinnitus. *Journal of Laryngology and Otology*, **98**, 1103–1109.

Marks, N. J., Karl, H. and Onisiphorou, C. (1985) A controlled trial of hypnotherapy in tinnitus. *Clinical Otolaryngology*, **10**, 43–46.

Marler, J., Elfenbein, J., Ryals, B., Urban, Z. and Netzloff, M. L. (2005) Sensorineural hearing loss in children and adults with Williams syndrome. *American Journal of Medical Genetics A*, **138**, 318–327.

Marler, J., Sitcovsky, J., Mervis, C., Kistler, D. and Wightman, F. (2010) Auditory function and hearing loss in children and adults with Williams syndrome: cochlear impairment in individuals with otherwise normal hearing. *American Journal of Medical Genetics C, Seminars in Medical Genetics*, 154C, 249–265.

Marlowe, F. I. (1973) Effective treatment of tinnitus through hypnotherapy. *American Journal of Clinical Hypnosis*, **15**, 162–165.

Marriage, J. and Barnes, N. M. (1995) Is central hyperacusis a symptom of 5-hydroxytryptamine (5-HT) dysfunction? *The Journal of Laryngology and Otology*, **109**, 915–921.

Martin, W. (1995) Spectral analysis of brain activity in the study of tinnitus. In *Mechanisms of tinnitus* (eds J. A. Vernon and A. R. Møller), London: Allyn & Bacon.

Martin, K. and Snashall, S. (1994) Children presenting with tinnitus: a retrospective study. *British Journal of Audiology*, **28**, 111–115.

Martinez-Devesa, P., Waddell, A., Perera, R. and Theodoulou, M. (2007) Cognitive behavioural therapy for tinnitus. *Cochrane Database of Systematic Reviews*, CD005233.

Martinez-Devesa, P., Waddell, A., Perera, R. and Theodoulou, M. (2010) Cognitive behavioural therapy for tinnitus. *Cochrane Database of Systematic Reviews*, Issue 9, Article CD005233. DOI: 10.1002/14651858.CD005233.pub3.

Mason, J. and Rogerson, D. (1995) Client-centered hypnotherapy for tinnitus: who is likely to benefit. *American Journal of Clinical Hypnosis*, **37**, 294–299.

Mason, J. D. T., Rogerson, D. R. and Butler, J. D. (1996) Client centered hypnotherapy in the management of tinnitus – is it better than counselling? *Journal of Laryngology and Otology*, **110**, 117–120.

Mathews, A. and Sebastian, S. (1993) Suppression of emotional Stroop effects by fear-arousal. *Cognition and Emotion*, **7**, 517–530.

Mathiesen, H. (1969) Phonophobia after stapedectomy. *Acta Oto-Laryngologica*, **68**, 73–77.

Matsuhira, T., Yamashita, K. and Yasuda, M. (1992) Estimation of the loudness of tinnitus from matching tests. *British Journal of Audiology*, **26**, 387–395.

Matsumoto, N., Kitani, R. and Kalinec, F. (2011) Linking LINK1 deficiency to hyperacusis and progressive hearing loss in individuals with Williams syndrome. *Communicative and Integrative Biology*, **4**, 208–210.

Mattox, D. and Reichert, M. (2008) Meniett device for Meniere's disease: use and compliance at 3 to 5 years. *Otology and Neurotology*, **29**, 29–32.

Maurizi, M., Ottaviani, F., Paludetti, G., Almadori, G. and Tassoni, A. (1985) Contribution to the differentiation of peripheral versus central tinnitus via auditory brain stem response evaluation. *Audiology*, **24**, 207–216.

Mazzolli, M., Sintoni, K., Stallato, A. et al. (2010) Mindfulness based stress reduction (MBSR) intervention in tinnitus therapy. *Symposium at the 4th International TRI Tinnitus Conference Frontiers in Tinnitus Research*.

McCall, A. A., Swan, E. E., Borenstein, J. T., Sewell, W. F., Kujawa, S. G. and McKenna, M. J. (2010) Drug delivery for treatment of inner ear disease: current state of knowledge. *Ear and Hearing*, **31**, 156–165.

McCombe, A., Baguley, D., Coles, R., McKenna, L., McKinney, C. and Windle-Taylor, P. (2001) Guidelines for the grading of tinnitus severity: the results of a working group commissioned by the British Association of Otolaryngologists, Head and Neck Surgeons. *Clinical Otolaryngology*, **26**, 388–393.

McDermott, A., Dutt, S., Irving, R., Pahor, A. and Chavda, S. (2003) Anterior inferior cerebellar artery syndrome: fact or fiction. *Clinical Otolaryngology*, **28**, 75–80.

McFadden, D. (1982) *Tinnitus. Facts, theories, and treatments*, Washington, DC: National Academy Press.

McFadden, D. and Pasanen, E. G. (1994) Otoacoustic emissions and quinine sulfate. *Journal of the Acoustical Society of America*, **95**, 3460–3474.

McFerran, D. J. and Baguley, D. M. (2007) Acoustic shock. *Journal of Laryngology and Otology*, **121**, 301–305.

McFerran, D. J. and Baguley, D. M. (2009) Is psychology really the best treatment for tinnitus? *Clinical Otolaryngology*, **34**, 99–101.

McKee, G. J. and Stephens, S. D. G. (1992) An investigation of normally hearing subjects with tinnitus. *Audiology*, **31**, 313–317.

McKenna, L. (1987) Goal planning in audiological rehabilitation. *British Journal of Audiology*, **21**, 5–11.

McKenna, L. (1997) *Audiological disorders: psychological state and cognitive functioning*. PhD Thesis, The City University, London.

McKenna, L. (2000) Insomnia and tinnitus. In *Tinnitus handbook* (ed. R. Tyler), Singular.

McKenna, L. (2004) Models of tinnitus suffering and treatment compared and contrasted. *Audiological Medicine*, **2**, 41–53.

McKenna, L. and Andersson, G. (2008) Changing reactions. In *The consumers handbook on tinnitus* (ed. R. Tyler), Sedona: Auricle Ink Publishers.

McKenna, L. and Daniel, H. C. (2006) The psychological management of tinnitus related insomnia. In *Tinnitus treatment. Clinical protocols* (ed. R. S. Tyler), New York: Thieme.

McKenna, L. and Hallam, R. (1999) A neuropsychological study of concentration problems in tinnitus patients. In *Proceedings of the Sixth International Tinnitus Seminar* (ed. J. Hazell), Cambridge, The Tinnitus and Hyperacusis Centre, pp. 108–113.

McKenna, L. and Love, J. (2011) Mindfulness based cognitive therapy for tinnitus; preliminary results. In *10th International Tinnitus Seminar*, Florianopolis, Brazil.

McKenna, L., Hallam, R. S. and Hinchcliffe, R. (1991) The prevalence of psychological disturbance in neuro-otology outpatients. *Clinical Otolaryngology*, **16**, 452–456.

McKenna, L., Hallam, R. S. and Shurlock, L. (1996) Cognitive functioning in tinnitus patients. In *Proceedings of the Fifth International Tinnitus Seminar 1995* (eds G. E. Reich and J. A. Vernon), Portland: American Tinnitus Association.

McKenna, L., Baguley, D. and McFerran, D. (2010) *Living with tinnitus and hyperacusis*, London: Sheldon Press.

McNeill, C. (ed.) (1993) *Temporomandibular disorders. Guidelines for classification, assessment, and management*, Chicago: Quintessence.

Meenemeir, M., Chelette, K., Allen , S., Bartel, T., Triggs, W., Kimbrell, T., Crew, J., Munn, T., Brown, G. and Dornhoffer, J. (2011) Variable changes in PET activity before and after rTMS treatment for tinnitus. *Laryngoscope*, **121**, 815–822.

Meeus, O., Spaepen, M., Ridder, D. and Heyning, P. (2010a) Correlation between hyperacusis measurements in daily ENT practice. *International Journal of Audiology*, **49**, 7–13.

Meeus, O., Heyndrickx, K., Lambrechts, P., De Ridder, D. and van de Heyning, P. (2010b) Phase-shift treatment for tinnitus of cochlear origin. *European Archives of Otorhinolaryngology*, **267**, 881–888.

Meeus, O., De Ridder, D. and van de Heyning, P. (2011) Administration of the combination clonazepam–Deanxit as treatment for tinnitus. *Otology and Neurootology*, **32**, 701–709.

Megwalu, U. C., Finnell, J. E. and Piccirillo, J. F. (2006) The effects of melatonin on tinnitus and sleep. *Otolaryngology, Head and Neck Surgery*, **134**, 210–213.

Meikle, M. B. and Griest, S. E. (1989) Gender-based differences in characteristics of tinnitus. *Hearing Journal*, **42**, 68–76.

Meikle, M. B. and Griest, S. E. (1992) Assymetry in tinnitus perceptions. Factors that may account for the higher prevalence of left-sided tinnitus, In *Tinnitus 91. Proceedings of the Fourth International Tinnitus Seminar* (eds J.-M. Aran and R. Dauman), Amsterdam/New York: Kugler Publications, pp. 231–237.

Meikle, M. B. and Taylor-Walsh, E. (1984) Characteristics of tinnitus and related observations in over 1800 tinnitus clinic patients. *Journal of Laryngology and Otology*, Suppl. 9, 17–21.

Meikle, M. B., Stewart, B. J., Griest, S. E., Martin, W. H., Henry, J. A., Abrams, H. B., McArdle, R., Newman, C. W. and Sandridge, S. A. (2007) Assessment of tinnitus: measurement of treatment outcomes. *Progress in Brain Research*, **166**, 511–521.

Meikle, M. B., Stewart, B. J., Griest, S. E. and Henry, J. A. (2008) Tinnitus outcomes assessment. *Trends in Amplification*, **12**, 223–235.

Meikle, M. B., Henry, J. A., Griest, S. E., Stewart, B. J., Abrams, H. B., McArdle, R., Myers, P. J., Newman, C. W., Sandridge, S., Turk, D. C., Folmer, R. L., Frederick, E. J., House, J. W., Jacobson, G. P., Kinney, S. E., Martin, W. H., Nagler, S. M., Reich, G. E., Searchfield, G., Sweetow, R. and Vernon, J. A. (2012) The Tinnitus Functional Index: development of a new clinical measure for chronic, intrusive tinnitus. *Ear and Hearing*, **32**, 153–176.

Melcher, J. R., Sigalosky, I. S., Guinan, J. J. and Levine, R. A. (2000) Lateralized tinnitus studied with functional magnetic resonance imaging: abnormal inferior colliculus activation. *Journal of Neurophysiology*, **83**, 1058–1072.

Melcher, J. R., Levine, R. A., Bergevin, C. and Norris, B. (2009) The auditory midbrain of people with tinnitus: abnormal sound-evoked activity revisited. *Hearing Research*, **257**, 63–74.

Melin, L., Scott, B., Lindberg, P. and Lyttkens, L. (1987) Hearing aids and tinnitus – an experimental group study. *British Journal of Audiology*, **21**, 91–97.

Meng, Z., Liu, S., Zheng, Y. and Phillips, J. S. (2011) Repetitive transcranial magnetic stimulation for tinnitus. *Cochrane Database of Systematic Reviews*, CD007946.

Ménière, P. (1861) Memoire sur des lesions de l'oreille interne donnant lieu a des symptomes des congestion cerebrale apoplectiforme. *Gazette Medical de Paris*, **16**, 597–601.

Merchant, S. N. and Rosowski, J. J. (2008) Conductive hearing loss caused by third-window lesions of the inner ear. *Otology and Neurotology*, **29**, 282–289.

Meric, C., Gartner, M., Collet, L. and Chéry-Croze, S. (1998) Psychopathological profile of tinnitus sufferers: evidence concerning the relationship between tinnitus features and impact on life. *Audiology and Neurootology*, **3**, 240–252.

Meric, C., Pham, E. and Chéry-Croze, S. (2000) Validation of a French version of the Tinnitus Reaction Questionnaire: a comparison between data from English and French versions. *Journal of Speech, Hearing, and Language Research*, **43**, 184–190.

Michikawa, T., Nishiwaki, Y., Kikuchi, Y., Saito, H., Mizutari, K., Okamoto, M. and Takebayashi, T. (2010) Prevalence and factors associated with tinnitus: a community-based study of Japanese elders. *Journal of Epidemiology*, **20**, 271–276.

Mihail, R. C., Crowley, J. M., Walden, B. E., Fishburne, J., Reinwall, J. E. and Zajtchuck, J. T. (1988) The tricyclic trimipramine in the treatment of tinnitus. *Annals of Otology, Rhinology and Laryngology*, **97**, 120–123.

Milhinch, J. (2002) Acoustic shock injury: real or imaginary. Audiology Online: http://www.audiologyonline.com/articles/article_detail.asp?article_id=351.

Miller, J. (1985) *CRC handbook of ototoxicity*, Roca Baton, FL: CRC Press.

Mills, R. P. and Cherry, J. R. (1984) Subjective tinnitus in children with otological disorders. *International Journal of Pediatric Otorhinolaryngology*, **7**, 21–27.

Mills, R. P., Albert, D. M. and Brain, C. E. (1986) Tinnitus in childhood. *Clinical Otolaryngology*, **11**, 431–434.

Mimeault, V. and Morin, C. M. (1999) Self-help treatment for insomnia: bibliotherapy with and without professional guidance. *Journal of Consulting and Clinical Psychology*, **67**, 511–519.

Min, S. K. and Lee, B. O. 1997. Laterality in somatization. *Psychosomatic Medicine*, **59**, 236–240.

Minor, L., Solomon, D., Zinreich, J. and Zee, D. (1998) Sound- and/or pressure-induced vertigo due to bone dehiscence of the superior semicircular canal. *Archives of Otolaryngology, Head and Neck Surgery*, **124**, 249–258.

Minton, J. P. (1923) Tinnitus and its relation to nerve deafness with application of the masking effect of pure tones. *Physical Review*, **22**, 506–509.

Mirz, F., Ovesen, T., Ishizu, K., Johannsen, P., Madsen, S., Gjedde, A. and Pedersen, C. B. (1999a) Stimulus-dependent central processing of auditory stimuli. A PET study. *Scandinavian Audiology*, **28**, 161–169.

Mirz, F., Pedersen, C. B., Ishizu, K., Johannsen, P., Ovesen, T., Søkilde-Jørgensen, H. and Gjedde, A. (1999b) Positron emission tomography of cortical centres of tinnitus. *Hearing Research*, **134**, 133–144.

Mirz, F., Støkilde-Jørgensen, H. and Pedersen, C. B. (1999c) Evidence of cortical networks subserving the perception of tinnitus: a fMRI study. *NeuroImage*, **9**, S794.

Mirz, F., Gjedde, A., Søkilde-Jørgensen, H. and Pedersen, C. B. (2000) Functional brain imaging of tinnitus-like perception induced by aversive auditory stimuli. *Neuroreport*, **11**, 633–637.

Mirz, F., Mortensen, M., Gjedde, A. and Pedersen, C. (2002) Positron emission tomography of tinnitus suppression by cochlear implantation. In *Proceedings of the Seventh International Tinnitus Seminar* (ed. R. Patuzzi), Freemantle, University of Western Australia.

Mitchell, P. L., Moffat, D. A. and Fallside, F. (1984) Computer-aided tinnitus characterization. *Clinical Otolaryngology*, **9**, 35–42.

Mitchell, C. R., Vernon, J. A. and Creedon, T. A. (1993) Measuring tinnitus parameters: loudness, pitch, and maskability. *Journal of the American Academy of Audiology*, **4**, 139–151.

Moffat, D., Hardy, D., Irving, R., Viani, L., Gj, B. and Baguley, D. (1995) Referral patterns in vestibular schwannomas. *Clinical Otolaryngology*, **20**, 80–83.

Moffat, G., Adjout, K., Gallego, S., Thai-Van, H., Collet, L. and Norena, A. J. (2009) Effects of hearing aid fitting on the perceptual characteristics of tinnitus. *Hearing Research*, **254**, 82–91.

Møller, A. (1984) Pathophysiology of tinnitus. *Annals of Otology*, **93**, 39–44.

Møller, A. R. (1997) Similarities between chronic pain and tinnitus. *American Journal of Otology*, **18**, 577–585.

Møller, A. (1998) Vascular compression of cranial nerves. 1: history of the microvascular decompression operation. *Neurological Research*, **20**, 727–731.

Møller, A. R. (2007) Tinnitus: pathology and treatment. *Progress in Brain Research*, **166**, 3–18.

Møller, A. R. (2011a) Cutaneous stimulation. In *Textbook of tinnitus* (eds A. R. Møller, B. Langguth, D. De Ridder and T. Kleinjung), New York: Springer.

Møller, A. R. (2011b) Different forms of tinnitus. In *Textbook of tinnitus* (eds A. R. Møller, B. Langguth, D. De Ridder and T. Kleinjung), New York: Springer.

Møller, A. R. (2011c) Similarities between tinnitus and pain. In *Textbook of tinnitus* (eds A. R. Møller, B. Langguth, D. De Ridder and T. Kleinjung), New York: Springer.

Møller, H. and Lydolf, M. (2002) A questionnaire survey of complaints of infrasound and low-frequency noise. *Low Frequency Noise, Vibration and Active Control*, **21**, 53–63.

Møller, A. R. and Shore, S. (2011) Interaction between somatosensory and auditory systems. In *Textbook of tinnitus* (eds A. R. Møller, B. Langguth, D. De Ridder and T. Kleinjung), New York: Springer.

Møller, A. R., Møller, M. B. and Yokota, M. (1992) Some forms of tinnitus may involve the extralemniscal auditory pathway. *Laryngoscope*, **102**, 1165–1171.

Møller, M., Møller, A., Jannetta, P. and Ito, H. (1993) Vascular decompression surgery for severe tinnitus: selection criteria and results. *Laryngoscope*, **103**, 421–427.

Moncrieff, J., Wessely, S. and Hardy, R. (2004) Active placebos versus antidepressants for depression. *Cochrane Database of Systematic Reviews*, CD003012.

Monzani, D., Genovese, E., Marrara, A., Gherpelli, C., Pingani, L., Forghieri, M., Rigatelli, M., Guadagnin, T. and Arslan, E. (2008) Validity of the Italian adaptation of the Tinnitus Handicap Inventory; focus on quality of life and psychological distress in tinnitus-sufferers. *Acta Otorhinolaryngology Italy*, **28**, 126–134.

Moore, B. C. J. (1998) *Cochlear hearing loss*, London: Whurr.

Moore, B. C. J. (2012) The psychophysics of tinnitus. In *Tinnitus* (eds J. Eggermont, F. Zeng, R. Fay and A. Popper), New York: Springer.

Moore, B. C. and Vinay, S. N. (2010) The relationship between tinnitus pitch and the edge frequency of the audiogram in individuals with hearing impairment and tonal tinnitus. *Hearing Research*, **261**, 51–56.

Mora, R., Salami, A., Barbieri, M., Mora, F., Passali, G., Capobianco, S. and Magnan, J. (2003) The use of sodium enoxaparin in the treatment of tinnitus. *International Tinnitus Journal*, **9**, 109–111.

Morgenstern, C. and Biermann, E. (2002) The efficacy of Ginkgo special extract EGb 761 in patients with tinnitus. *International Journal of Clinical Pharmacology Therapy*, **40**, 188–197.

Morin, C. M. (1993) *Insomnia. Psychological assessment and management*, New York, Guilford press.

Morin, C. M., Culbert, J. P. and Schwartz, S. M. (1994) Nonpharmacological interventions for insomnia: a meta-analysis of treatment efficacy. *American Journal of Psychiatry*, **151**, 1172–1180.

Morin, C. M., Hauri, P. J., Espie, C. A., Spielman, A. J., Buysse, D. J. and Bootzon, R. R. (1999) Nonpharmacological treatment of chronic insomnia. *Sleep*, **22**, 1134–1156.

Morrison, A. and Bundey, S. (1970) The inheritance of otosclerosis. *Journal of Laryngology and Otology*, **84**, 921–932.

Morrison, G. and Sterkers, J. (1996) Unusual presentations of acoustic tumours. *Clinical Otolaryngology*, **21**, 80–83.

Muehlmeier, G., Biesinger, E. and Maier, H. (2011) Safety of intratympanic injection of AM-101 in patients with acute inner ear tinnitus. *Audiology and Neurootology*, **16**, 388–397.

Mühlau, M., Rauschecker, J. P., Oestreicher, E., Gaser, C., Rottinger, M., Wohlschlager, A. M., Simon, F., Etgen, T., Conrad, B. and Sander, D. (2006) Structural brain changes in tinnitus. *Cerebral Cortex*, **16**, 1283–1288.

Mühlnickel, W., Elbert, T., Taub, E. and Flor, H. (1998) Reorganization of the auditory cortex in tinnitus. *Proceedings of the National Academy of Science*, **95**, 10340–10343.

Muñoz, D., Aedo, C. and Der, C. (2010) Patulous Eustachian tube in bariatric surgery patients. *Otolaryngology, Head and Neck Surgery*, **143**, 521–524.

Munro, K. and Blount, J. (2009) Adaptive plasticity in brainstem of adult listeners following earplug-indiced deprivation. *Journal of the Acoustical Society of America*, **126**, 568–571.

Murai, K., Tyler, R. S., Harker, L. A. and Stouffer, J. L. (1992) Review of pharmacological treatment of tinnitus. *The American Journal of Otology*, **13**, 454–464.

Murtagh, D. R. R. and Greenwood, K. M. (1995) Identifying effective psychological treatments for insomnia. *Journal of Consulting and Clinical Psychology*, **63**, 79–89.

Myrseth, E., Møller, P., Pedersen, P. H., Lund-Johansen, M. (2009) Vestibular schwannoma: surgery or gamma knife radiosurgery? A prospective, nonrandomized study. *Neurosurgery*, **64**(4), April, 654–661.

Nagel, D. and Drexel, M. K. A. (1989) Epidemiologische untersuchungen zum tinnitus aurium. *Auris Nasus Larynx*, **16**.

Nageris, B. I., Attias, J. and Raveh, E. (2010) Test-retest tinnitus characteristics in patients with noise-induced hearing loss. *American Journal of Otolaryngology*, **31**, 181–184.

Nahas, R. and Sheikh, O. (2011) Complementary and alternative medicine for the treatment of major depressive disorder. *Canadian Family Physician*, **57**, 659–663.

Nakashima, T., Ueda, H., Misawa, H., Suzuki, T., Tominaga, M., Ito, A., Numata, S., Kasai, S., Asahi, K., Vernon, J. A. and Meikle, M. B. (2002) Transmeatal low-power laser irridation for tinnitus. *Otology and Neurootology*, **23**, 296–300.

Nam, E., Handzel, O. and Levine, R. A. (2010a) Carbamazepine responsive typewriter tinnitus from basilar invagination. *Journal of Neurology, Neurosurgery, and Psychiatry*, **81**, 456–458.

Nam, E. C., Lewis, R., Nakajima, H. H., Merchant, S. N. and Levine, R. A. (2010b) Head rotation evoked tinnitus due to superior semicircular canal dehiscence. *Journal of Laryngology and Otology*, **124**, 333–335.

Nebeska, M., Rubinstein, B. and Wenneberg, B. (1999) Influence of acupuncture on tinnitus in patients with signs and symptoms of temporomandibular disorders: a placebo-controlled study. In *Proceedings of the Sixth International Tinnitus Seminar* (ed. J. Hazell), Cambridge, The Tinnitus and Hyperacusis Centre.

Nelken, I. and Young, E. D. (1996) Why do cats need a dorsal cochlear nucleus? *Journal of Basic Clinical Physiology and Pharmacology*, **7**, 199–220.

Nelting, M., Rienhoff, N. K., Hesse, G. and Lamparter, U. (2002) The assessment of subjective distress related to hyperacusis with a self-rating questionnaire on hypersensitivity to sound. *Laryngorhinootlogie*, **81**, 32–34.

Neri, G., Baffa, C., De Stefano, A., Poliandri, A., Kulamarva, G., Di Giovanni, P., Petrucci, A., Castriotta, A., Citraro, L., D, C., D' Orazio, F. and Croce, A. (2009) Management of tinnitus: oral treatment with melatonin and sulodexide. *Journal of Biologica Regulation and Homeostatic Agents*, **23**, 103–110.

Newman, C. W. and Sandridge, S. A. (2006) Incorporating group and individual sessions into a tinnitus management clinic. In *Tinnitus treatment. Clinical protocols* (ed. R. S. Tyler), New York: Thieme.

Newman, C. W. and Sandridge, S. A. (2012) A comparison of benefit and economic value between two sound therapy tinnitus management options. *Journal of the American Academy of Audiology*, **23**, 126–138.

Newman, C. W., Weinstein, B. E., Jacobson, G. P. and Hug, G. A. (1990) The hearing handicap inventory for adults: psychometric adequacy and audiometric correlates. *Ear and Hearing*, **11**, 430–433.

Newman, C. W., Jacobson, G. P. and Spitzer, J. B. (1996) Development of the tinnitus handicap inventory. *Archives of Otolaryngology, Head and Neck Surgery*, **122**, 143–148.

Newman, C. W., Jacobson, G. P., Hug, G. A. and Sandridge, S. A. (1997a) Perceived hearing handicap of patients with unilateral or mild hearing loss. *Annals of Otology, Rhinology and Laryngology*, **106**, 210–214.

Newman, C. W., Wharton, J. A. and Jacobson, G. P. (1997b) Self-focused and somatic attention in patients with tinnitus. *Journal of the American Academy of Audiology*, **8**, 143–149.

Newman, C. W., Sandridge, S. A. and Jacobson, G. (1998) Psychometric adequacy of the Tinnitus Handicap Inventory (THI) for evaluating treatment outcome. *Journal of the American Academy of Audiology*, **9**, 153–160.

Newman, C. W., Sandridge, S. A. and Bolek, L. (2008) Development and psychometric adequacy of the screening version of the tinnitus handicap inventory. *Otology and Neurotology*, **29**, 276–281.

Niedermeyer, H. P. and Arnold, W. (2008) Otosclerosis and measles virus – association or causation? *ORL Journal of Otorhinolaryngology and Related Specialities*, **70**, 63–69; Discussion, 69–70.

Nields, J. A., Fallon, B. A. and Jastreboff, P. J. (1999) Carbamazepine in the treatment of Lyme disease-induced hyperacusis. *Journal of Neuropsychiatry and Clinical Neuroscience*, **11**, 97–99.

Nieschalk, M., Hustert, B. and Stoll, W. (1998) Auditory reaction times in patients with chronic tinnitus with normal hearing. *American Journal of Otology*, **19**, 611–618.

Noble, W. (1998) *Self-assessment of hearing and related functions*, London: Whurr.

Noble, W. (2000) Self-reports about tinnitus and about cochlear implants. *Ear and Hearing*, **21**, 50S–59S.

Noble, W. (2008) Treatments for tinnitus. *Trends in Amplification*, **12**, 236–241.

Noble, W. (2010) Assessing binaural hearing: results using the speech, spatial and qualities of hearing scale. *Journal of the American Academy of Audiology*, **21**, 568–574.

Noble, W. and Tyler, R. (2007) Physiology and phenomenology of tinnitus: implications for treatment. *International Journal of Audiology*, **46**, 569–574.

Nodar, R. H. (1972) Tinnitus aurium in school age children. *Journal of Auditory Research*, **12**, 133–135.

Nodar, R. H. (1996) Tinnitus reclassified: new oil in an old lamp. *Otolaryngology, Head and Neck Surgery*, **114**, 582–585.

Nodar, R. H. and Lezak, M. H. W. (1984) Paediatric tinnitus: a thesis revisited. *Journal of Laryngology and Otology*, **98**, 234–235.

Nondahl, D. M., Cruickshanks, K. J., Wiley, T. L., Klein, R., Klein, B. E. and Tweed, T. S. (2002) Prevalence and 5-year incidence of tinnitus among older adults: the epidemiology of hearing loss study. *Journal of the American Academy of Audiology*, **13**, 323–331.

Nondahl, D. M., Cruickshanks, K. J., Wiley, T. L., Klein, B. E., Klein, R., Chappell, R. and Tweed, T. S. (2010) The ten-year incidence of tinnitus among older adults. *International Journal of Audiology*, **49**, 580–585.

Nondahl, D. M., Cruickshanks, K. J., Huang, G. H., Klein, B. E., Klein, R., Javier Nieto, F. and Tweed, T. S. (2011) Tinnitus and its risk factors in the Beaver Dam offspring study. *International Journal of Audiology*, **50**, 313–320.

Norena, A. J. (2011) An integrative model of tinnitus based on a central gain controlling sensititivity. *NeuroScience Biobehavior Review*, **35**, 1089–1109.

Norena, A. and Chéry-Croze, S. (2007) Enriched acoustic environment rescales auditory sensitivity. *Neuroreport*, **18**, 1251–1255.

Norena, A. J. and Eggermont, J. (2005) Enriched acoustic environment after noise trauma reduces hearing loss and prevents cortical map reorganization. *Journal of Neuroscience*, **25**, 699–705.

Norena, A. J. and Eggermont, J. (2006) Enriched acoustic environment after noise trauma abolishes neural signs of tinnitus. *Neuroreport*, **17**, 559–563.

Norena, A., Cransac, H. and Chéry-Croze, S. (1999) Towards an objectification by classification of tinnitus. *Clinical Neurophysiology*, **110**, 666–675.

Nowé, V., De Ridder, D., van de Heyning, P., Wang, X., Gielen, J., van Goethem, J., Ozsarlak, O., De Schepper, A. and Parizel, P. (2004) Does the location of a vascular loop in the cerebellopontine angle explain pulsatile and non-pulsatile tinnitus? *European Radiology*, **14**, 2282–2829.

Ochi, K., Ohasi, T. and Kinoshita, H. (1997) Serum zinc levels in patients with tinnitus and the effect of zinc treatment. *Annals of Otology, Rhinology and Laryngology (Japan)*, **100**, 915–919.

Ochi, K., Kinoshita, H., Kenmochi, M., Nishino, H. and Ohasi, T. (2003) Zinc defiency and tinnitus. *Auris Nasus Larynx*, **30**, 25–28.

Office of Population Census and Surveys (1983) General household survey: the prevalence of tinnitus 1981. *OPCS Monitor*, Reference GHS83/1.

Ogata, Y., Sekitani, T., Moriya, K. and Watanabe, K. (1993) Biofeedback therapy in the treatment of tinnitus. *Auris Nasus Larynx*, **20**, 95–101.

Ogawa, K., Takei, S., Inoue, Y. and Kanzaki, J. (2002) Effect of prostaglandin E1 on idiopathic sudden sensorineural hearing loss: a double-blinded clinical study. Otology and Neurootology, **23**, 665–668.

Ogles, B. M., Lunnen, K. M. and Bonesteel, K. (2001) Clinical significance: history, application, and current practice. *Clinical Psychology Review*, **21**, 421–446.

Okada, D. M., Onishi, E. T., Chami, F. I., Borin, A., Cassola, N. and Guereiro, V. M. (2006) Acupuncture for immediate tinnitus relief. *Revista Brasileira De Otorrinolaringologia*, **72**, 182–186.

Okamoto, H., Stracke, H., Stoll, W. and Pantev, C. (2010) Listening to tailor-made notched music reduces tinnitus loudness and tinnitus-related auditory cortex activity. *Proceedings of the National Academy of Sciences*, **107**, 1207–1210.

Ooms, E., Vanheule, S., Meganck, R., Vinck, B., Watelet, J. B. and Dhooge, I. (2011) Tinnitus severity and its association with cognitive and somatic anxiety: a critical study. *European Archives of Oto-Rhino-Laryngology*. Epub.

Oort, H. (1918) Uber die verastellung des nervus octavus bei sautetieren. *Anat Anz*, **51**, 272–280.

Oron, Y., Shushan, S., Kreitler, S. and Roth, Y. (2011) A Hebrew adaptation of the tinnitus handicap inventory. *International Journal of Audiology*, **50**, 426–430.

Osaki, Y., Nishimura, H., Takasawa, M., Imaizumi, M., Kawashima, T., Iwaki, T., Oku, N., Hashikawa, K., Doi, K., Nishimura, T., Hatazawa, J. and Kubo, T. (2005) Neural mechanism of residual inhibition of tinnitus in cochlear implant users. *Neuroreport*, **16**, 1625–1628.

Öst, L.-G. (1987) Applied relaxation: description of a coping technique and review of controlled studies. *Behaviour Research and Therapy*, **25**, 379–409.

Öst, L.-G. (1997) Rapid treatments of specific phobias. In *Phobias. A handbook of theory, research and treatment* (ed. G. C. L. Davey), Chichester: John Wiley & Sons, Ltd.

Oster, G. (1973) Auditory beats in the brain. *Scientific American*, **229**, 94–102.

Paaske, P., Pedersen, C., Kjems, G. and Sam, I. (1991) Zinc in the management of tinnitus. Placebo-controlled trial. *Annals of Otology Rhinology and Laryngology*, **100**, 647–649.

Paglialonga, A., Barozzi, S., Brambila, D., Soi, D., Cesarani, A., Gaglardi, Comiotto, E., Spreafico, E. & Tognola, G. 2011. Cochlear active mechanisms in young normal-hearing subjects affected by Williams syndrome: time-frequency analysis of otoacoustic emissions. *Hearing Research*, **272**, 157–167.

Palmer, K. T., Griffin, M. J., Syddall, H. E., Davis, A., Pannett, B. and Coggon, D. (2002) Occupational exposure to noise and the attributable burden of hearing difficulties in Great Britain. *Occupational and Environmental Medicine*, **59**, 634–639.

Pan, T., Tyler, R. S., Ji, H., Coelho, C., Gehringer, A. K. and Gogel, S. A. (2009) The relationship between tinnitus pitch and the audiogram. *International Journal of Audiology*, **48**, 277–294.

Pantev, C., Hoke, M., Lütkenhöner, B., Lehnertz, K. and Kumpf, W. (1989) Tinnitus remission objectified by neuromagnetic measurements. *Hearing Research*, **40**, 216–264.

Papez, J. W. (1937) A proposed mechanism of emotion. *Archives of Neurology and Psychiatry*, **38**, 725–743.

Park, J., White, A. R. and Ernst, E. (2000) Efficacy of acupuncture as a treatment for tinnitus. A systematic review. *Archives of Otolaryngology, Head and Neck Surgery*, **126**, 489–492.

Park, C. E., Park, B., Lim, Y. and Yeo, S. (2011) Functional outcomes in retrosigmoid approach microsurgery and gamma knife stereotactic radiosurgery in vestibular schwannoma. *European Archives of Otorhinolaryngology*, **268**, 955–959.

Park, S. S., Grills, I., Bojrab, D., Pieper, D., J, K., Maitz, A., Martin, A., Perez, E., Hahn, Y., Ye, H., Martinez, A. and Chen, P. (2011) Longitudinal assessment of quality of life and audiometric test outcomes in vestibular schwannoma patients treated with gamma knife surgery. *Otology and Neurootology*, **32**, 676–679.

Parnes, L. S. and McCabe, B. F. (1987) Perilymph fistula: an important cause of deafness and dizziness in children. *Pediatrics*, **80**, 524–528.

Parving, A., Hein, H. O., Suadicani, B., Ostri, B. and Gyntelberg, F. (1993) Epidemiology of hearing disorders. *Scandinavian Audiology*, **22**, 101–107.

Patuzzi, R. (2011) Ion flow in cochlear hair cells and the regulation of hearing sensitivity. *Hearing Research*, **280**, 3–20.

Patuzzi, R. B., Brown, D. J., McMahon, C. M. and Halliday, A. F. (2004) Determinants of the spectrum of the neural electrical activity at the round window: transmitter release and neural depolarisation. *Hearing Research*, **190**, 87–108.

Pavlov, I. P. (1927) *Conditioned reflexes*, New York: Oxford University Press.

Pearce, J. M. (2008) Palatal myoclonus (syn. Palatal tremor). *European Neurology*, **60**, 312–315.

Pearson, M. M. and Barnes, L. J. (1950) Objective tinnitus aurium: report of two cases with good results after hypnosis. *Journal of Philadelphia General Hospital*, **1**, 134–138.

Peck, J. E. (2011) *Pseudohypacusis: false and exaggerated hearing loss*, San Diego, CA, Plural.

Pedersen, C. S., Møller, H. and Waye, K. P. (2008) A detailed study of low-frequency noise complaints. *Low Frequency Noise, Vibration and Active Control*, **27**, 1–33.

Penner, M. J. (1983a) The annoyance of tinnitus and the noise required to mask it. *Journal of Speech and Hearing Research*, **26**, 73–76.

Penner, M. J. (1983b) Variability in matches to subjective tinnitus. *Journal of Speech and Hearing Research*, **26**, 263–267.

Penner, M. J. (1986) Magnitude estimation and the 'paradoxical' loudness of tinnitus. *Journal of Speech and Hearing Research*, **29**, 407–412.

Penner, M. J. (1987) Masking of tinnitus and central masking. *Journal of Speech and Hearing Research*, **30**, 147–152.

Penner, M. J. (1990) An estimate of the prevalence of tinnitus caused by spontaneous otoacoustic emissions. *Archives of Otolaryngology, Head and Neck Surgery*, **116**, 418–423.

Penner, M. J. (1993) Synthesizing tinnitus from sine waves. *Journal of Speech and Hearing Research*, **36**, 1300–1305.

Penner, M. J. (1996) Rating the annoyance of synthesized tinnitus. *International Tinnitus Journal*, **2**, 3–7.

Penner, M. J. and Bilger, R. C. (1988) Adaption and the masking of tinnitus. *Journal of Speech and Hearing Research*, **32**, 339–346.

Penner, M. J. and Burns, E. (1987) The dissociation of SOAEs and tinnitus. *Journal of Speech and Hearing Research*, **30**, 396–403.

Penner, M. and Coles, R. (1992) Aspirin as a palliative for SOAE-caused tinnitus. *British Journal of Audiology*, **26**, 91–96.

Penner, M. J. and Jastreboff, P. J. (1996) Tinnitus: psychophysical observations in humans and an animal model. In: (eds.) *Clinical aspects of hearing* (eds T. R. van de Water, A. N. Popper and R. R. Fay), New York: Springer Verlag.

Penner, M. J. and Klafter, E. J. (1992) Measures of tinnitus: step size, matches to imagined tones, and masking patterns. *Ear and Hearing*, **13**, 410–416.

Penner, M. J., Brauth, S. and Hood, L. (1981) The temporal course of the masking of tinnitus as a basis for inferring its origin. *Journal of Speech and Hearing Research*, **24**, 257–261.

Penney, S., Bruce, I. and Saeed, S. (2006) Botulinum toxin is effective and safe for palatal tremor: a report of five cases and a review of the literature. *Journal of Neurology*, **253**, 857–860.

Perlman, H. B. (1938) Hyperacusis. *Annals of Otology, Rhinology and Laryngology*, **47**, 947–953.

Persons, J. B. and Davidson, J. (2001) Cognitive-behavioral case formulation. In *Handbook of cognitive-behavioral therapies*, (ed. K. S. Dobson), New York: Guilford Press.

Persons, J. B., Davidson, J. and Tompkins, M. A. (2001) *Essential components of cognitive-behavior therapy for depression*, Washington, DC: American Psychological Association.

Peters, M. L., Vlaeyen, J. W. S. and van Drunen, C. (2000) Do fibromyalgia patients display hypervigilance for innocuous somatosensory stimuli? Application of a body scanning reaction time paradigm. *Pain*, **86**, 283–292.

Philippot, P., Nef, F., Clauw, L., Romree, M. and Segal, Z. (2011) A randomized controlled trial of mindfulness-based cognitive therapy for treating tinnitus. *Clinical Psychology and Psychotherapy*. DOI: 10.1002/cpp.756.

Phillips, D. P. and Carr, M. M. (1998) Disturbances of loudness perception. *Journal of the American Academy of Audiology*, **9**, 371–379.

Phillips, J. S. and McFerran, D. (2010) Tinnitus Retraining Therapy (TRT) for tinnitus. *Cochrane Database of Systematic Reviews*, Article CD007330.

Phillips, J. and Westerberg, B. (2011) Intratympanic steroids for Ménière's disease or syndrome. *Cochrane Database of Systematic Reviews*, Issue 7, Article CD008514.

Piccirillo, J. F., Finnell, J., Vlahiotis, A., Chole, R. A. and Spitznagel Jr, E. (2007) Relief of idiopathic subjective tinnitus: is gabapentin effective? *Archives of Otolaryngology, Head and Neck Surgery*, **133**, 390–397.

Pierce, K. J., Kallogjeri, D., Piccirillo, J. F., Garcia, K. S., Nicklaus, J. E. and Burton, H. (2012) Effects of severe bothersome tinnitus on cognitive function measured with standardized tests. *Journal of Clinical and Experimental Neuropsychology*, **34**, 126–134.

Pilgramm, M., Rychlick, R., Lebisch, H., Siedentop, H., Goebel, G. and Kirchoff, D. (1999) Tinnitus in the Federal Republic of Germany: a representative epidemiological study. In *Proceedings of the Sixth International Tinnitus Seminar* (ed. J. Hazell), Cambridge, The Tinnitus and Hyperacusis Centre, pp. 64–67.

Pinchoff, R. J., Burkard, R. F., Salvi, R. J., Coad, M. L. and Lockwood, A. H. (1998) Modulation of tinnitus by voluntary jaw movements. *American Journal of Otology*, **19**, 785–789.

Pineda, J. A., Moore, F. R. and Viirre, E. (2008) Tinnitus treatment with customized sounds. *International Tinnitus Journal*, **14**, 17–25.

Plath, P. and Olivier, J. (1995) Results of combined low-power laser therapy and extracts of Ginko biloba in cases of sensorineural hearing loss and tinnitus. *Advances in Otorhinolaryngology*, **49**, 101–104.

Plewnia, C. (2011) Brain stimulation: new vistas for the exploration and treatment of tinnitus. *CNS Neuroscience and Therapeutics*, **17**, 449–461.

Plewnia, C., Reimold, M., Najib, A., Brehm, B., Reischl, G., Plontke, S. K. and Gerloff, C. (2007) Dose-dependent attenuation of auditory phantom perception (tinnitus) by PET-guided repetitive transcranial magnetic stimulation. *Human Brain Mapping*, **28**, 238–246.

Pober, B. R. (2010) Williams-Beuren syndrome. *New England Journal of Medicine*, **362**, 239–252.

Podoshin, L., Ben-David, Y., Fradis, M., Gerstel, R. and Felner, H. (1991) Idiopathic subjective tinnitus treated by biofeedback, acupuncture and drug therapy. *Ear, Nose and Throat Journal*, **70**, 284–289.

Podoshin, L., Fradis, M. and Ben-David, Y. (1992) Treatment of tinnitus by intratympanic instillation of lignocaine (lidocaine) 2 per cent through ventilation tubes. *Journal of Laryngology and Otology*, **106**, 603–606.

Poe, D. S. (2007) Diagnosis and management of the patulous Eustachian tube. *Otology and Neurotology*, **28**, 668–677.

Poreisz, C., Boros, K., Antal, A. and Paulus, W. (2007) Safety aspects of transcranial direct current stimulation concerning healthy subjects and patients. *Brain Research Bulletin*, **72**, 208–214.

Postema, R., Kingma, C., Wit, H., Albers, F. and Bf, V. D. L. (2008) Intratympanic gentamicin therapy for control of vertigo in unilateral Meniere's disease: a prospective, double-blind, randomized, placebo-controlled trial. *Acta Oto-Laryngologica*, **128**, 876–880.

Pratt, H. (2003) Human auditory electrophysiology. In *Textbook of audiological medicine. Clinical aspects of hearing and balance* (eds L. Luxon, J. M. Furman, A. Martini and D. Stephens), London: Martin Dunitz Publishers.

Prezant, T. R., Chaltraw Jr, W. E. and Fischel-Ghodsian, N. (1996) Identification of an over-expressed yeast gene which prevents aminoglycoside toxicity. *Microbiology*, **142** (12), December, 3407–3414.

PriyadarshI, S., Panda, K., Panda, A. and Pv, R. (2010) Lack of association between SNP rs3914132 of the RELN gene and otosclerosis in India. *Genetic and Molecular Research*, **9**, 1914–1920.

Puel, J. L. (1995) Chemical synaptic transmission in the cochlea. *Progress in Neurobiology*, **47**, 449–476.

Puel, J. L. (2007) Cochlear NMDA receptor blockade prevents salicylate-induced tinnitus. *B-ENT*, **3** (Suppl. 7), 19–22.

Puel, J. and Guitton, M. J. (2007) Salicylate-induced tinnitus: molecular mechanisms and modulation by anxiety. *Progress in Brain Research*, **166**, 141–146.

Puel, J. L., Bobbin, R. P. and Fallon, M. (1990) Salicylate, mefenamate, meclofenamate, and quinine on cochlear potentials. *Otolaryngology, Head and Neck Surgery*, **102**, 66–73.

Puel, J. L., Ruel, J., Gervais D'Aldin, C. and Pujol, R. (1998) Excitotoxicity and repair of cochlear synapses after noise-trauma induced hearing loss. *Neuroreport*, **9**, 2109–2114.

Pugh, R., Budd, R. J. and Stephens, S. D. G. (1995) Patients' reports of the effect of alcohol on tinnitus. *British Journal of Audiology*, **29**, 279–283.

Pugh, R., Stephens, S. D. G. and Budd, R. (2004) The contribution of spouse responses and marital satisfaction to the experience of chronic tinnitus. *International Journal of Audiology*, **2**, 60–73.

Pulec, J. L. (1967) Abnormally patent Eustachian tubes: treatment with injection of poly-tetrafluoroethylene (teflon) paste. *Laryngoscope*, **77**, 1543–1554.

Pulec, J. L. (1995) Cochlear nerve section for intractable tinnitus. *Ear, Nose and Throat Journal*, **74**, 468–476.

Pullens, B. and Van Benthem, P. (2011) Intratympanic gentamicin for Ménière's disease or syndrome. *Cochrane Database of Systematic Reviews*, Issue 3, Article CD008234.

Pullens, B., Giard, J., Verschuur, H. and Van Benthem, P. (2010) Surgery for Ménière's disease. *Cochrane Database of Systematic Reviews*, Issue 1, Article CD005395.

Punte, A., Meeus, O. and van der Heyning, P. (2011) Cochlear implants and tinnitus. In *Textbook of tinnitus* (eds A. R. Møller, B. Langguth, D. De Ridder and T. Kleinjung), New York: Springer.

Quaranta, A., Assennato, G. and Sallustio, V. (1996) Epidemiology of hearing problems among adults in Italy. *Scandinavian Audiology*, **25** (Suppl. 42), 7–11.

Quaranta, N., Wagstaff, S. and Baguley, D. M. (2004) Tinnitus and cochlear implantation. *International Journal of Audiology*, **43**, 245–251.

Quaranta, N., Baguley, D. and Moffat, D. (2007) Change in hearing and tinnitus in conservatively managed vestibular schwannomas. *Skull Base*, **17**, 223–228.

Quick, C. (1973) Chemical and drug effects on the inner ear. In *Otolaryngology* (eds M. Paparella and D. Shumrick), Volume 2, Philadelphia, PA: WB Saunders.

Rajah, V. (1992) Tinnitus related to eyelid blinking. *Journal of Laryngology and Otology*, **106**, 44–45.

Raj-Koziak, D., Piłka, A., Bartnik, G., Fabijańska, A., Kochanek, K. and Skarzyńsk, I. H. (2011) The prevalence of tinnitus in 7-year-old children in the eastern of Poland (in Polish). *Otolaryngologia Polska*, **65**, 106–910.

Rapaport, M. H., Nierenberg, A. A., Howland, R., Dording, C., Schettler, P. and Mishoulon, D. (2011) The treatment of minor depression with St John's Wort or citalopram: failure to show benefit over placebo. *Journal of Psychiatric Research*, **45**, 931–941.

Rasmussen, G. L. (1946) The olivary peduncle and other fiber projections of the superior olivary complex. *Journal of Comparative Neurology*, **99**, 61–74.

Rauschecker, J. P. (1999) Auditory cortical plasticity: a comparison with other sensory systems. *Trends in Neuroscience*, **22**, 74–80.

Rauschecker, J. P., Leaver, A. M. and Mühlau, M. (2010) Tuning out the noise: limbic-auditory interactions in tinnitus. *Neuron*, **66**, 819–826.

Reavis, K. M., Chang, J. E. and Zeng, F.-G. (2010) Patterned sound therapy for the treatment of tinnitus. *Hearing Journal*, **63**, 21–22,24.

Rechtshaffen, A. and Siegel, J. (2000) Sleep and dreaming. In *Principles of neural science* (eds E. R. Kandel, J. H. Schwartz and T. M. Jessel), New York: McGraw-Hill.

Reed, G. F. (1960) An audiometric study of two hundred cases of subjective tinnitus. *Archives of Otolaryngology*, **71**, 94–104.

Reed, H. T., Meltzer, J., Crews, P., Norris, C. H., Quine, D. B. and Guth, P. S. (1985) Amino oxyacetic acid as a palliative in tinnitus. *Archives of Otolaryngology, Head and Neck Surgery*, **111**, 803–805.

Reich, G. E. and Johnson, R. M. (1984) Personality characteristics of tinnitus patients. *Journal of Laryngology and Otology*, **97**, 228–232.

Reiss, S., Peterson, R. A., Gurksy, D. M. and McNally, R. J. (1986) Anxiety sensitivity, anxiety frequency and the prediction of fearfulness. *Behaviour Research and Therapy*, **34**, 1–8.

Reiter, R., Tan, D., Korkmaz, A. and Fuentes-Broto, L. (2011) Drug-mediated ototoxicity and tinnitus: alleviation with melatonin. *Journal of Physiology and Pharmacology*, **62**, 151–157.

Rejali, D., Sivakumar, A. and Balaji, N. 2004. Ginko biloba does not benefit patients with tinnitus: a randomized placebo-controlled double-blind trial and meta-analysis of randomized trials. *Clinical Otolaryngology*, **29**, 226–231.

Rendell, R. J., Carrick, D. G., Fielder, C. P., Callaghan, D. E. and Thomas, K. J. (1987) Low-powered ultrasound in the inhibition of tinnitus. *British Journal of Audiology*, **21**, 289–293.

Repacholi, M., Lerchl, A., Röösli, M., Sienkiewicz, Z., Auvinen, A., J, B., d'Inzeo, G., Elliott, P., Frei, P., Heinrich, S., Lagroye, I., Lahkola, A., McCormick, D., Thomas, S. and Vecchia, P. (2012) Systematic review of wireless phone use and brain cancer and other head tumors. *Bioelectromagnetics*, **33** (3), April, 187–206.

Reyes, S., Salvi, R., Burkard, R., Coad, M., Wack, D., Galantowicz, P. and Lockwood, A. (2002) Brain imaging of the effects of lidocaine on tinnitus. *Hearing Research*, **171**, 43–50.

Reynolds, P., Gardner, D. and Lee, R. (2004) Tinnitus and psychological morbidity: a cross-sectional study to investigate psychological morbidity in tinnitus patients and its relationship with severity of symptoms and illness perceptions. *Clinical Otolaryngology*, **29**, 628–634.

Rief, W., Sanders, E., Gunther, M. and Nanke, A. (2004) Aufmerksamkeitslenkung bei Tinnitus – eine experimentelle psychophysiologische Untersuchung. *Zeitschrift für Klinische Psychologie und Psychotherapie*, **33**, 230–236.

Rief, W., Weise, C., Kley, N. and Martin, A. (2005) Psychophysiologic treatment of chronic tinnitus: a randomized clinical trial. *Psychosomatic Medicine*, **67**, 833–838.

Rienhoff, N., Thimm, L., Pöllmann, H. Nelting. M. and Hesse, G. (2002) Irrationale Einstellungen bei chronisch komplexem Tinnitus (Irrational beliefs and chronic complex tinnitus). *Zeitschrift für Klinische Psychologie und Psychotherapie*, **31** (1), 47–52.

Ringdahl, A., Eriksson-Mangold, M. and Andersson, G. (1998) Psychometric evaluation of the Gothenburg Profile for measurement of experienced hearing disability and handicap: applications with new hearing aid candidates and experienced hearing aid users. *British Journal of Audiology*, **32**, 375–385.

Risey, J., Briner, W., Guth, P. S. and Norris, C. H. (1989) The superiority of the Goodwin procedure over the traditional procedure in measuring the loudness level of tinnitus. *Ear and Hearing*, **10**, 318–322.

Rizzardo, R., Savastano, M., Maron, M. B., Mangialaio, M. and Salvadori, L. (1998) Psychological distress in patients with tinnitus. *Journal of Otolaryngology*, **27**, 21–25.

Roberts, L. E., Eggermont, J. J. Caspary. D. M., Shore, S. E., Mecher, J. R. and Kaltenbach, J. A. (2010) Ringing ears: the neuroscience of tinnitus. *Journal of Neuroscience*, **45**, 14972–14979.

Roberts, C., Inamdar, A., Koch, A., Kitchiner, P., Dewit, O., Merlo-Pich, E., Fina, P., McFerran, D. J. and Baguley, D. M. (2011) A randomized, controlled study comparing the effects of vestipitant or vestipitant and paroxetine combination in subjects with tinnitus. *Otology and Neurootology*, **32**, 721–727.

Robertson, D. and Irvine, D. (1989) Plasticity of frequency organization in auditory cortex of guinea pigs with partial unilateral deafness. *Journal of Comparative Neurology*, **282**, 456–471.

Robinson, P. J. and Hazell, J. (1989) Patulous Eustachian tube syndrome: the relationship with sensorineural deafness: treatment by Eustachian tube diathermy. *Journal of Laryngology and Otology*, **103**, 739–742.

Robinson, S. K., Viirre, E. S., Bailey, K. A., Gerke, M. A., Harris, J. P. and Stein, M. B. (2005) Randomized placebo-controlled trial of a selective serotonin reuptake inhibitor in the treatment of nondepressed tinnitus subjects. *Psychosomatic Medicine*, **67**, 981–988.

Ronis, M. (1984) Alcohol and dietary influences on tinnitus. *Journal of Laryngology and Otology*, Suppl. 9, 242–246.

Rosen, S. (1953) Mobilization of the stapes to restore hearing in otosclerosis. *New York Journal of Medicine*, **53**, 2650–2653.

Rosenberg, S., Silverstein, H., Rowan, P. T. and Olds, M. J. (1998) Effect of melatonin on tinnitus. *Laryngoscope*, **108**, 305–310.

Rosenhall, U. and Axelsson, A. (1995) Auditory brainstem response latencies in patients with tinnitus. *Scandinavian Audiology*, **24**, 97–100.

Rosenhall, U., Nordin, V., Sandstrom, M., Ahlsen, G. and Gillberg, C. (1999) Autism and hearing loss. *Journal of Autism and Developmental Disorders*, **29**, 349–357.

Rosenstiel, A. K. and Keefe, F. J. (1983) The use of coping strategies in chronic low back pain patients: relationship to patient characteristics and current adjustment. *Pain*, **17**, 33–44.

Rosowski, J. J. (2010) External and middle ear function. In *The Oxford handbook of auditory science*, Volume 1, *The Ear* (ed. P. A. Fuchs), Oxford: Oxford University Press.

Rossi, S., Hallett, M., Rossini, P. M. and Pascaul-Leone, A. (2009) Saftey, ethical considerations, and application guidelines for the use of transcranial magnetic stimulation in clinical practice and research. *Clinical Neurophysiology*, **120**, 2008–2039.

Rossiter, S., Stevens, C. and Walker, G. (2006) Tinnitus and its effect on working memory and attention. *Journal of Speech, Hearing, and Language Research*, **49**, 150–160.

Rubinstein, B. (1993) Tinnitus and craniomandibular disorders – is there a link? *Swedish Dental Journal*, **95** (Suppl.), 1–46.

Rubinstein, B. and Carlsson, G. E. (1987) Effects of stomatognathic treatment on tinnitus: a retrospective study. *Journal of Craniomandibular Practice*, **5**, 254–259.

Rubinstein, B., Axelsson, A. and Carlsson, G. E. (1990) Prevalence of signs and symptoms of craniomandibular disorders in tinnitus patients. *Journal of Craniomandibular Disorders: Facial and Oral Pain*, **4**, 186–192.

Rubinstein, B., Österberg, T. and Rosenhall, U. (1992) Longitudinal fluctuations in tinnitus as reported by an elderly population. *Journal of Audiological Medicine*, **1**, 149–155.

Rubinstein, B., Ahlqwist, M. and Bengtsson, C. (1996) Hyperacusis, headache, temporomandibular disorders and amalgam fillings – an epidemiological study. In *Proceedings of the Fifth International Tinnitus Seminar 1995* Portland, OR: American Tinnitus Association.

Rubinstein, J., Tyler, R., Johnson, A. and Brown, C. (2003) Electrical suppression of tinnitus with high-rate pulse trains. *Otology and Neurotology*, **24**, 478–485.

Russell, D. and Baloh, R. W. (2009) Gabapentin responsive audiovestibular paroxysmia. *Journal of the Neurological Sciences*, **281**, 99–100.

Russo, J. E., Katon, W. J., Sullivan, M. D., Clark, M. R. and Buchwald, D. (1994) Severity of somatization and its relationship to psychiatric disorders and personality. *Psychosomatics*, **35**, 546–556.

Sadlier, M. and Stephens, S. D. G. (1995) An approach to the audit of tinnitus management. *Journal of Laryngology and Otology*, **109**, 826–829.

Sadlier, M., Stephens, S. D. and Kennedy, V. (2008) Tinnitus rehabilitation: a mindfulness meditation cognitive behavioural therapy approach. *Journal of Laryngology and Otology*, **122**, 31–37.

Saeed, S. R. and Brookes, G. B. (1993) The use of clostridium botulinum toxin in palatal myoclonus. A preliminary report. *Journal of Laryngology and Otology*, **107**, 208–210.

Sahley, T., Nodar, R. and Musiek, F. (1997) *Efferent auditory system: structure and function*, San Diego, Singular.

Sahley, T. L. and Nodar, R. H. (2001) A biochemical model of peripheral tinnitus. *Hearing Research*, **152**, 43–54.

Salembier, L., De Ridder, D. and van de Heyning, P. (2006) The use of flupirtine in treatment of tinnitus. *Acta Otolaryngologica*, **126**, 93–95.

Saltzman, M. and Ersner, M. S. (1947) A hearing aid for the relief of tinnitus aurium. *Laryngoscope*, **57**, 358–366.

Salvi, R. J., Wang, J. and Powers, N. L. (1996) Plasticity and reorganization in the auditory brainstem. In *Proceedings of the Fifth International Tinnitus Seminar* (eds G. E. Reich and J. A. Vernon), Portland, OR, American Tinnitus Association.

Salvi, R. J., Lockwood, A. H. and Burkard, R. (2000) Neural plasticity and tinnitus. In *Tinnitus handbook* (ed. R. S. Tyler), San Diego, CA: Singular, Thomson Learning.

Salvi, R., Lobarinas, E. and Sun, W. (2009) Pharmacological treatments for tinnitus: new and old. *Drugs Future*, **34**, 381–400.

Sammeth, C. A., Preves, D. A. and Brandy, W. T. (2000) Hyperacusis: case studies and evaluation of electronic loudness suppression devices as a treatment approach. *Scandinavian Audiology*, **29**, 28–36.

Sanchez, T. and Rocha, C. (2011) Diagnosis of somatosensory tinnitus. In *Textbook of tinnitus* (eds A. R. Møller, B. Langguth, D. De Ridder and T. Kleinjung), New York: Springer.

Sanchez, L. and Stephens, D. (1997) A tinnitus problem questionnaire. *Ear and Hearing*, **18**, 210–217.

Sanchez, T. G., Balbani, A. P. S., Bittar, R. S. M., Bento, R. F. and Camara, J. (1999) Lidocaine test in patients with tinnitus: rationale of accomplishment and relation to the treatment with carbamazepine. *Auris Nasus Larynx*, **26**, 411–417.

Sanchez, T. G., Guerra, G. C., Lorenzi, M. C., Brandao, A. L. and Bento, R. F. (2002) The influence of voluntary muscle contractions upon the onset and modulation of tinnitus. *Audiology and Neurootology*, **7**, 370–375.

Sanchez, T. G., Rocha, S. C., Knobel, K. A., Kii, M. A., Santos, R. M. and Pereira, C. B. (2011) Musical hallucination associated with hearing loss. *Arquivos de Neuro-Psiquiatria*, **69**, 395–400.

Sand, P. G., Langguth, B., Kleinjung, T. and Eichhammer, P. (2007) Genetics of chronic tinnitus. *Progress in Brain Research*, **166**, 159–168.

Santos Filha, V. A. and Matas, C. G. (2010) Late auditory evoked potentials in individuals with tinnitus. *Brazilian Journal of Otorhinolaryngology*, **76**, 263–270.

Saper, C. B. (2000) Brain stem, reflexive behavior, and the cranial nerves. In *Principles of neural science* (eds E. R. Kendel, J. H. Schwartz and T. M. Jessel), New York: McGraw-Hill.

Sataloff, R. T., Mandel, S., Muscal, E., Park, C. H., Rosen, D. C., Kim, S. M. and Spiegel, J. R. (1996) Single-photon-emission computed tomography (SPECT) in neurotologic assessment: a preliminary report. *American Journal of Otology*, **17**, 909–916.

Sataloff, R. T., Dentchev, D. I. and Hawkshaw, M. J. (2007) *Tinnitus: source readings*, San Diego, CA: Plural Publishing.

Sato, T., Kawase, T., Yano, H., Suetake, M. and Kobayashi, T. (2005) Trans-tympanic silicone plug insertion for chronic patulous Eustachian tube. *Acta Oto-Laryngologica*, **125**, 1158–1163.

Savastano, M., Brescia, G. and G, M. (2007) Antioxidant therapy in idiopathic tinnitus: preliminary outcomes. *Archives of Medical Research*, **38**, 456–459.

Schaette, R. and Kempter, R. (2006) Development of tinnitus-related neuronal hyperactivity through homeostatic plasticity after hearing loss: a computational mode. *European Journal of Neuroscience*, **11**, 3124–3138.

Schaette, R. and McAlpine, D. (2011) Tinnitus with a normal audiogram: physiological evidence for hidden hearing loss and computational model. *Journal of Neuroscience*, **31**, 13452–13457.

Scharf, B., Magnan, J. and Chays, A. (1997) On the role of the olivocochlear bundle in hearing: 16 case studies. *Hearing Research*, **103**, 101–122.

Schecklmann, M., Landgrebe, M., Poeppl, T. B., Kreuzer, P., Manner, P., Marienhagen, J., Wack, D. S., Kleinjung, T., Hajak, G. and Langguth, B. (2011) Neural correlates of tinnitus duration and distress: a positron emission tomography study. *Human Brain Mapping*, **22**, October. DOI: 10.1002/hbm.21426. Epub ahead of print.

Scheier, M. F. and Carver, C. S. (1985) Optimism, coping, and health: assessment and implications of generalized outcome expectancies. *Health Psychology*, **4**, 219–247.

Schellenberg, K., Bedlack, R. and Tucci, D. (2010) Roaring in the ears: patulous Eustachian tube in bulbar amyotrophic lateral sclerosis. *Amyotrophic Lateral Sclerosis*, **11**, 395–396.

Schloth, E. and Zwicker, E. (1983) Mechanical and acoustical influences on spontaneous oto-acoustic emissions. *Hearing Research*, **11**, 285–293.

Schmidt, J. and Huizing, E. (1992) The clinical drug trial in Menière's disease with emphasis on the effect of betahistine SR. *Acta Otolaryngologica Supplement*, **497**, 1–189.

Schmidt, L. P., Teixeira, V. N., Dall'igna, C., Dallagnol, D. and Smith, M. M. (2006) Brazilian Portuguese Language version of the 'Tinnitus Handicap Inventory': validity and reproducibility. *Brazilian Journal of Otorhinolaryngology*, **72**, 808–810.

Schmidtt, C., Patak, M. and Kröner-Herwig, B. (2000) Stress and the onset of sudden hearing loss and tinnitus. *International Tinnitus Journal*, **6**, 41–49.

Schneer, H. I. (1956) Psychodynamics of tinnitus. *Psychoanalytic Quarterly*, **25**, 72–78.

Schneider, P., Andermann, M., Wengenroth, M., Goebel, R., Flor, H., Rupp, A. and Diesch, E. (2009) Reduced volume of Heschl's gyrus in tinnitus. *NeuroImage*, **45**, 927–939.

Schuknecht, H. F. (1993) *Pathology of the ear*, Philadelphia, PA: Lea & Febiger.

Schulman, A. (1985) External electrical stimulation in tinnitus control. *American Journal of Otology*, **6**, 110–115.

Schulman, A. (1995) A final common pathway for tinnitus – the medial temporal lobe system. *International Tinnitus Journal*, **1**, 115–126.

Schutte, N. S., Noble, W., Malouff, J. M. and Bhullar, N. (2009) Evaluation of a model of distress related to tinnitus. *International Journal of Audiology*, **48**, 428–432.

Schwaber, M. K. and Whetsell, W. O. (1992) Cochleovestibular nerve compression syndrome. II. Vestibular nerve histopathology and theory of pathophysiology. *Laryngoscope*, **102** (9), 1030–1036.

Schwartz, N. (1999) Self-reports. How the questions shape the answers. *American Psychologist*, **54**, 93–105.

Schwartz, B., Wasserman, E. A. and Robbins, S. J.(2002) *Psychology of learning and behavior*, New York: Norton.

Scott, B. (1989) *A behavioural treatment approach to tinnitus*, Acta Universitas Upsaliensis, Comprehensive Summaries of Uppsala Dissertations from the faculty of Social Sciences, 13 (Dissertation), 44 pp.

Scott, B. (1993) A graded exposure treatment for patients with hyperacusis. Paper presented at the 19th Annual Convention of the Association for Behavior Analysis, Chicago, May.

Scott, B. and Lindberg, P. (2000) Psychological profile and somatic complaints between help-seeking and non-help-seeking tinnitus subjects. *Psychosomatics*, **41**, 347–352.

Scott, B., Lindberg, P., Melin, L. and Lyttkens, L. (1985) Psychological treatment of tinnitus. An experimental group study. *Scandinavian Audiology*, **14**, 223–230.

Scott, B., Lindberg, P., Melin, L. and Lyttkens, L. (1990) Predictors of tinnitus discomfort, adaption and subjective loudness. *British Journal of Audiology*, **24**, 51–62.

Searchfield, G. D. (2005) Hearing aids and tinnitus. In *Tinnitus treatment* (ed. R. Tyler), New York: Thieme.

Seely, D. R., Quigley, S. M. and Langman, A. W. (1996) Ear candles – efficacy and safety. *Laryngoscope*, **10**, 1226–1229.

Segal, Z. V., Teasdale, J. D. and Williams, J. M. G. (2002) *Mindfulness-based cognitive therapy. A new approach to preventing relapse*, New York: Guilford Press.

Seltzer, Z. and Devor, M. (1979) Ephaptic transmission in chronically damaged peripheral nerves. *Neurology*, **29**, 1061–1064.

Senge, P. M. (1990) *The fifth discipline*, London: Random House.

Sereda, M., Hall, D. A., Bosnyak, D. J., Edmondson-Jones, M., Roberts, L. E., Adjamian, P. and Palmer, A. R. (2011) Re-examining the relationship between audiometric profile and tinnitus pitch. *International Journal of Audiology*, **50**, 303–312.

Shailer, M. J., Tyler, R. S. and Coles, R. R. A. (1981) Critical masking bands for sensorineural tinnitus. *Scandinavian Audiology*, **10**, 157–162.

Shambaugh, G. E. (1986) Zinc for tinnitus, imbalance and hearing loss in the elderly. *American Journal of Otology*, **7**, 476–477.

Shargorodsky, J., Curhan, G. C. and Farwell, W. R. (2010) Prevalence and characteristics of tinnitus among US adults. *American Journal of Medicine*, **123**, 711–718.

Shea, J. (1958) Fenestration of the oval window. *Annals of Otology, Rhinology and Laryngology*, **67**, 932–951.

SHemirani, N., Tang, D. and Friedland, D. (2010) Acute auditory and vestibular symptoms associated with heat and transdermal lidocaine. *Clinical Journal of Pain*, **26**, 58–59.

Shergill, S. S., Brammer, M. J., Williams, S. C. R., Murray, R. M. and McGuire, P. K. (2000) Mapping auditory hallucinations in schizophrenia using functional magnetic resonance imaging. *Archives of General Psychiatry*, **57**, 1033–1038.

Sherlock, L. P. and Formby, C. (2005) Estimates of loudness, loudness discomfort, and auditory dynamic range: normative estimates, comparison of procedures, and test–retest reliability. *Journal of the American Academy of Audiology*, **16**, 85–100.

Shetye, A. and Kennedy, V. (2010) Tinnitus in children: an uncommon symptom? *Archives of Disability in Children*, **95**, 645–648.

Shim, H., Song, S., Choi, A., Hyung Lee, R. and Yoon, S. (2011) Comparison of various treatment modalities for acute tinnitus. *Laryngoscope*, **121**, 2619–2625.

Shiraishi, T., Sugimoto, K., Kubo, T. and Matsunaga, T. (1990) Depressive condition and double blind study of anti-depressant drug (Sulpiride) for tinnitus patients. *Audiology Japan*, **33**, 303–309.

Shore, S. (2011) Plasticity of somatosensory inputs to the cochlear nucleus – implications for tinnitus. *Hearing Research*, **281**, 38–46.

Shore, S., Zhou, J. and Koehler, S. (2007) Neural mechanisms underlying somatic tinnitus. *Progress in Brain Research*, **166**, 107–124.

Siedentopf, C. M., Ischebeck, A., Haala, I. A., Mottaghy, F. M., Schikora, D., Verius, M., Koppelstaetter, F., Buchberger, W., Schlager, A., Felber, S. R. and Golaszewski, S. M. (2007) Neural correlates of transmeatal cochlear laser (TCL) stimulation in healthy human subjects. *Neuroscience Letters*, **411**, 189–193.

Siedman, M. D. and Babu, S. (2003) Alternative medications and other treatments for tinnitus: facts from fiction. *Otolaryngologic Clinics of North America*, **36**, 359–382.

Silberstein, S. D. (1995) Migraine symptoms: results of a survey of self-reported migraineurs. *Headache*, **35**, 387–396.

Simpson, J. J. and Davies, W. E. (1999) Recent advances in the pharmacological treatment of tinnitus. *Trend in Pharmacological Sciences*, **20**, 12–18.

Simpson, J. J. and Davies, W. E. (2000) A review of evidence in support of a role for 5-HT in the perception of tinnitus. *Hearing Research*, **145**, 1–7.

Simpson, R. B., Nedzelski, J. M., Barber, H. O. and Thomas, M. R. (1988) Psychiatric diagnoses in patients with psychogenic dizziness or severe tinnitus. *Journal of Otolaryngology*, **17**, 325–330.

Simpson, J. J., Donaldson, I. and Davies, W. E. (1998) Use of homeopathy in the treatment of tinnitus. *British Journal of Audiology*, **32**, 227–233.

Simpson, J., Gilbert, A., Weiner, G. and Davies, W. (1999) The assessment of lamotrigine, an anti-epileptic drug in the treatment of tinnitus. *American Journal of Otology*, **20**, 627–631.

Sindhusake, D., Mitchell, P., NewalL, P., Rochtchina, E. and Rubin, G. (2003) Prevalence and characteristics of tinnitus in older adults: the Blue Mountains hearing study. *International Journal of Audiology*, **42**, 289–294.

Singh, S., Munjal, S. K. and Panda, N. K. (2011) Comparison of auditory electrophysiological responses in normal-hearing patients with and without tinnitus. *Journal of Laryngology and Otology*, **125**, 668–672.

Sismanis, A. (1987) Otologic manifestations of benign intracranial hypertension syndrome: diagnosis and management. *Laryngoscope*, **97**, 1–17.

Sismanis, A. and Smoker, W. R. (1994) Pulsatile tinnitus: recent advances in diagnosis. *Laryngoscope*, **104**, 681–688.

Smith, P. and Coles, R. (1987) Epidemiology of tinnitus: an update. In *Proceedings of the III International Tinnitus Seminar* (ed. H. Feldmann), Karlsruhe: Harsch Verlag.

Smith, S. L. and Fagelson, M. (2011) Development of the self-efficacy for tinnitus management questionnaire. *Journal of the American Academy of Audiology*, **22**, 424–440.

Smith, P. A., Parr, V. M., Lutman, M. E. and Coles, R. R. A. (1991) Comparative study of four noise spectra as potential tinnitus maskers. *British Journal of Audiology*, **25**, 25–34.

Smith, M. T., Perlis, M. L., Park, A., Smith, M. S., Pennington, J., Giles, D. E. and Buysse, D. J. (2002) Comparative meta-analysis of pharmacotherapy and behavior therapy for persistent insomnia. *American Journal of Psychiatry*, **159**, 5–11.

Smithies, O. (2007) http://www.nobelprize.org/nobel_prizes/medicine/laureates/2007/smithies-speech_en.html.

Smits, M., Kovacs, S., De Ridder, D., Peeters, R. R., van Hecke, P. and Sunaert, S. (2007) Lateralization of functional magnetic resonance imaging (fMRI) activation in the auditory pathway of patients with lateralized tinnitus. *Neuroradiology*, **49**, 669–679.

Sobrinho, P. G., Oliveira, C. A. and Venosa, A. R. (2004) Long-term follow-up of tinnitus in patients with otosclerosis after stapes surgery. *International Tinnitus Journal*, **10**, 197–201.

Sood, S. K. and Coles, R. R. A. (1988) Hyperacusis and phonophobia in tinnitus patients. *British Journal of Audiology*, **22**, 228.

Spielberger, C. D., Gorsuch, R. L. and Lushene, R. E. (1970) *Manual for the State-Trait Anxiety Inventory,* Palo Alto, CA: Consulting Psychologists Press.

Spitzer, J. and Ventry, I. (1980) Central auditory dysfunction among chronic alcoholics. *Archives of Otolaryngology*, **106**, 224–229.

Stacey, J. S. G. (1980) Apparent total control of severe bilateral tinnitus by masking, using hearing aids. *British Journal of Audiology*, **14**, 59–60.

Staffen, W., Biesinger, E., Trinka, E. and Ladurner, G. (1999) The effect of lidocaine on chronic tinnitus: a quantative cerebral perfusion study. *Audiology*, **38**, 53–57.

Stahle, J., Stahle, C. and Arenberg, I. (1978) Incidence of Ménière's disease. *Archives of Otolaryngology*, **104**, 99–102.

Stangerup, S., Tos, M., Thomsen, J. and Caye-Thomasen, P. (2010) True incidence of vestibular schwannoma? *Neurosurgery*, **67**, 1335–1340.

Stansfeld, S. A. (1992) Noise, noise sensitivity and psychiatric disorder: epidemiological and psychophysiological studies. *Psychological Medicine,* Monograph Supplement 22, 1–44.

Stansfeld, S. A., Clark, C. A., Jenkins, L. M. and Tarnopolsky, A. (1985) Sensitivity to noise in a community sample. 1. The measurement of psychiatric disorder and personality. *Psychological Medicine*, **15**, 243–254.

Staples, S. L. (1996) Human response to environmental noise. *American Psychologist*, **51**, 143–150.

St Claire, L., Stothart, G., McKenna, L. and Rogers, P. J. (2010) Caffeine abstinence: an ineffective and potentially distressing tinnitus therapy. *International Journal of Audiology*, **49**, 24–29.

Steigerwald, D. P., Verne, S. V. and Young, D. (1996) A retrospective evaluation of the impact of temporomandibular joint arthroscopy on the symptoms of headache, neck pain, shoulder pain, dizziness, and tinnitus. *Journal of Craniomandibular Practice*, **14**, 46–54.

Stephens, S. D. G. (1987) Historical aspects of tinnitus. In *Tinnitus* (ed. J. W. P. H. Hazell), London: Churchill Livingstone.

Stephens, D. (1999) Detrimental effects of alcohol on tinnitus. *Clinical Otolaryngology*, **24**, 114–116.

Stephens, D. (2000) A history of tinnitus. In *Tinnitus handbook* (ed. R. S. Tyler), San Diego, CA: Singular, Thomson Learning.

Stephens, S. D. G. and Corcoran, A. L. (1985) A controlled study of tinnitus masking. *British Journal of Audiology*, **19**, 159–167.

Stephens, S. D. G. and Hallam, R. S. (1985) The Crown-Crisp Experiental Index in patients complaining of tinnitus. *British Journal of Audiology*, **19**, 151–158.

Stephens, S. D., Blegvad, B. and Krogh, H. J. (1977) The value of some suprathreshold auditory measures. *Scandinavian Audiology*, **6**, 213–221.

Stephens, S. D. G., Hallam, R. S. and Jakes, S. C. (1986) Tinnitus: a management model. *Clinical Otolaryngology and Allied Sciences*, **11**, 227–238.

Stevens, C., Walker, G., Boyer, M. and Gallagher, M. (2007) Severe tinnitus and its effect on selective and divided attention. *International Journal of Audiology*, **46**, 208–216.

Stidham, K. R., Solomon, P. H. and Roberson, J. B. (2005) Evaluation of botulinum toxin A in treatment of tinnitus. *Otolaryngology, Head and Neck Surgery*, **132**, 883–889.

Stokroos, R. and Kingma, H. (2004) Selective vestibular ablation by intratympanic gentamicin in patients with unilateral active Meniere's disease: a prospective, double-blind, placebo controlled, randomized clinical trial. *Acta Oto-Laryngologica*, **124**, 172–175.

Stouffer, J. L. and Tyler, R. S. (1990) Characterization of tinnitus by tinnitus patients. *Journal of Speech and Hearing Research*, **55**, 493–453.

Stouffer, J. L. and Tyler, R. S. (1992) Ratings of psychological changes pre-and post-tinnitus onset. In *Tinnitus 91. Proceedings of the Fourth International Tinnitus Seminar* (eds J.-M. Aran and R. Dauman), Amsterdam/New York: Kugler Publications.

Stouffer, J. L., Tyler, R. S., Kileny, P. R. and Dalzell, L. E. (1991) Tinnitus as a function of duration and etiology: counselling implications. *American Journal of Otolaryngology*, **12**, 188–194.

Stouffer, J. L., Tyler, R. S., Booth, J. C. and Buckrell, B. (1992) Tinnitus in normal-hearing and hearing-impaired children. In *Proceedings of the Fourth International Tinnitus Seminar* (eds J.-M. Aran and R. Dauman), Amsterdam/New York: Kugler Publications.

Strangerup, S. E., Tos, M., Thomsen, J. and Caye-Thomasen, P. (2010) True incidence of vestibular schwannoma? *Neurosurgery*, **67** (5), November, 1335–1340.

Sturmey, P. (1996) *Functional analysis in clinical psychology*, Chichester: John Wiley & Sons, Ltd.

Stypulkowski, P. H. (1990) Mechanisms of salicylate ototoxicity. *Hearing Research*, **46**, 113–145.

Su, Y., Luo, B. and Wang, H. (2009) Differential effects of sodium salicylate on current-evoked firing of pyramidal neurons and fast-spiking interneurons in slices of rat auditory cortex. *Hearing Research*, **253**, 60–66.

Suckfüll, M., Althaus, M., Ellers-Lenz, B., Gebauer, A., Görtelmeyer, R., Jastreboff, P., Moebius, H., Rosenberg, T., Russ, H., Wirth, Y. and Krueger, H. (2011) A randomized, double-blind, placebo-controlled clinical trial to evaluate the efficacy and safety of neramexane in patients with moderate to severe subjective tinnitus. *BMC Ear, Nose and Throat Disorders*, **11**, 1.

Sullivan, M. D., Katon, W. J., Russo, J. E., Dobie, R. A. and Sakai, C. (1993) A randomized trial of nortriptyline for severe chronic tinnitus. *Archives of Internal Medicine*, **153**, 2251–2259.

Sullivan, M., Katon, W., Russo, J., Dobie, R. and Sakai, C. (1994) Coping and marital support as correlates of tinnitus disability. *General Hospital Psychiatry*, **16**, 259–266.

Sullivan, M. D., Katon, W., Dobie, R., Sakai, C., Russo, J. and Harrop-Griffiths, J. (1988) Disabling tinnitus. Association with affective disorders. *General Hospital Psychiatry*, **10**, 285–291.

Sundell, M. and Sundell, S. S. (1999) *Behavior change in the human services. An introduction to principles and applications*, Thousand Oaks, CA: Sage.

Surr, R. K., Montgomery, A. A. and Mueller, H. G. (1985) Effect of amplification of tinnitus among new hearing aid users. *Ear and Hearing*, **6**, 71–75.

Surr, R. K., Kolb, J. A., Cord, M. T. and Garrus, N. P. (1999) Tinnitus Handicap Inventory (THI) as a hearing aid outcome measure. *Journal of the American Academy of Audiology*, **10**, 489–495.

Sweetow, R. W. (1984) Cognitive-behavioral modification in tinnitus management. *Hearing Instruments*, **35**, 14–52.

Sweetow, R. W. and Levy, M. C. (1990) Tinnitus severity scaling for diagnostic/therapeutic usage. *Hearing Instruments*, **41**, 20–21,46.

Szczepaniak, W. S. and Møller, A. R. (1996) Effects of (-)-baclofen, clonazepam, and diazepam on tone exposure-induced hyperexcitability of the inferior colliculus in the rat: possible therapeutic implications for pharmacological management of tinnitus and hyperacusis. *Hearing Research*, **97**, 46–53.

Sziklai, I., Szilvassy, J. and Szilvassy, Z. (2011) Tinnitus control by dopamine agonist pramipexole in presbycusis patients: a randomized, placebo-controlled, double-blind study. *Laryngoscope*, **121**, 888–893.

Takano, A., Takahashi, H., Hatachi, K., Yoshida, H., Kaieda, S., Adachi, T., Takasaki, K., Kumagami, H. and Tsukasaki, N. (2007) Ligation of Eustachian tube for intractable patulous Eustachian tube: a preliminary report. *European Archives of Oto-Rhino-Laryngology*, **264**, 353–357.

Takasaki, K., Kumagami, H., Umeki, H., Enatsu, K. and Takahashi, H. (2008) The patulous Eustachian tube complicated with amyotrophic lateral sclerosis: a video clip demonstration. *Laryngoscope*, **118**, 2057–2058.

Tan, C. M., Lecluyse, W., McFerran, D. and Meddis, R. (in press) Tinnitus is a marker for a specific pattern of hearing loss. *Journal of Association for Research in Otolarngology* (submitted).

Tass, P., Adamchic, I., Fruend, H. J., von Stakelberg, T. and Hauptmann, C. (2012) Counteractiong tinnitus by acoustic co-ordinated rest stimulation. *Restorative Neurology and Neuroscience*, **30**, 137–159.

Tecchio, F., Benassi, F., Zappasodi, F., Gialloreti, L. E., Palermo, M., Seri, S. and Rossini, P. M. (2003) Auditory sensory processing in autism: a magnetoencephalographic study. *Biological Psychiatry*, **54**, 647–654.

Teggi, R., Bellini, C., Piccioni, L. O., Palonta, F. and Bussi, M. (2009) Transmeatal low-level laser therapy for chronic tinnitus with cochlear dysfunction. *Audiology and Neurotology*, **14**, 115–120.

Teismann, H., Okamoto, H. and Pantev, C. (2011) Short and intense tailor-made notched music training against tinnitus: the tinnitus frequency matters. *Public Library of Science*, **6**, e24685.

Telischi, F. F., Rodgers, G. K. and Balkany, T. J. (1994) Dizziness in childhood. In *Neurotology* (eds R. K. Jackler and D. E. Brackmann), New York: Mosby Year Book.

Terry, A. M. P., Jones, D. M., Davis, B. R. and Slater, R. (1983) Parametric studies of tinnitus masking and residual inhibition. *British Journal of Audiology*, **17**, 245–256.

Thai-Van, H., Micheyl, C., Moore, B. C. and Collet, L. (2003) Enhanced frequency discrimination near the hearing loss cut-off: a consequence of central auditory plasticity induced by cochlear damage? *Brain*, **126**, 2235–2245.

Thai-Van, H., Micheyl, C., Norena, A., Veuillet, E., Gabriel, D. and Collet, L. (2007) Enhanced frequency discrimination in hearing-impaired individuals: a review of perceptual correlates of central neural plasticity induced by cochlear damage. *Hearing Research*, **233**, 14–22.

Tharpe, A. M., Bess, F. H., Sladen, D. P., Schissel, H., Couch, S. and Schery, T. (2006) Auditory characteristics of children with autism. *Ear and Hearing*, **27**, 430–441.

Theopold, H.-M. (1985) Nimodipine (Bayer 9736). A new concept in the treatment of inner ear disease. *Laryngology, Rhinology and Otology*, **64**, 609–913.

Thompson, R. C. (1931) Assyrian prescriptions for diseases of the ear. *Journal of the Royal Asiatic Society*, 1–25.

Thompson, G. C., Thompson, A. M., Garrett, K. M. and Britton, B. H. (1994) Serotonin and serotonin receptors in the central auditory system. *Otolaryngology Head and Neck Surgery*, **100**, 93–102.

Thompson, A. M., Thompson, G. C. and Britton, B. H. (1998) Serotoninergic innervation of stapedial and tensor tympani motoneurons. *Brain Research*, **787**, 175–178.

Topak, M., Sahin-Yilmaz, A., Ozdoganoglu, T., Yilmaz, H. B., Ozbay, M. and Kulekci, M. J. (2009) Intratympanic methylprednisolone injections for subjective tinnitus. *Journal of Laryngology and Otology*, **123**, 1221–1225.

Trotter, M. I. and Donaldson, I. (2008) Hearing aids and tinnitus therapy: a 25-year experience. *Journal of Laryngology and Otology*, **122**, 1052–1056.

Tucker, D. A., Phillips, S. L., Ruth, R. A., Clayton, W. A., Royster, E. and Todd, A. D. (2005) The effect of silence on tinnitus perception. *Otolaryngology Head, and Neck Surgery*, **132**, 20–24.

Tullberg, M. and Ernberg, M. (2006) Long-term effect on tinnitus by treatment of temporomandibular disorders: a two-year follow-up by questionnaire. *Acta Odontologica Scandinavica*, **64**, 89–96.

Turk, D. C., Meichenbaum, D. and Genest, M. (1983) *Pain and behavioral medicine. A cognitive-behavioral perspective*, New York: Guilford Press.

Turk, D. C., Rudy, T. E., Kubinski, J. A., Zaki, H. S. and Greco, C. M. (1996) Dysfunctional patients with temporomandibular disorders: evaluating the efficacy of a tailored treatment protocol. *Journal of Consulting and Clinical Psychology*, **64**, 139–146.

Tye-Murray, N. (1991) Repair strategy usage by hearing-impaired adults and changes following communication therapy. *Journal of Speech and Hearing Research*, **34**, 921–928.

Tyler R. S. (1984) Does tinnitus originate from hyperactive nerve fibers in the cochlea? *Journal of Laryngology and Otology*, Suppl. 9, 38–44.

Tyler, R. S. (1987) Tinnitus maskers and hearing aids for tinnitus. *Seminars in Hearing*, **8**, 49–61.

Tyler, R. S. (1993) Tinnitus disability and handicap questionnaires. *Seminars in Hearing*, **14**, 377–383.

Tyler, R. S. (2000) The psychoacoustical measurement of tinnitus. In *Tinnitus handbook* (ed. R. S. Tyler), San Diego, CA: Singular, Thomson Learning.

Tyler, R. S. and Babin, R. W. (1993) Tinnitus. In *Otolaryngology – head and neck surgery* (eds C. W. Cummings, J. M. Fredrickson, L. A. Harker, C. J. Krause and D. E. Schuller), St Louis, MI: CV Mosby.

Tyler, R. S. and Baker, L. J. (1983) Difficulties experienced by tinnitus sufferers. *Journal of Speech and Hearing Disorders*, **48**, 150–154.

Tyler, R. S. and Conrad-Armes, D. (1983a) The determination of tinnitus loudness considering the effects of recruitment. *Journal of Speech and Hearing Research*, **26**, 59–72.

Tyler, R. S. and Conrad-Armes, D. (1983b) Tinnitus pitch: a comparison of three measurement methods. *British Journal of Audiology*, **17**, 101–107.

Tyler, R. S. and Conrad-Armes, D. (1984) Masking of tinnitus compared to masking of pure tones. *Journal of Speech and Hearing Research*, **27**, 106–111.

Tyler, R. S. and Stouffer, J. L. (1989) A review of tinnitus loudness. *Hearing Journal*, **42**, 52–57.

Tyler, R., Haskell, G., Preece, J. and Bergan, C. (2001) Nurturing patient expectations to enhance the treatment of tinnitus. *Seminars in Hearing*, **22**, 15–21.

Tyler, R. S., Coelho, C. and Noble, W. (2006) Tinnitus: standard of care, personality differences, genetic factors. *ORL: Journal for Oto-Rhino-Laryngology and Its Related Specialties*, **68**, 14–19.

Valente, M., Potts, L. G. and Valente, M. (1997) Differences and intersubject variability of loudness discomfort levels measured in sound pressure level and hearing level for TDH-50P and ER-3A earphones. *Journal of the American Academy of Audiology*, **8**, 59–67.

Vallianatou, N., Christodoulou, P., Nestoros, J. and Helidonis, E. (2001) Audiologic and psychological profile of Greek patients with tinnitus – preliminary findings. *American Journal of Otolaryngology*, **22**, 33–37.

van Borsel, J., Curfs, L. M. G. and Fryns, J. P. (1997) Hyperacusis in Williams syndrome: a sample survey study. *Genetic Counselling*, **8**, 121–126.

Vandenbroucke, J. P. (1997) Homoeopathy trials: going nowhere. *Lancet*, **350**, 824.

van de Heyning, P., Vermeire, K., Diebl, M., Nopp, P., Anderson, I. and De Ridder, D. (2008) Incapacitating unilateral tinnitus in single-sided deafness treated by cochlear implantation. *Annals of Otology, Rhinology and Laryngology*, **117**, 645–652.

Vanneste, S. and De Ridder, D. (2011) Transcranial direct current stimulation (tDCS): A new tool for the treatment of tinnitus? In *Textbook of tinnitus* (eds A. R. Møller, B. Langguth, D. De Ridder and T. Kleinjung), New York: Springer.

Vanneste, S., Plazier, M., Ost, J., van der Loo, E., van de Heyning, P. and De Ridder, D. (2010) Bilateral dorsolateral prefrontal cortex modulation for tinnitus by transcranial direct current stimulation: a preliminary clinical study. *Experimental Brain Research*, **202**, 779–785.

Vanneste, S., Focquaert, F., van de Heyning, P. and De Ridder, D. (2011) Different resting state brain activity and functional connectivity in patients who respond and not respond to bifrontal tDCS for tinnitus suppression. *Experimental Brain Research*, **210**, 217–227.

Verbeek, J. H., Kateman, E., Morata, T. C., Dreschler, W. and Sorgdrager, B. (2009) Interventions to prevent occupational noise induced hearing loss. *Cochrane Database of Systematic Reviews*, CD006396.

Vermeire, K., Heyndrickx, K., De Ridder, D. and van de Heyning, P. (2007) Phase-shift tinnitus treatment: an open prospective clinical trial. *B-ENT*, **3** (Suppl. 7), 65–69.

Vermeire, K. and van de Heyning, P. (2009) Binaural hearing after cochlear implantation in subjects with unilateral sensorineural deafness and tinnitus. *Audiology and Neurootology*, **14**, 163–171.

Vernon, J. (1977) Attempts to relieve tinnitus. *Journal of the American Audiology Society*, **2**, 124–131.

Vernon, J. (1987a) Assessment of the tinnitus patient. In *Tinnitus* (ed. J. W. P. Hazell), London: Churchill Livingstone.

Vernon, J. A. (1987b) Pathophysiology of tinnitus: a special case – hyperacusis and a proposed treatment. *American Journal of Otology*, **8**, 201–202.

Vernon, J. A. (ed.) (1998) *Tinnitus. Treatment and relief*, Boston, MA: Allyn & Bacon.

Vernon, J. V. and Johnson, R. (1980) The characteristics and natural history of tinnitus in Meniere's disease. *Otolaryngolic Clinics of North America*, **13**, 611–619.

Vernon, J. A. and Meikle, M. B. (2000) Tinnitus masking. In *Tinnitus handbook* (ed. R. S. Tyler), San Diego, CA: Singular, Thomson Learning.

Vernon, J., Greist, S. and Press, L. (1990) Attributes of tinnitus and the acceptance of masking. *American Journal of Otolaryngology*, **11**, 44–50.

Veuillet, E., Collet, L., Disnat, F. and Morgon, A. (1992) Tinnitus and medial cochlear efferent system. *Tinnitus 91. Proceedings of the Fourth International Tinnitus Seminar* (eds J.-M. Aran and R. Dauman), Amsterdam/New York: Kugler Publications.

Viani, L. G. (1989) Tinnitus in children with hearing loss. *Journal of Laryngology and Otology*, **103**, 142–145.

Vilholm, O. J., Møller, K. and Jørgensen, K. (1998) Effect of traditional Chinese acupuncture on severe tinnitus: a double-blind, placebo-controlled, clinical investigation with open therapeutic control. *British Journal of Audiology*, **32**, 197–204.

Vlaeyen, J. W. and Linton, S. J. (2000) Fear-avoidance and its consequences in chronic musculoskeletal pain: a state of the art. *Pain*, **85**, 317–332.

Vlaeyen, J., De Jong, J., Geilen, M., Heuts, P. H. T. G. and van Breukelen, G. (2001) Graded exposure *in vivo* in the treatment of pain-related fear: a replicated single-case experimental design in four patients with chronic low back fear. *Behaviour Research and Therapy*, **39**, 151–166.

Vogt, J. and Kastner, M. (2002) Tinnituskrankungen be fluglotsen: eine klinisch–arbeitspsycho-logischestudie. (Tinnitus in air traffic controllers: a clinical–ergonomical pilot study). *Zeitschrift für Arbeits und Organisationpsychologie*, **46**, 35–44.

von Wedel, H., Calero, L., Walger, M., Hoenen, S. and Rutwalt, D. (1995) Soft-laser/Ginkgo biloba therapy in chronic tinnitus. A placebo controlled study. *Advances in Otorhinolaryngology*, **49**, 105–108.

Wahlström, B. and Axelsson, A. (1996) The description of tinnitus sounds. In *Proceedings of the Fifth International Tinnitus Seminar, 1995* (eds G. E. Reich and J. A. Vernon), Portland, OR: American Tinnitus Association, pp. 298–301.

Wall, M. (2010) Idiopathic intracranial hypertension. *Neurologic Clinics*, **28**, 593–617.

Wall, M., Rosenberg, M. & Richardson, D. 1987. Gaze-evoked tinnitus. *Neurology*, **37**, 1034–1036.

Wallhäusser-Franke, E. and Langner, G. (1999) Central activation patterns after experimental tinnitus induction in an animal model. In *Proceedings of the Sixth International Tinnitus Seminar* (ed. J. Hazell), Cambridge, The Tinnitus and Hyperacusis Centre, pp. 155–162.

Wallhäusser-Franke, E., Braun, S. and Langner, G. (1996) Salicylate alters 2-DG uptake in the auditory system: a model for tinnitus? *NeuroReport*, **7**, 1585–1588.

Walpurger, V., Hebing-Lennartz, G., Denecke, H. and Pietrowsky, R. (2003) Habituation deficit in auditory event-related potentials in tinnitus complainers. *Hearing Research*, **181**, 57–64.

Walsh, W. M. and Gerley, P. P. (1985) Thermal biofeedback and the treatment of tinnitus. *Laryngoscope*, **95**, 987–989.

Wang, H., Luo, B. and Zhou, K. (2006) Sodium salicylate reduces inhibitory postsynaptic currents in neurons of rat auditory cortex. *Hearing Research*, **215**, 77–83.

Wang, K., Bugge, J. and Bugge, S. (2010) A randomized, placebo-controlled trial of manual and electrical acupuncture for the treatment of tinnitus. *Complementary Therapies in Medicine*, **18**, 249–255.

Wangemann, P. and Schact, J. (1996) Homeostatic mechanisms in the cochlea. In *The cochlea* (eds P. Dallos, A. N. Popper and R. R. Fay), New York: Springer.

Ward, L. M. and Baumann, M. (2009) Measuring tinnitus loudness using constrained psychophysical scaling. *American Journal of Audiology*, **18**, 119–128.

Ware, J. E. (1993) *The SF36 health survey: manual and interpretation*, Boston, MA: Nimrod Press.

Watanabe, I., Kumagami, H. and Tsuda, Y. (1974) Tinnitus due to abnormal contraction of stapedial muscle. An abnormal phenomenon in the course of facial nerve paralysis and its audiological significance. *ORL: Journal for Oto-rhinolaryngology and Its Related Specialties*, **36**, 217–226.

Watkins, P. L. and Clum, G. A. (eds) (2008) *Handbook of self-help therapies*, New York: Routledge.

Watson, J. B. (1913/1994) Psychology as the behaviorist views it. *Psychological Review*, **20** (101), 248–253.

Wazen, J. J., Foyt, D. and Sisti, M. (1997) Selective cochlear neurectomy for debilitating tinnitus. *Annals of Otology, Rhinology and Laryngology*, **106**, 568–570.

Weber, C., Arck, P., Mazureck, B. and Klapp, B. F. (2002a) Impact of relaxation training on psychometric and immunologic parameters in tinnitus sufferers. *Journal of Psychosomatic Research*, **52**, 29–33.

Weber, H., K, P., Stohr, M. and Rosler, A. (2002b) Central hyperacusis with phonophobia in multiple sclerosis. *Multiple Sclerosis*, **8**, 505–509.

Wegel, R. L. (1931) A study of tinnitus. *Archives of Otolaryngology*, **14**, 158–165.

Wegner, D. M. (1994) *White bears and other unwanted thoughts*, New York: Guilford Press.

Wei, L. J. and Lachin, J. M. (1988) Properties of the urn randomization in clinical trials. *Controlled Clinical Trials*, **9**, 345–364.

Wei, B. P. C., Mubiru, S. and O'Leary, S. (2006) Steroids for idiopathic sudden sensorineural hearing loss. *Cochrane Database of Systematic Reviews*, Issue 1, Article CD003998. DOI: 10.1002/14651858.CD003998.pub2.

Weiner, I. B. and Bornstein, R. F. (2009) *Principles of psychotherapy. Promoting evidence-based psychodynamic practice*, New Jersey: John Wiley & Sons, Inc.

Weinmeister, K. (2000) Prolonged suppression of tinnitus after peripheral nerve block using bupivacaine and lidocaine. *Regional Anesthesia and Pain Medicine*, **25**, 67–68.

Weinshel, E. M. (1955) Some psychiatric considerations in tinnitus. *Journal of the Hillside Hospital*, **4**, 67–92.

Weinstein, N. D. (1980) Individual differences in critical tendencies and noise annoyance. *Journal of Sound and Vibration*, **68**, 241–248.

Weir, N. (1990) *Otolaryngology: an Illustrated history*, London: Butterworths.

Weise, C., Heinecke, K. and Rief, W. (2008a) Stability of physiological variables in chronic tinnitus sufferers. *Applied Psychophysiology and Biofeedback*, **33**, 149–159.

Weise, C., Heinecke, K. and Rief, W. (2008b) Biofeedback-based behavioral treatment for chronic tinnitus: results of a randomized controlled trial. *Journal of Consulting and Clinical Psychology*, **76**, 1046–1057.

Weissman, J. L. and Hirsch, B. E. (2000) Imaging of tinnitus: a review. *Radiology*, **216**, 342–349.

Weisz, N., Wienbruch, C., Dohrmann, K. and Elbert, T. (2005) Neuromagnetic indicators of auditory cortical reorganization of tinnitus. *Brain*, **128**, 2722–2731.

Weisz, N., Hartmann, T., Dohrmann, K., Schlee, W. and Norena, A. (2006) High-frequency tinnitus without hearing loss does not mean absence of deafferentation. *Hearing Research*, **222**, 108–114.

Westcott, M. (2002) Case study: management of hyperacusis associated with post-traumatic stress disorder. In *Proceedings of the Seventh International Tinnitus Seminar* (ed. R. Patuzzi), Freemantle, University of Western Australia.

Westcott, M. (2006) Acoustic shock injury (ASI). *Acta Otolaryngologica*, **126**, 54–58.

Westerberg, B. D., Roberson Jr, J. B. and Stach, B. A. (1996) A double-blind placebo-controlled trial of baclofen in the treatment of tinnitus. *American Journal of Otolology*, **17**, 896–903.

Westin, V., Hayes, S. C. and Andersson, G. (2008a) Is it the sound or your relationship to it? The role of acceptance in predicting tinnitus impact. *Behaviour Research and Therapy*, **46**, 1259–1265.

Westin, V., Östergren, R. and Andersson, G. (2008b) The effects of acceptance versus thought suppression for dealing with the intrusiveness of tinnitus. *International Journal of Audiology*, **47** (Suppl. 2), S184–S190.

Wewers, M. E. and Lowe, N. K. (1990) A critical review of visual analogue scales in the measurement of clinical phenomena. *Research in Nursing and Health*, **13**, 227–236.

White, T. P., Hoffman, S. R. and Gale, E. N. (1986) Psychophysiological therapy for tinnitus. *Ear and Hearing*, **7**, 397–399.

Whittaker, C. K. (1982) Letter to the editor. *American Journal of Otology*, **4**, 188.

Williams, J. M. G. and Broadbent, K. (1986) Autobiographical memory in suicide attempters. *Journal of Abnormal Psychology*, **95**, 144–149.

Williams, J. M. G., Watts, F. N., MacLeod, C. and Mathews, A. (1997) *Cognitive psychology and emotional disorders*, Chichester: John Wiley & Sons, Ltd.

Williams, J. M. G., Barnhofer, T., Crane, C., Herman, D., Raes, F., Watkins, E. and Dalgleish, T. (2007) Autobiographical memory specificity and emotional disorder. *Psychological Bulletin*, **133**, 122–148.

Wilson, B. A. (2008) Neuropsychological rehabilitation. *Annual Review of Clinical Psychology*, **4**, 141–162.

Wilson, P. H. and Henry, J. L. (1998) Tinnitus cognitions questionnaire: development and psychometric properties of a measure of dysfunctional cognitions associated with tinnitus. *International Tinnitus Journal*, **4**, 23–30.

Wilson, J. and Sutton, G. J. (1981) Acoustic correlates of tonal tinnitus. In *Tinnitus, Ciba Foundation Symposium 85* (eds D. Evered and G. Lawrenson), London: Pitman Books.

Wilson, P. H., Henry, J., Bowen, M. and Haralambous, G. (1991) Tinnitus reaction questionnaire: psychometric properties of a measure of distress associated with tinnitus. *Journal of Speech and Hearing Research*, **34**, 197–201.

Wilson, P. H., Henry, J. L., Andersson, G., Hallam, R. S. and Lindberg, P. (1998) A critical analysis of directive counselling as a component of tinnitus retraining therapy. *British Journal of Audiology*, **32**, 273–286.

Wilson, C., Lewis, P. and Stephens, D. (2002) The short form 36 (SF36) in a specialist tinnitus clinic. *International Journal of Audiology*, **41**, 216–220.

Witsell, D. L., Hannley, M. T., Stinnet, S. and Tucci, D. L. (2007) Treatment of tinnitus with gabapentin: a pilot study. *Otology and Neurotology*, **28**, 11–15.

Wolraich, D. and Zur, K. (2010) Use of calcium hydroxylapatite for management of recalcitrant otorrhea due to a patulous Eustachian tube. *International Journal of Pediatric Otorhinolaryngology*, **74**, 1455–1457.

Wood, K. A., Webb, W. L., Orchik, D. J. and Shea, J. J. (1983) Intractable tinnitus: psychiatric aspects of treatment. *Psychosomatics*, **24**, 559–565.

Woodhouse, A. and Drummond, P. D. (1993) Mechanisms of increased sensitivity to noise and light in migraine headache. *Cephalgia*, **13**, 417–421.

World Health Organization (WHO) (2001) *International classification of functioning, disability and health*, Geneva: WHO.

Wright, E. F. and Bifano, S. L. (1997) Tinnitus improvement through TMD therapy. *Journal of the American Dental Association*, **128**, 1424–1432.

Wunderlich, A. P., Schonfeldt-Lecuona, C., Wolf, R. C., Dorn, K., Bachor, E. and Freund, W. (2010) Cortical activation during a pitch discrimination task in tinnitus patients and controls – an fMRI study. *Audiology and Neurotology*, **15**, 137–148.

Xie, J., Talaska, A. E. and Schacht, J. (2011) New developments in aminoglycoside therapy and ototoxicity. *Hearing Research*, **281**, 28–37.

Xu, Z. and Xiong, Y. (1999) Effect of decompression of blood vessel on vascular compressive tinnitus. *Lin Chuang Er Bi Yan Hou Ke Za Zhi*, **13**, 155–156.

Yanez, C., Pirron, J. A. and Mora, N. (2011) Curvature inversion technique: a novel tuboplastic technique for patulous Eustachian tube – a preliminary report. *Otolaryngology, Head and Neck Surgery*, **145**, 446–451.

Yetiser, S., Tosun, F., Satar, B., Arslanhan, M., Akcam, T. and Ozakapta, Y. (2002) The role of zinc in management of tinnitus. *Auris Nasus Larynx*, **29**, 329–333.

Yilmaz, I., Akkuzu, B., Cakmak, O. and Ozlüoglu, L. (2004) Misoprostol in the treatment of tinnitus: a double-blind study. *Otolaryngology, Head and Neck Surgery*, **130**, 604–610.

Young, D. W. (2000) Biofeedback training in the treatment of tinnitus. In *Tinnitus handbook* (ed. R. S. Tyler), San Diego, CA: Singular, Thomson Learning.

Young, E. D. (2010) Level and spectrum. In: REES, A. & PALMER, A. (eds.) *The Oxford handbook of auditory science*, Volume 2, *The auditory brain*. Oxford: Oxford University Press.

Young, Y. H., Cheng, P. W. and Ko, J. Y. (1997) A 10-year longitudinal study of tubal function in patients with nasopharyngeal carcinoma after irradiation. *Archives of Otolaryngology, Head and Neck Surgery*, **123**, 945–948.

Yu, N., Zhu, M., Johnson, B., Liu, Y., Jones, R. and Zhao, H. (2008) Prestin up-regulation in chronic salicylate (aspirin) administration: an implication of functional dependence of prestin expression. *Cell and Molecular Life Sciences*, **65**, 2407–2418.

Zachariae, R., Mirz, F., Johansen, L. V., Andersen, S. E., Bjerring, P. and Pedersen, C. B. (2000) Reliability and validity of a Danish adaption of the tinnitus handicap inventory. *Scandinavian Audiology*, **29**, 37–43.

Zadikoff, C., Lang, A. E. and Klein, C. (2006) The 'essentials' of essential palatal tremor: a reappraisal of the nosology. *Brain*, **129**, 832–840.

Zapp, J. J. (2001) Gabapentin for the treatment of tinnitus: a case report. *Ear, Nose and Throat Journal*, **80**, 114–116.

Zarchi, O., Attias, J. and Gothelf, D. (2010) Auditory and visual processing in Williams syndrome. *Israelian Journal of Psychiatry and Related Sciences*, **47**, 125–131.

Zatorre, R. J. and Binder, J. R. (2000) Functional and structural imaging of the human auditory system. In *Brain mapping. The systems* (eds A. W. Toga and J. C. Mazziotta), San Diego, CA: Academic Press.

Zehlicke, T., Punke, C., Dressler, D. and Pau, H. W. (2008) Intratympanic application of botulinum toxin: experiments in guinea pigs for excluding ototoxic effects. *European Archives of Otorhinolaryngology*, **265**, 167–170.

Zelman, S. (1973) Correlation of smoking history with hearing loss. *Journal of the American Medical Association*, **233**, 920.

Zeman, F., Koller, M., Figueiredo, R., Aazevedo, A., Rates, M., Coelho, C., Kleinjung, T., De Ridder, D., Langguth, B. and Landgrebe, M. (2011) Tinnitus handicap inventory for evaluating treatment effects: which changes are clinically relevant? *Otolaryngology, Head and Neck Surgery*, **145**, 282–287.

Zeng, F. G., Tang, Q., Dimitrijevic, A., Starr, A., Larky, J. and Blevins, N. H. (2011) Tinnitus suppression by low-rate electric stimulation and its electrophysiological mechanisms. *Hearing Research*, **277**, 61–66.

Zenner, H. P. and Ernst, A. (1993) Cochlear-motor, transduction and signal-transfer tinnitus: models for three types of cochlear tinnitus. *European Archives of Otorhinolaryngology*, **249**, 447–454.

Zetterqvist-Westin, V., Schulin, M., Hesser, H., Karlsson, M., Zare Noe, R., Olofsson, U., Stalby, M., Wisung, G. and Andersson, G. (2011) Acceptance and commitment therapy versus tinnitus retraining therapy in the treatment of tinnitus distress: a randomized controlled trial. *Behaviour Research and Therapy*, **49**, 737–747.

Zhang, J. S. and Kaltenbach, J. A. (1998) Increases in spontaneous activity in the dorsal cochlear nucleus of the rat following exposure to high intensity sound. *Neuroscience Letters*, **250**, 197–200.

Zigmond, A. S. and Snaith, R. P. (1983) The hospital anxiety and depression scale. *Acta Psychiatrica Scandinavia*, **67**, 361–370.

Zimmer, K. and Ellermeier, W. (1999) Psychometric properties of four measures of noise sensitivity: a comparison. *Journal of Environmental Psychology*, **19**, 295–302.

Zlomke, K. and Davis III, T. E. (2008) One-session treatment of specific phobias: a detailed description and review of treatment efficacy. *Behavior Therapy*, **39**, 207–223.

Zöger, S., Holgers, K.-M. and Svedlund, J. (2001) Psychiatric disorders in tinnitus patients without severe hearing impairment: 24 month follow-up of patients at an audiological clinic. *Audiology*, **40**, 133–140.

Zöger, S., Svedlund, J. and Holgers, K.-M. (2004) Relationship between tinnitus severity and psychiatric disorders. *Psychosomatics*, **47**, 282–288.

Zöger, S., Svedlund, J. and Holgers, K.-M. (2006) The effects of sertraline on severe tinnitus suffering – a randomized, double-blind, placebo-controlled study. *Journal of Clinical Psychopharmacology*, **26**, 32–39.

Index

Note: Page references in *italics* refer to Figures; those in **bold** refer to Tables

ultrasonic stimulation of the ear 206
unilateral sudden sensorineural hearing
    loss 64–5
    investigations **65**
unilateral vestibular schwannoma
    surgery 74

vascular compression syndrome 57
vascular loops 57–8
vascular pulsatile tinnitus 59
vasodilators 156
ventral acoustic stria 25
ventral cochlear nucleus (VCN) 36
vertigo 16, 158
    benign paroxysmal positional 51, 58
    in otosclerosis 45
    post-operative 148
vestibular evoked myogenic potentials
    (VEMPs) 58
vestibular failure *see* patulous Eustachian
    tube syndrome
vestibular nerves 23
vestibular schwannoma (acoustic
    neuroma) 16, 30, 40, 41, 51–4, *52*,
    118, 148, 151, 211

vestipitant 152
Veterans Affairs Programme,
    US 220
visual analogue scales 125,
    125, 182
visual field testing 56
vitamin B complex supplements 205
vitamin C 205
vitamin deficiencies, pulsatile tinnitus
    and 56
vitamin E 205
vomiting, post-operative 148
voxel-based morphometry
    (VBM) 78

wax, impacted 47
Weinstein's Noise Sensitivity Scale 139
Williams Syndrome (Williams-Beuren
    Syndrome) 141, **142**,
    143, 212, 213
work 98
working memory 107

zinc deficiency 205
zinc supplementation 205

Printed and bound by CPI Group (UK) Ltd, Croydon, CR0 4YY

27/10/2024

14580387-0005